SABRINA'S SUIT

A Novel

William Stuart Gould M.D.

WMG LTD.

New York

WMG
WMG Ltd. Publisher
288 Lexington Avenue
Suite 6-F
New York, New York
10016
wmg.ltd.publishing@gmail.com

For information about WMG Ltd.'s Speakers Bureau or discounts for
bulk purchases, please email: wmg.ltd.publishing@gmail.com
ISBN 978-0-9979804-5-5 (pbk)
ISBN 978-0-9979804-4-8 (ebook)

Cover image compliments of:
Prof. A. Abdel-Gadir MBBS, PhD, FRCOG

ALSO BY BILL GOULD

At Yonah Mountain

Captain Iron Mustache

In Black Granite

C.O.L.A.

A Heart Wind from the Desert

Raphael's Blanket

Lincoln Friday

Marlene

SABRINA'S SUIT

The Anatomy of a Medical Malpractice Case

Sabrina Friday, a striking Doctor of Psychology, was born with a spinal defect, the result of her father's exposure to Agent Orange in Viet Nam. Nonetheless, she easily adapts and leads a perfectly normal life until a pregnancy leaves her with medical challenges so profound, her soul is changed forever. She and her husband bring suit against the doctor and hospital they believe responsible for the tragedy. This is the narrative of that medical malpractice lawsuit.

PART ONE

CHAPTER ONE

Her course through the lobby was blocked by a half dozen, thick-necked proto-primates, the usuals who lolled between classes blocking the front doors. As on most days, their brash repartee intensified with the approach of a comely co-ed, that jabber obliging most women to pivot and wend their way around them. Today, though, a smaller man in their midst shushed them, stepped aside, and waved his arm gallantly through the roadblock. He was not alone gaping at the deep blue eyes that sparkled in the brilliance of central Pennsylvania's winter sun. At the doors, her auburn hair took on a shimmer that further muted the men's boorishness. Not one, though, noticed the left thumb hooked into the belt of her overcoat, schoolbooks wedged precariously under that arm.

She bent toward the grand glass doors of Bouche Building and nudged the panic bar with her right hip. While the doors parted a crack, a burst of December wind blew them closed, whacking her back into the hall. In a trice, though, her jaw clenched, and she dropped a shoulder forcefully against the glass. Still, the doors remained nearly vacuumed shut, so the man who had cleared the path lunged forward to jam a forearm against the exit. The door opened, but the torrent of freezing air caused the woman to stumble. Her hefty textbooks arched from under the hanging arm through the door, finally landing on the snow-coated steps. She sighed and shook her head resignedly, but straightened, pursed her lips, and took a pace toward the closest volume. The young man, though, was not done. He darted through the door, raised a palm to her face, and gushed, "Hey, I'm sorry, I really am. I'll get 'em for ya." Still

1

numbed by her eyes, he let his foot drop onto the first icy step. As arms and legs thrashed, an errant shoe punted the closest book into an ellipse that expired under the tire of a passing campus patrol car. With a single revolution of the front wheel, frazzled sheets of developmental psychology skittered into the winds thrashing off central Pennsylvania's Nittany Mountain. By the time the man rose to his feet, paper and cardboard fragments had been blown far up Pollack Road to heap against the HUB.

The campus cop jammed his brakes but skidded another thirty feet before stopping. He bellowed back toward the man, "Hey, you throw those books at me?" When there was only a raised middle finger in reply, the chubby sentinel jammed the patrol car in reverse to start a U-turn, but the back tires were quickly mired in a snowbank. A gaggle of laughing students gathered in front of the car howling in derisive laughter before giving him the finger and tramping off through the snow to their next classes.

The crew cut man collected what he could of the errant pages, slipping them sheepishly into the shredded cover, his eyes cast down as he presented the jumble to the co-ed. "Oh, man. I'm really sorry. I was just trying to open the door, and then it was the ice, and..."

She laughed softly, "It's okay. My fault. I'm so clumsy," forgiving him more for his gentle smile than his words. She hooked her left thumb back on the belt of her coat and asked, "Could you put what remains of my library under my arm, please?"

Gently, he replaced the books, cautious not to touch even her coat. He looked back into her eyes and blurted. "I'm really sorry. Really, I was just trying to open the door for you. Give me your name and number, and I'll pay for the books I ruined."

"No, you won't. And I don't pay for my books."

"Huh. You on a football scholarship or somethin'? Never seen you at practice."

"No, I don't have to go. I'm so good, I only need to show up for the games. But let me guess. You're a football player."

"Yeah. How'd you know?"

She nodded over her shoulder. "By the company you keep. I imagine those young men are your teammates."

"Yeah, defensive line. Ignore them. Meat without mentality. Hey, my name's Mike Maddingly. What's yours?"

He paused as if waiting for her to recognize him, but she shook her head and laughed then turned and worked her way down the stairs. At the bottom, she called over her shoulder, "Sabrina Friday, 415 East Halls A."

CHAPTER TWO

They were married on July 4th the next year, days before relocating to Boston. Sabrina had been accepted to do a PhD in psychology at Harvard. They moved hurriedly into a shabby apartment in Somerville, two miles from the university. Furnished with hand-me-downs and selections from the St. Vincent De Paul, they had enough left over to buy a second car, a beater for Mike, leaving the Mazda for Sabrina to drive to school.

In late July, though his presence had been unsolicited, Mike armed himself with videos of his college football exploits, tucked them into a backpack, and drove to the New England Patriots' pre-season camp in Foxborough. On the seventeenth morning of his sojourn, the defensive coordinator, Russ Roberts, came to Mike's room at 6 AM. With a hard rap on the door, Coach Roberts let himself in. He ran his fingers through his gray hair as he limped to the edge of Mike's bed.

"This goddamn hip's killing me. Need to get the sumbitch fixed." Mike's heart burst into his throat, for this was the same preamble he'd given ear to three mornings before when Coach Roberts came to tell Mike's roommate to pack his bags. "You been cut, son."

The speech went on unaltered, save for the name of the castaway. "Meanwhile, Maddingly, thanks for helping us get the team ready. It's not only the guys on the field on game day that make the Patriots who we are. It's guys like you, too. Thanks for being here. There's a check waitin' for you in the office. If you need anything, let me know. And you got to clear out of the room

4

and get your equipment into Mel by seven-thirty." When Mike did not move, Roberts stared for a moment and added, "You need to pack your bags, son. You been cut."

"Coach," Mike barely choked, "I got no job, nowhere to work. Haven't had time to apply for a teaching job. I got a family."

Roberts sighed as if those words had played like a broken record in his head for the past thirty years. He opened Mike's file and looked through a few pages. "Says here, you got a teaching degree. You got a trade far as I can see. You'll do fine. Most of these guys got diddly in their back pocket."

Mike nodded. "K-12—science, math, but I just moved here. Don't know a soul."

Coach Roberts mumbled, "Well, lemme call one of my teacher friends in Boston. Heard they need a JV coach. Who knows, may turn into a real job." He tapped Mike on the shoulder. "Who knows?"

Mike had four years as a science teacher and junior coach at Boston Catholic under his belt when Sabrina graduated third in her class as a Doctor of Psychology. They stayed another two years for Sabrina to do a fellowship, which she finished at the top of the program. Recruited by the medical schools at Harvard, Penn, and Cornell, she and Mike sat each evening over glasses of wine trying to decide where to spend the rest of their lives. Mike was happy teaching at Boston Catholic, and particularly loved coaching football there. They were settled, and both agreed Sabrina would never find a position with the depth Harvard offered. But they also knew that as Protestants, and not from Boston, there was no doubt Mike would remain a lesser teacher and an assistant coach, at best, for the rest of his career.

He swore he didn't care as long as Sabrina was where she belonged, though each night, she shook her head, smiling, "I will be fine anywhere. What we are going to do is find a place where you can become who *you* are." The discussion went on until a late summer Friday evening when the phone rang during the cocktail hour. Mike laughed, "Screw 'em," but he growled and leaned forward to lift the receiver. He muttered, "Hello," and hadn't even begun to tip back in his chair before a man's voice boomed on the other end.

"Mike, that you?" He started to answer, but the voice pushed on, "God, I'm glad I got ahold of you two."

Mike asked abruptly, "Excuse me, but who is this?"

"Sorry, Mike. I got ahead of myself. It's Peter Hegge. You remember, Sabrina's advisor at the NIH?"

"Peter, oh man, what a surprise."

"Hey, look, I don't have a lot of time. Could you put Sabrina on?"

She took the phone and gushed, "Peter, how are..." but he cut her off.

"Hey, Sabrina, so glad to hear your voice. Look, we're in a meeting and I need to ask you something and I need an answer kind of quickly." When there was only silence, he took a breath. "Hey, I'm sorry. Let me stop for a moment. You see, I'm not at NIH anymore. They got tired of me. I'm all of a sudden Dean of the School of Medicine at the University of Washington. Been here six months. Ran into Carmen DeSoto. She told me you just finished her program hovering around the top of the class at Haaaavahd. Also, that they offered you an assistant professorship and decent salary. Look, I told the search committee here about you, and they're meeting as we speak, or should I say as I speak. I regaled them with tales of your many talents when you did the three months down in Bethesda with me for your fellowship. I told them you were the best I ever mentored at the NIH, or anywhere else for that matter.

"Let me get down to brass tacks. University of Washington's willing to offer you an assistant professorship, and we'll beat the Harvard salary. And, more bang for your buck out here. Problem is, like I hinted, we have to know right away. Got two others being considered, but far as I'm concerned, it's no contest. But we have to play the game."

Sabrina had placed the conversation on speakerphone. She chuckled, "Hinted?" But she and Mike looked at each other, shrugged, giggled, and nodded in concert. "Well, we talked it over quite seriously and for some time. The answer is," she paused and laughed, "yes, why not."

Hegge gushed, "Great. We'll find Mike a teaching position. And we pay moving expenses."

Mike interviewed at several Seattle high schools but was taken by the fresher faces and slower life in Evanston, thirty miles from of the city proper. The former farming area had morphed into a bedroom community serving the cities of McKinley and Seattle, but the prices were a third of those in the metropolitan area. They found a log home on two acres of old growth forest a mile from the Community Transit bus stop where Sabrina would park for free and ride to the University in a little over thirty minutes. She was excited to know she'd get her paperwork done on the trip, promising Mike she'd never again bring home a patient chart.

When the superintendent of schools in Evanston heard that his new science and math teacher had been in the NFL, Mike was instantly anointed assistant varsity football coach. A month after school started, the head coach, who had gone to the local walk-in clinic for a flu shot on the Friday morning of a home game, was found to have a blood pressure of 236 over 178. The doctor tried what she could to lower the critically high pressure, but nothing worked. Despite the coach's protests and then bellowed threats, she had him transported to the hospital in McKinley. There, he howled ever more frenzied intimidations as the emergency room doctor declared the man was to be admitted, but as the orderly began to push his gurney toward the elevator, the coach screamed, "Like hell you'll lock me up." He sprang from the stretcher and dashed toward the hospital exit, though got only as far as the main doors before he grasped his chest and collapsed. At the cardiac cath lab, a stent was placed in the left anterior descending coronary artery of his damaged heart. With the sudden shot of blood to an organ that had been starved for oxygen over the past decade or two, he was out of bed by mid-afternoon, demanding to be released to coach that night.

The cardiologist called the superintendent of the Evanston School District and warned him the coach would likely die if he showed up at the game. "It'll be right on the old grid iron, my friend. And who are they going to blame? Not me. I wrote in his chart that I ordered him not to go back to school for a month. Had a nurse and a resident co-sign it." The superintendent called the high school that afternoon and ordered Mike be elevated to temporary head coach.

The old coach was placed on involuntary sick leave. He argued there was no such thing, but the superintendent told him he just made it a rule. Over that weekend, the coach's wife prevailed, and the man retired with 42 years of service to the district. By the third week of watching the soaps, pacing the house, grumbling, snapping at his wife on the half-hour, and gaining half a pound a day, he grabbed his keys and sped to the stadium for the annual game against the cross-town rivals. He tried to push his way past security, but when three of the guards lined up in front of him, he stood stark upright, howled, "Jesus Christ!" clutched his chest, and tumbled to the turf. He died before the game ambulance had gone the two miles from the field to the hospital.

The next day, Mike was made permanent head coach, for, after all, he had played in the NFL.

CHAPTER THREE

In late November of that first year, Sabrina and Mike invited the high school athletic staff home for Thanksgiving dinner. Forewarned of the abrupt storms that blacked out most of the Northwest in late fall, Sabrina started preparing the meal at eight on Wednesday evening. She opened the oven door and slid the turkey off the counter with her right arm, pushing the roasting pan into her gut to balance it. As she bent forward to glide it onto the rack, a deep, searing pain clutched her innards. Her back froze in reflex, and the Pyrex slipped free, sending shattered glass skittering across the tile floor. She fell to one knee before collapsing onto the shards, her crash louder than the clatter of the bursting dish. Mike felt and heard the thud of Sabrina's fall over the drone of the vacuum cleaner.

He had never seen her grumble, despite the pain she tolerated constantly in her left arm, but now her eyes reddened, and her breathing came in short puffs. "Oh, man, you did your back. I told you not to lift stuff like that. You can't do that, Honey. You know that."

Though Mike helped her off the ground, she could not straighten her spine. He half-carried her to the living room couch, where she lay back wordlessly as he picked spicules of glass from her arms and legs. After bandaging the superficial cuts, Mike glided a pillow under her head and wrapped her in a blanket. In the kitchen, he wiped grit and glass from the turkey and called out with a sour laugh, "What's a little extra pepper?" When she did not laugh, he quickly dropped the bird into a new Pyrex dish, snapped it into the oven, and brought her a glass of wine and two aspirins. He sat at the foot of the couch, stunned to see tears on her cheeks.

"What the... Honey, you're crying. I'm taking you to the doctor. We'll get some pain pills. And if that doesn't do it, we'll cancel tomorrow."

"No way. No doctors. I've had enough of them. And no pain pills. They make me sick. Just let me rest here for a few minutes. It always goes away in a few minutes."

"What goes away?"

"The pain in my stomach."

"I thought it was in your back. You've had this before?"

"Last couple of days. It's nothing. Probably just a rough period. I've been spotting a little." Her body tensed, and she snapped, "Please just let me rest for a few minutes, I said. I'll be fine."

Mike stood bewildered, but when tears splashed in rosettes onto the couch, he lifted her gently and took her to the car. They rode in silence to the tiny urgent care clinic a mile from their home. Sabrina, though, would not allow Mike to carry her inside.

Barely looking up at Mike, the receptionist warned, "There's a long wait. Seems like the night before a holiday, everybody's got something going on."

"How long? Look, my wife's in a lot of pain."

"An hour at lea...," the receptionist started to answer, but she raised her eyes to Sabrina's, sucked air between her teeth, and came to her feet uneasily. She finally mumbled, "Wait here for a second. Let me get the nurse."

A woman in a soiled white pants suit followed the receptionist back to the waiting room. She glanced at Sabrina, then at the clock. "You know, we close in a few minutes. The best thing for you is to go to the ER. Yeah, we're just about closed." This time, she squinted at the clock again and nodded.

Mike's shoulders drooped, and his head shook sadly. He took a deep breath to protest, but scanning the nurse's vacuous eyes and yellow, neglected teeth, he nodded Sabrina toward the door. They turned to leave but got only as far as the door before a tall woman in a white lab coat appeared from the innards of the converted, small, 50s ranch-style house. She called out, "Excuse me, folks. Hang on a second. I'm Dr. Weathersby, Khai Weathersby. May I help you?"

Mike was buoying Sabrina as he answered over his shoulder, "Yeah. my wife's got a lot of pain in her stomach. Bent over to put a turkey in the oven and fell down, right into broken glass."

As the doctor took a few steps toward them, her eyes passed irritably over the nurse, though softened as she placed her palm soothingly against Sabrina's lower back. With that touch, Sabrina's shoulders relaxed faintly, as did Mike's, and both turned to the pretty blond.

Mike queried sharply. "Do you know what's wrong?"

A thin smile crossed Khai Weathersby's eyes. "Well, let's get your wife checked in. You go ahead and do that while we take her back. Sharon, please help Mrs. ah..."

"It's Dr. Maddingly," Mike appended less than meekly.

"Well, Dr. Maddingly, come on back. Where do you practice?"

"Nah, I'm just a psychologist at the U."

"Ah ha. So, the real truth is, you've come here to examine *me*. Who sent you? State Medical Board?" When Sabrina tried to smile but couldn't, the doctor added, "Come on back. We'll get on top of things. Not to worry." She turned, and Sabrina took a few steps to follow but gulped and flexed forward in pain. Khai Weathersby swung around. "Sharon, why don't we get the wheelchair for Dr. Maddingly."

Poker-faced, the nurse disappeared, returning sluggishly to the waiting room pushing a still-folded wheelchair which she jerked to a stop in front of Sabrina. In the same breath, she spun about and stomped toward the back of the clinic. The doctor shook her head subtly as she opened the chair, set the brake, and leaned forward to guide her wilting patient into the seat.

At the door to Room 1, Sabrina sat hunched forward, nearly silent, save for the softest groan when the wheelchair jolted over the sill. The doctor helped her out of the chair and onto the exam table, then turned to wash her hands. Sensing it was taking longer than usual to get settled, Khai faced around quickly and stared into Sabrina's eyes, pulled a few tissues from the desk, and handed them to her gently. She noticed that her new patient was barely able to use her left arm to steady herself on the exam table as she reached forward for the tissues.

Khai Weathersby muttered, "First things first. Let's get a blood pressure." As the cuff deflated, the doctor spoke with a bit of relief in her voice. "Pressure, 132 over 88, pulse 88, not bad. Dr. Maddingly, tell me, where do you hurt?"

Sabrina placed her right hand slowly on her left abdomen then slid it down on to her pelvis."

11

"Is it sharp or dull?"

"Deep, dull."

"Does it come and go, or is it there all the time?"

"The bad pain comes and goes, but some of it's there all the time."

"When did it start, again?"

"Less than an hour ago. I bent forward, and it was sharp at first. I couldn't stand up. I thought it was my back."

"Did you ever have this before?"

"Not like this. Sometimes, but almost never, I have painful periods in the same area, but my monthly isn't due until late next week or maybe the next."

"Last period was when?"

Sabrina pulled a tiny notebook from her purse. "First day was two weeks ago."

"Was it totally normal?"

"I guess. Normal for me, which means it comes every three to four weeks. I can't ever be sure like some of my friends. And that one was not really heavy at first. But sometimes that's the way it is. Got problems down there, apparently. Also, I've had a little spotting this week, and that's pretty unusual. It's only happened a few times in the past."

The doctor's eyes drifted uncomfortably toward the ceiling as she thought about what might be unfolding in front of her. Whatever it turned out to be, it was already crystal clear she would not be treating and streeting this one. It was an uncomfortable feeling, for, while every patient, every single patient, held the potential for catastrophe, this woman was, she sensed, already halfway there.

At first blush, it seemed to Khai Weathersby that her patient was showing signs of gynecologic disease, and she went through the list of common women's problems. She mouthed under her breath that it could be a twisted ovary; possibly PID, pelvic inflammatory disease, from a sexually transmitted infection; or maybe a tubal pregnancy. She dug deeper in her memory to ponder the signs and symptoms of an ovarian cyst but warned herself, as she took a mental step backwards, not to forget a garden variety pregnancy gone bad. Then, again, it could be as simple as a foreign body festering deep in the vagina, usually a forgotten tampon or diaphragm. Anything was possible. After all, *people* were involved.

She could not, though, allow herself to ignore the worst-case scenario. It was every doctor's job to go there first. She thought back to her residency when

12

everyone, including the professors, had been fooled by a young woman who had complained of cramps during her period for years. And each time she was seen, she got a pat on the back then was sent home on ibuprofen. She died months later of ovarian cancer. Khai's chest clutched at the endless, critical, gynecologic possibilities brewing in a patient enduring such distress, though quietly. Perhaps, that was what disturbed Khai the most—Sabrina was quiet; the pain reflected in her face, not in moans or escalating shrieks. She'd learned early on that the screamers were generally nowhere near as sick as the patients who cried, but softly, as they bore the pain and fear.

And she took another step back. What about the usual suspects in people, male or female, doubled over with belly pain? That opened a different drop-down box, one that included appendicitis, kidney stones, inflammatory bowel disease, an inguinal hernia, blood clots in the abdomen, a twisted bowel, a bowel telescoping in on itself, the dread of cancer, and as was always the greatest fear with acute debilitating abdominal pain, an aortic aneurism, which often killed in seconds. She winced at the work ahead on a holiday evening to puzzle out what was wrong with this woman.

Then Khai Weathersby's eyes relaxed as she reminded herself of what had been beaten into her head over the years of medical school and residency: common things happened commonly, and that the most common source of anything unusual in a young woman's pelvis was pregnancy. "You have any kids?"

"No. I can't."

Khai smiled to herself—famous last words.

Sabrina spoke softly. "We tried for a long time, but the doctors at Mass General told me my birth defect must have affected my ovaries, because I had such irregular periods at that time."

"Birth defect? Tell me about that."

"When I was born, I was diagnosed with a neural tube defect. I'm sure you know about those."

Khai nodded but tensed inwardly. Certainly, she had heard of neural tube defects somewhere along the line, but where in the greater scheme of disease processes they fell was probably a bigger mystery to her than her patient. But she did know that where there was one congenital defect, there were sure to be others. "Did they find anything else?"

"Nothing but my irregular periods."

"Did they tell you more about the defect itself?"

"They couldn't say at the time, but my folks claimed it was from my father's exposure to Agent Orange in Viet Nam, and if it was, the doctors told them there were sure to be other problems. My dad sprayed that stuff all over the country to kill the vegetation so they could see the enemy." Khai's shoulders tightened and Sabrina queried nervously, "Do you think the Agent Orange has anything to do with this?"

Khai paused for a moment. "Wish I could answer that. Don't know if anyone can."

Sabrina added quickly, "Okay, but there's another chapter to the story. When I was born, the doctor who was supposed to be delivering me was still washing his hands and flirting with a nurse when my head delivered. I guess I popped into the world instead of glided. Another nurse saw the whole thing and made a note in the chart. She was the star witness for the Veterans Administration when my parents tried to get the VA to pay for my special care after birth."

Khai looked at Sabrina questioningly. "Not sure I understand the connection."

"It seems the government claimed it was the doctor's fault, that I had had a stroke at birth from the trauma of my head popping. That's why I didn't, don't, have much use of my left arm. Veterans Administration lawyers claimed my paralysis had nothing to do with the Agent Orange, that neural tube defects didn't affect arms. All my troubles were because of the obstetrician. I guess, in those days, there weren't any MRIs, so our lawyers couldn't prove it was a neural tube defect that weakened my arm and not a stroke.

"But my folks found doctors who suggested some new tests and statistical analyses to show it was more likely than not a spinal cord defect, not a stroke, and most likely due to the Agent Orange. But the government refused to send me to the NIH for those studies, so the VA ruled I was not eligible for care. Said Agent Orange killed plants, not people, and it certainly did not cause strokes. But then a bunch of neurologists back home in Philadelphia convinced my folks to take the VA to court. They testified for free, but the government doctors stood up one after the other to back the VA's claim that maybe the Dioxin in Agent Orange caused leukemia, but nothing else. My parents lost. Of course, we know better, now."

"Wow, what a story. I would never have guessed. But I'm not sure I understand what that has to do with an inability to conceive. On the other hand," she twisted her lips, "if they told you at Mass General, they must know. They know everything back there. It's where I did my residency." Khai smiled sarcastically then thought for a minute before mumbling, "Listen, I think we need to do a pelvic exam. Would you like your husband in here?"

"Yes."

"You've never, ever been pregnant?"

"No."

"Breasts tender recently?"

"You know, a little."

"Increased urination."

"A little."

"I'm sorry to be asking so many personal questions. I hope you don't mind."

"That's all I do for a living is ask questions, and a lot more probing than yours. Actually, I appreciate you taking the time."

Khai Weathersby cracked the closed door and called out, "Sharon."

When the nurse didn't appear, Khai opened the door and called a bit more stridently. After a few seconds, Sharon sauntered out of the kitchenette, a fleck of popcorn hanging from her lower lip. Khai hesitated, then ordered quietly, "Let's set up for a pelvic. You get Dr. Maddingly into a gown. I'll get her husband."

Mike sat quietly in the corner as Khai began her examination by just looking at Sabrina's abdomen. She noted three small, well-healed, barely visible surgical scars over her patient's right lower quadrant. "Dr. Maddingly, what are these from?"

"I had an appendectomy when I was three or four."

"Looks like they did it via laparoscope."

"Yes."

"Any complications?"

"No. Went home the next morning. Back to pre-school the next Monday."

Mike looked away as Khai then probed slowly with both hands on the outside of Sabrina's middle. Finding her abdomen not terribly hard, she pushed a bit deeper, and when there was no resistance, deeper still. Abruptly, and without warning, she withdrew both hands from her patient's belly. Sabrina did not lift off the table or screech in pain, a welcome sign her patient was not suffering from an "acute" abdomen. That lowered, but did not eliminate, Khai warned herself, the chance that her patient needed emergency surgery. Her heart slowed, but just a bit.

Then Khai put two fingers deep inside Sabrina. On the left side, she sensed a thickening, but one so subtle, Khai wondered if it was just her imagination. It was enough, though, to erase the fleeting moment of confidence that nothing ominous was brewing inside her patient. This opened a new set of unpleasant possibilities. With rising concern, she pushed less gently, seeking to sandwich the possible mass between the fingers inside Sabrina and those of the other hand pushing from the outside. Still not sure, Khai used the tips of her fingers for a final prod, this time snaring the thickening. Something was there— she was sure. To drive Khai's heart farther toward her mouth, Sabrina's face tensed almost as rigidly as did her right fist. Though Sabrina remained silent, her quiet distress did not escape Khai's notice, and the young doctor fought to keep her eyes from widening. Slowly gazing up at the ceiling as if in relaxed thought, Khai swallowed hard and pushed one last time, just to convince herself. With that, Sabrina groaned and brought a fist to her mouth.

Mike jumped up. "Doctor, is all this necessary?"

"Nah, we're done. I'm sorry. I had to see what was going on."

Mike bristled, "Well, what is it?"

"Let me ask a few more questions. Dr. Maddingly, feel free to just lay there, if that's more comfortable."

"No, I'm better when I'm sitting up, better standing, actually."

Khai Weathersby realized all that she had heard and found meant Sabrina's pain was almost certainly associated with a pelvic organ, and probably was an ectopic pregnancy, where the blood flow to the pelvis, and to the damaged organ, decreased when the body was upright."

"You've never been pregnant?"

"For sure, not."

"Have you ever had, and I'm sorry to ask but I have to, any venereal infections?"

Mike's eyes tightened. Sabrina shook her head at him. "Mike, please." She turned to Khai, "No, absolutely not."

"Did you ever have a D&C, say for heavy menstrual bleeding?"

"No. Never had any test there except yearly Paps."

16

"No tests or even the most minor surgery for anything in your abdomen other than the appendicitis?"

Sabrina thought for a moment. "You know, when I was a baby my folks say the doctors in Philly did months and months of tests on my neural tube defect, but all those medical records are long gone."

"Ever been a smoker?"

"Took a drag of a Marlboro in college once. That was enough for me."

Khai forced a giggle. "Ever been told you have endometriosis?"

"No."

"Ever had ovarian torsion? That's twisting of the ovary—terribly painful."

"Not as far as a I can remember.

"Ever been fitted with an IUD?" Mike rolled his eyes. Sabrina shook her head. "Ever had assisted reproductive technology? You know, artificial insemination, or in vitro?"

"No."

"And, last question, do you think your mom was exposed to DES when she was pregnant?"

"No, not unless there's DES in Agent Orange."

Khai Weathersby thought again. "I don't know, but, thinking back, it hasn't been used in the U.S. since 1970, DES that is; and you were born after that. Do you have any siblings?"

"No."

"Do you know if your mother was pregnant before 1970?"

"I'm sure not. She's pretty straightlaced."

"Mike was wiggling in his seat. "Doctor, do you know what's going on? You don't seem to think it's her back."

"Very perceptive of you. I think, but I am not sure, that your wife has a thickening in her pelvis. It could be an ovarian cyst, a cyst in the fallopian tube, rupture of a cyst on the ovary, even a urinary tract infection. But all that doesn't matter. What we have to do is rule out an ectopic pregnancy, then we can think about the other things. I hate to hassle you, but I'm going to ask you to go down to the hospital in McKinley for a pregnancy test."

Mike snapped, "Well, the hospital probably won't be open tomorrow. Can it wait until Monday, after the holiday?"

"No, no. I mean you need to go right now. If it's positive, even a little, we'll get an ultrasound to see where the pregnancy is located."

Mike was halfway out of his chair, his palm outstretched toward Khai's face. "Wait a minute, Doctor. I don't know what an ec...what was the pregnancy?"

"Ectopic."

"I don't know what that means. All I know is that Sabrina can't get pregnant. A nurse told us that at Mass General. And that's a good thing, because if she did, it would mean a possible stroke during delivery. She can't afford that."

"And who told you that, again?"

"A GYN nurse."

"Well, I understand, and it's probably just a cyst, but there's no way to tell unless we get a pregnancy test. If it is an ectopic, we don't want it to start bleeding internally, especially if you're in your own car. Let me call medical transport."

"Honey," Mike shook his head, "we know you can't be pregnant. Come on up, and let's get you dressed. I think it's in your back. You bent over. Your back suddenly started to hurt. Common sense says it's in your spine. You've had back problems in the past. Remember when we were moving last summer? Let's just go home and let you rest. Take a couple of aspirins. If it gets worse, we'll go down to the ER in McKinley." He grimaced at Khai. "Doctor you just said it wasn't an emergency."

Sabrina sat up slowly and stretched. "You know, I'm feeling a little better. Actually, I'm much better when I'm sitting up. Maybe it was a cyst and ruptured when you pushed on it. Is that possible? Really, I feel much better." She turned to Mike. "Honey, we have a turkey in the oven and twenty-five people coming over in a few hours. Let's not burn down the house."

Mike's face relaxed and as he nodded, Sabrina started to slide off the table, but Khai Weathersby raised her hands, palms toward her patients. "Folks, look, like I said, I'm not trying to stress you out, but if you refuse an ambulance, at the very least you need to drive down to the hospital in McKinley and get this figured out. If it's an ovarian cyst, and it feels better for a while, it's coming back, and, Mr. Maddingly, you're going to wind up running down there in the middle of the night, driving crazy. And if it's a tubal pregnancy, and that ruptures, it's going to be too late to do any driving."

Mike hesitated, then nodded. "Let's just get it over with, Honey. We'll go home, take the turkey out of the oven, and head down to McKinley."

She whispered reluctantly, "Okay."

18

"No," Khai scolded. "Dr. Maddingly, I'll call an ambulance. Mr. Maddingly, you go home and deal with the turkey, or you can call someone to go to your house, a neighbor. If the both of you go home, you'll find thirty things to do. Dr. Maddingly's tough. She'll tell you she's fine, and you'll never go. I have to make sure it's not an ectopic."

Mike drew a deep, impatient breath. "I still don't know what you're talking about."

Khai spoke softly. "Please, please, just sit down. Dr. Maddingly is stable for the moment, so let me explain. You're educated people. Listen to the facts, then make your decision." Sabrina nodded to calm Mike, but he drew an angry breath, which brought a tightening of Sabrina's jaw and an invisible hand that dropped Mike back into his chair.

Khai Weathersby went on softly. "Let me explain the biology." When Mike dared not protest, she went on. "An unfertilized egg is produced in the ovaries each month. One month in the left ovary, the next month on the right. In the middle of that cycle, due to some impossibly convoluted hormonal reactions, the egg bursts free, floats into this really lacy funnel, is captured, and pushed down a tube that leads to the uterus. That's the fallopian tube. It is named after Gabriello Fallopio—Italian anatomy professor who first discovered it in the 1500s. Anyway, the tube is lined with tiny hairs that beat in one direction from the funnel and carry the egg down toward the uterus. At the end of the top third of the tube, if sperm is there waiting, fertilization takes place.

"After intercourse, semen is squeezed by vaginal contractions through the tiny opening in the cervix into the uterus. The uterus is basically a muscular pouch. It's always contracting, but those contractions increase as the woman approaches mid-month fertility. That forces the semen into the fallopian tube, and amazingly, only on the side that is active that month. The sperm has to swim upstream against the beating hairs."

Mike leaned forward and asked, "Is that why they have tails, so they can get to where they want?"

"Exactly. But only the strongest make it, like salmon swimming upriver, birds migrating thousands of miles. The same biologic process repeating itself over and over in every species, survival of the fittest. At the top third of the fallopian tube, the few sperm that make it that far sit and wait. Can even be several days. When the egg appears, one and only one sperm is allowed into the egg. The instant that sperm enters, a hard wall forms around the egg. The fertilized egg then sits right there in the tube for a few days, doubling in size over and over as the process of a new life begins. Eventually, when it gets to a certain size, it's carried down the rest of the tube into the uterus, where it hooks onto the inside wall and implants itself for the rest of the pregnancy. Each month, through a lot of complicated hormonal stuff, the body has already caused a thick buildup of blood vessels inside the uterus to prepare for the fetus's arrival. Like stocking the fridge in anticipation of guests." Mike's face tightened again. Khai smiled sheepishly. "Poor metaphor, huh?"

Sabrina smiled weakly. "No, it was perfect. Please go on, Doctor."

"Okay, if there is no tiny fetus to implant, a different set of hormones gets released, and these are designed to do the opposite, that is, stop the growth of new blood vessels. Those that were there awaiting the fetus die and flow out. That's what the period is. At least, that's the normal sequence of events.

"Sometimes, rarely, the egg gets stuck partway down the fallopian tube and implants there instead of the uterus. Maybe it's because the hairs don't beat properly, or maybe there's scar tissue from an old infection, or maybe a defect in the tube due to the Agent Orange. The causes go on and on. And, maybe, the tube *is* damaged, but only to the point that, by crazy chance, just one in a thousand times, a few sperm get up that far. Doesn't sound like much of a possibility, does it?"

They both nodded, and Khai spoke more forcefully. "But it's still one in a thousand, and that means it can happen. No, no, that means it *will* happen, someday. How long have you been together?"

Mike answered, "About eight years."

Khai smiled. "Okay, say intercourse two to three times a week for eight years. There's your one thousand. And it doesn't matter what the cause of the low odds, because once the fetus starts to develop there, it's not going to stop. But, and it's a big but, the defect that lowered the odds of conception so much, then turns around and wildly increases the odds that the embryo will not make its way down into the uterus normally. In other words, that it will get stuck there.

"Problem is, the fallopian tube isn't the thick, strong muscled sac the uterus is, and soon the stuck, developing fetus stretches the thin walls of the fallopian tube and starts pulling apart the blood vessels that are suddenly growing to nourish the fetus. And there are a lot of these very delicate, new blood vessels which, if they're ripped open, bleed like crazy. At first, just a few tear, and while there may be a little pain, there's not much bleeding. But in a couple of weeks, as the embryo gets bigger, you can lose a lot of blood very quickly and, after a certain point, there's no way to stop it unless you operate right away. So, not knowing what stage Dr. Maddingly is at, not even knowing if it is really an ectopic, I can't send you home, wait patiently, watch, and cross my fingers that it'll magically fix itself like a small leak from a rusty water pipe sometimes does."

"But Doctor, we know Sabrina can't conceive."

"Mr. Maddingly, I don't mean to doubt you, but we don't know that for sure, and you guys are sexually active, right?"

"Yes."

"Dr. Maddingly, have you had a hysterectomy or had your ovaries removed?"

She answered softly, "No."

Khai nodded, and with a gentle smile and asked, "Are you using any form of birth control?"

Mike mumbled, "I told you, we don't need to."

"Good, so you're not using any birth control, and you had a not-so-normal last period. You're spotting—confused hormones. Breasts are tender, peeing more frequently. Bottom line: far as I am concerned, you are pregnant until proven otherwise, and that pregnancy is an ectopic until you can prove to me it isn't."

"Doctor," Mike snapped, "She can't be pregnant. And we're about to burn our house down. Sabrina, we need to go home."

Mike stepped forward to take his wife's hand and lead her out of the room, but Khai Weathersby placed herself in the doorway. "Sharon," she called loudly over her shoulder, "Please have an AMA printed out with the Maddinglys' info on it." She turned back to Mike and spoke impatiently. "Mr. Maddingly, if you choose to leave this clinic against my orders, you'll have to sign out AMA first. I'm trying to help you, protect your wife, not badger you. I'm telling you, do not go home. It's time to go to the hospital."

"Mike snapped, "What the hell does the AMA have to do with it?"

"No, it's a form. Against Medical Advice. You have to sign it."

Sharon brought the document and handed it to the doctor without looking at her. Mike took the pen proffered by Khai, scribbled a line at the bottom, and lead Sabrina out the door. Khai watched from the waiting room window as the Maddinglys drove east on Highway 4, in the opposite direction of the hospital.

The patients who had been sitting in the waiting room when the Maddinglys arrived had long since walked out muttering. The receptionist locked the door behind the Maddinglys. Khai, head down, gathered her pile of thirty undone charts and retreated into the x-ray room to sit at a tiny table in the corner and chastise herself to get started writing notes. Though she lifted the first chart from the stack, she could not even open it as her mind raced with thoughts of the warnings she had been issued over the past two decades; that no matter how much she applied herself, when push came to shove, she was still a woman in man's world. That no matter her medical school class had been nearly half women, the nurses and doctors, even lowly residents, had treated her and the other women as second-class healers, ignoring them, or worse, purposely involving them in procedures that were already headed south, co-opting the women apprentices as stooges upon whom they would heap the eventual blame for bollixed treatments. Though she had known, in those dark days of residency, that by the end of the week the doctors and nurses would forget the frightening blunders, she also understood that the mistakes would steam inside her mind forever. It was just part of her soul, a peculiarity she had tried to sugarcoat, but one that had been honed to a saber's point during the years leading up to that night.

So, she was not surprised that a football coach from the local high school, the second one in three months, came in to push his weight around, refusing to accept her professional advice. "Screw 'em," she hissed, but then clutched inside when she thought of the likely coming death of the beautiful, regal, professional woman who'd just struggled out of her clinic.

Her chest grabbed even harder as she pictured the inevitable lawsuit, and the Against Medical Advice form tossed out of court the moment Sharon testified that Dr. Weathersby had neither explained the gravity of Dr. Maddingly's situation, nor done anything other than shrug and hand the pen angrily to Mr. Maddingly. "Yeah, that Dr. Weathersby sure has a chip on her shoulder. Must not like football coaches. Scared they're more macho than she is, or something. All I know is that if it's a coach, they always leave angry. Try to tell her anything, and all you get back is snot."

Was she, she wondered, that unprofessional looking and acting that even patients in extremis could not trust her? And with that, the wounds of her recent years began their daily percolation, though tonight it was worse, for the nurse had sassed her publicly, and there was nothing on earth she could do to retaliate, or even stop it from happening again. She considered contacting the clinic owners, four doctors in Bellevue who'd tired of seeing patients and gone over to the dark side; businessmen now, tallying the number of gauze pads each of their employees squandered. But one word of rebellion and she would be out on her ear by morning. It was far easier these days to stumble upon a wayward healer willing to work as a doc-in-a-box, for a quarter of what most physicians were making, than lure a proper registered nurse away from a safe, high-paying floor job in a hospital, even a slovenly nurse with awful teeth. Though Khai Weathersby's pedigree was quite unusual in the world of walk-in medicine, she laughed sardonically, thinking that scarcely a patient she'd seen in Evanston had ever heard of the places she'd spent her twenties.

But here she was, and as on every night for the past many months, she began slipping along the usual path, cursing herself for having given up after the tragedy. Though it wasn't how she'd been trained to deal with misfortune, she justified the pity party with sudden flashes, assurances that her paralysis was but temporary, and that she had been wise to move slowly until the pain ebbed. Time would heal what reason could not. Or so she stilled herself for just seconds until the chastisement flowed back even more vociferously.

As the back door closed softly, the receptionist leaving, Khai tightened, anticipating the nightly slam as Sharon departed. When it came with the predictable chorus of grumbles, Khai shuffled to the kitchenette to reheat her half-eaten dinner. Eventually, she made her way dejectedly through the eerily silent clinic, chuckling cynically at the sign in the parking lot with its blazing neon:

EVANSTON MEDICAL CENTER
EMERGENCY CARE

"Medical Center," she whispered sarcastically. "I am the CENTER! Huh. If they only knew."

As she switched off the signage, her form flashed as a great silhouette against the back wall of the waiting room. She hoped it was just the headlights of a car using the parking lot to turn around. The shadow, though, became sharper, and she turned to look through the front window. A car was approaching the building, and Khai turned away to slip deeper into the clinic, hoping she had not been seen. And even if she had, there was no choice but to ignore the coming knock, for the practice was closed, and her malpractice insurance covered her only during normal clinic hours. Then it dawned upon her that whoever it was, it was sure to be not a trivial medical concern, and without an answer at the door, they would speed away west toward the hospitals in McKinley. Maybe she would be struck with only short-lasting pangs of conscience for having turned away a fellow traveler.

But once the banging started, it was insistent, hard, clearly a man's hand, and one who was not sick. So, it was a woman or a child who needed her, and she cursed under her breath as she turned back from the hallway and opened the front door.

"Mr. Maddingly!"

"She's not getting any better. I think she should go to the hospital. Tell me what to do."

Khai walked to the car. Sabrina sat quietly but looked up and whispered, "I'm so sorry to bother you again."

Khai ran back into the clinic and grabbed a blood pressure cuff. "You just sit there, Dr. Maddingly. I'll take a blood pressure to make sure you're not bleeding." It was done quickly, and Khai mumbled, "One-nineteen over seventy-five; pulse, eighty-four. Mr. Maddingly, things are stable, so I want you to get back in your car and drive immediately to McKinley, to Mitchie-Sterling Hospital. Do you know where that is?"

"Yes."

The wind had begun to howl, and the rain swirled around Khai and Mike. She wiped the water from her face. "I'll call ahead and make arrangements. Go to the emergency room entrance. We'll get a pregnancy test first, then do an ultrasound, and when we have a diagnosis, I'll have the emergency room doctor give Dr. Maddingly something for pain. She doesn't have to suffer like this. And we'll get the proper specialist to do something definitive. I'll be coordinating from right here until things get fixed. Now, go ahead. Don't speed, but don't dawdle."

Mike opened the driver's side door but stopped abruptly and stood up straight. "I'm sorry for the way I acted. It wasn't right. We want you to take care of Sabrina in the hospital."

"Thanks, but I can't. Don't have privileges there. What I can do is coordinate her care over the phone and make sure you're in the best of hands. So, please, don't worry." She smiled, took a few steps toward him, tapped him on the shoulder, and smiled warmly. "Now get goin'."

CHAPTER FOUR

K hai called the hospital lab and spoke with the night director, who agreed to meet the car in the parking lot and hand-carry the Maddinglys into the hospital. Minutes later, the tech directed Mike to the admitting desk and walked Sabrina downstairs to the basement lab. She drew blood and started the pregnancy test, then walked Sabrina back upstairs and across the hospital to Radiology for an ultrasound. At 11:00, the lab tech called Evanston to report a positive pregnancy test. Khai called Radiology and asked for them to go ahead with the ultrasound to rule out an ectopic pregnancy. As the last image came up on her screen, the tech entered the study into the computer, checked that it had been saved onto the hospital's hard drive, then transferred the images to the radiologist in the reading room. He keyed the intercom, acknowledging he had received them, and asked the tech to escort Sabrina back across the hospital to the emergency room. Mike joined them at the ER doors, and the tech walked him to the admitting clerk.

At 11:20, the phone rang again in Evanston. Khai apologized to the radiologist for having dragged him in on Thanksgiving Eve. He laughed. "No problem, Doctor. According to the husband, sounds like you've gone the extra mile for these folks. They are very appreciative."

"Thanks. We don't hear that too often, do we?"

The man took a deep breath. "Anyway, I didn't see a fetal sac in the uterus, but I can't rule out a thickening in the left fallopian tube. Actually, I'm pretty sure it's there. Good news is, I didn't see any free blood in the pelvis. If it's there, it's hiding in the corners, and that means it's likely insignificant, at least for the time being."

Khai mumbled, "I was afraid of an ectopic. Looks pretty clear, huh?"

"I'd bet on it. And before I forget, she has a bicornate uterus. Looks like the typical variant, though. No big deal."

Khai repeated, "Thanks for coming in."

"Hey, don't worry about me. Had to be up anyway. I'm off in three hours. Going to Bellingham with my wife and kids—see my mom. Dad just passed away. She's not handling it all that well." He paused and choked, "Doctor or not, guess I'm not either. Life, huh?"

Khai spoke softly. "I'm so sorry. Hug your mom for me."

"That's sweet. You new here?"

"Pretty. Fairly fresh from the East Coast." Khai sighed, "Okay, let me give the ER a call. I feel for your mom...and you. Hitting pretty close to home for me, too."

"Glad to sort of meet you. Come on over to the office on a weekday. Meet our staff. You sound like a good doc; they'll be happy you're around."

Khai called Mike's cell phone. "Dr. Maddingly has a tubal pregnancy. She may need surgery. Where are you in the hospital right now?"

Mike spoke softly, "Sitting in the ER. Checked in. They told us to take a seat. Just waiting."

"Okay. Stay there, please. I'll call the ER doc and tell him what's going on. Now that we've defined the problem, it's cool. Everything's going to be fine. You made a good decision coming back here. Your wife'll be fine in no time. Soon enough you'll be eating that turkey of yours. And I expect some—drumstick, if you don't mind."

Khai phoned the emergency room back line. She was put on hold. After several Christmas carols, she hung up and called again, snapping, "Look, this is Dr. Weathersby. Do not put me on hold. Put me through to the ER doctor immediately. This is an emergency." The line died. She called again, hissing, "This is Dr. Khai Weathersby. We got disconnected, again. Just put me through to the emergency room doctor immediately."

After several additional Christmas carols, a male voice came on the line. "He's not available at the moment. Do you want to wait, or I can have him call you when he gets back?"

"Just get 'em right now. This is an emergency."

27

"Hey, lady, cool your jets. I'll try to find him."

Khai's ire deepened during "Hark the Herald Angles Sing" and "Silent Night," until a click and an irritated voice interrupted "Little Drummer Boy." "This is Dr. Cardozo. What's the problem?"

"Dr. Cardozo, this is Dr. Khai Weathersby from the Evanston Medical Center. Thank you for taking my call. I've got a thirty-some-year-old, white female with an ectopic sitting in your waiting ro..."

The screeched, "What the hell do you want me to do with her? She needs an OB," blew Khai back in her chair.

"Sir, I'm just telling you, you've got an atom bomb percolating in your waiting room. You might want to have someone take her blood pressure every few minutes in case she starts to bleed. And are you telling me *I'm* supposed to find an OB to see her in *your* emergency room?"

"You know, goddamnit, I'm so tired of you quacks up in Evanston ripping off patients and then sending them down to me to patch up your mistakes."

Khai spoke evenly, though made no attempt to hide her fury. "Look Doctor, we'll take care of your attitude with the state medical commission in the morning, but for right now, you've got a sick patient in your ER. I didn't ask for anything more than for you to do your jo..."

The man fumed, "You can go to hell..." Khai was sure she heard him snort, "cunt." under his breath, then, "If you want to talk to someone here, call my secretary."

The phone slammed down. Khai phoned back and asked the ER secretary who was on call for OB. Khai dialed that number. Dr. Klicpera had been asleep. She growled, "I'm on ER call, not call for the whole world. If they call me, I'll go in, not otherwise." Khai started to explain, but she realized the line had gone silent on the other end.

Khai phoned several more local obstetricians listed in the Medical Society's membership guide, and when one finally answered, probably by reflex, she got a, "Jesus, it's Thanksgiving. What kind of insurance does she have?"

"I don't know. She's works at the U. Husband teaches here in Evanston. Should be good."

"Okay, I'll come in, but you better be right, I mean about it being an ectopic."

"Are you going to contact the ER and tell Cardozo you're coming in?"

"Cardozo's on duty?"

"Yes."

"Then you call."

Khai phoned the ER again and told the receptionist an OB was on the way in. She asked if the Maddinglys had checked in. The woman said they had, but Sabrina had not yet been screened. Khai asked to speak to the triage nurse, but the woman would not take the call, and Khai heard her snap at the receptionist to take a message. Khai went over the situation once again. The receptionist read it back and promised to take it to the triage nurse as soon as she could get away from her desk. "No," Khai barked, "you need to get it to her right now. Is that clear?" There was silence on the other end of the line, but a second later, Khai was sure she heard quiet sniveling. "Miss, look," Khai pleaded, "please have the triage nurse call me. This is critical." There was no answer.

She tried to call Mike, but he had turned off his cell phone as the posters in the waiting room demanded. She called the lab; there was no answer. She tried the radiologist; the phone rang and rang. As she leaned forward to hang up, she was, once again, nearly blown from her chair, this time by a barrage of lightning and rolls of thunder that shook the building. A moment later, the clinic lights flashed off, and the phone went dead. She walked out the back door into the zephyr blowing off Puget Sound. There were no lights in Evanston. And gone, too, was the night glow over McKinley. She sat for a few moments in the dark of the kitchenette before packing charts, dozens still undone. She considered stopping at the hospital on her way home to Seattle but knew well she would not be welcomed in a facility at which she did not have, or want, privileges.

And what was she going to do about Cardozo? "Just forget it, girl. No different than anything you've ever seen in medicine." She stopped and, trying to quell the anger, grumbled aloud, "You're pounding sand." But she shook her head, smiling caustically, for she knew herself far better than that.

She slowed along I-740 to peer out at McKinley's darkened, clapboard homes, the silhouette of their uneven gables juddering through sheets of whipping rain. Closer to the river rose the monolith of Mitchie-Sterling Hospital, its grand tower imprecise in the storm, a barely lit buoy undulating in an angry sea of shake roofs. Lights flickered on the hospital floors, a tired, 1980's generator doing yeoman's service to meet the needs of the technological explosion in hospital medicine. Suddenly, though, streetlights came to life, neighborhood by neighborhood, resurrecting McKinley. An instant later, the hospital's light flashed off, and then back on, this time a steady glow. Khai saw one bright floor in particular, the Intensive Care Unit, its signature disco of red blips dancing off smudged windows, thirty monitors broadcasting the final secrets of the dying. She wondered if Sabrina was out of surgery, if there had been complications, and how long she would live in the never-never land of the ICU, half-alive, eating and drinking and sleeping at the whim of the staff.

At the last exit for McKinley, Khai worried again that Sabrina was far more vulnerable than the average patient to the unavoidable errors that marked every surgery, no matter how carefully planned and well executed. After all, Sabrina had already shouted to the world that deep within her were loci of fragility the most cautious surgeon on Earth could not predict, ones that invariably emerged when an already-flawed body was stressed. It was a law of medicine.

Though she tried to convince herself it was not intentional, her car eased off the highway toward the hospital. As she drove the two miles on flooded streets, she asked herself what surgeon at a community hospital, no matter how well read or experienced, could be aware of the potential for disaster that lurked inside Sabrina? What she did remember of the Agent Orange controversy was that the Veterans Administration policy on research into the extent of chromosomal delinquencies had been contrived deep within the Pentagon, skunk-work agencies, sub-basement hideaways, from which even the President was banned. What did surface from those dens of corruption was the suffocation of government grants for research into what was causing the unprecedented levels of bizarre cancers in GIs who had served in Viet Nam. It was a strategy honed to a fare-thee-well by VA bean counters and lawyers, concocted to insulate the agency from a coming avalanche of medical and disability benefit claims. The potential cost of treating two and a half million aging men, and now their children, for the rest of their lives, was impractical. The government had no choice but to absorb the political hit and abandon ailing veterans to their own devices. They had, though, softened the blow by co-opting a sufficient number of government-subsidized scientists to trumpet publicly the paucity of cold hard facts to prove that Agent Orange was a menace.

In fact, it turned out to be not that much of a political hit. After all, seventy-year-old vets weren't likely to band together and burn cities to the ground in petition for governmental benefits and programs, nor were they likely to stage elaborate, shrill, vulgar parades to demand research on bizarre diseases that affected an insignificantly small percent of society. Actually, these hardened combat veterans were so docile in real life, so programmed for obedience, they received their mortal diagnoses with a nod and a grateful, "Thank you, sir," to the VA doctor as they rose to drive home and die quietly.

But then came the UN figures from post-war Viet Nam. Peasants in the countryside who had been exposed to Agent Orange demonstrated the same percentage and types of unusual cancers being reported by the dying Viet Nam vets at home. And then, a generation of Vietnamese children were suddenly being born with never-before-seen deformities that soon also began appearing across America. That kindled a bit of pressure on the VA, and to calm the growing rumbles from veteran activists, a few diagnoses were grudgingly accepted by the government, but only for ill former combatants. After years of further haggling, a paltry death payment was paid to widows for these cancers, but the VA remained steadfast in dismissing, out of hand, any hint that Agent Orange could cause birth defects in the children of soldiers.

Urged on by a hometown attorney, Sabrina Friday's parents, though, went to court to plead that their daughter was born with a neural tube defect, not a stroke resulting from a difficult birth. The attorney, a Holocaust survivor, mistrusted political power so completely, he took the case pro bono and went on to recruit several local physicians to testify without compensation.

"Hog wash," the government doctors grunted after each of the Friday's physicians took the stand in Philadelphia Federal Court. For every one of the medical witnesses called by the Fridays, the Veterans Administration presented two that pronounced Sabrina's parents greedy freeloaders and their doctors small town GPs who would say anything to keep locals coming to their meager clinics. The government's experts swore under oath that Sabrina's neural tube defect was the product of shoddy prenatal care and poor lifestyle choices. After three years of litigation, Lincoln and Isabelle accepted defeat and went home quietly to raise their daughter.

Dr. Khai Weathersby was as ignorant of the medical complications of exposure to Agent Orange as the rest of the healers in her community, and even those in the big city hospitals across the country. Though she had heard of Dioxin, the assumed guilty party in Agent Orange, her medical training had begun long after the Army had retired the defoliant. The experts were mostly VA doctors who had treated veterans exposed to the toxin, and most of those physicians had since passed, their medical records long ago shredded.

Khai fretted that, like most doctors, she could not know if Sabrina harbored aberrations deep within that made her ectopic pregnancy perilously atypical. Had Khai lulled herself into believing that, with a normal blood pressure at the clinic, it was safe to allow Sabrina to ride with her husband to the hospital? With her underlying damaged genetic profile, was she already on the verge of a fatal hemorrhage before she had even arrived at the clinic?

As the usual misgivings began percolating, Khai convinced herself Sabrina likely harbored a bizarre anatomy that made ectopic pregnancies even more fragile, more treacherous, than in the general population. Had she pushed too hard on Sabrina's belly? Was she already filling with blood because of Khai's ignorance? The feeling of dread welled up from deep within her chest. It was almost the worst emotion in life, that you had harmed a patient. A nurse once described it as if the bottom had just fallen out of your life. And each time it happened, it was more throbbing than the last, nothing to soothe it, not a colleague's arm around your shoulder, not a call to your husband. Even time did not expunge those heart-seizing moments, at least not for good doctors.

Her Lexus, the present Perry had had shining in the driveway the day she finished residency, ground slowly along Azores Avenue, her foot reflexively seeking the brake as she came to Mitchie-Sterling Hospital. The wheel, again, verily turned of its own will into the parking lot, the Lexus coming to a stop just outside the ER. She sat shivering for a moment, having forgotten to turn on the heat as she rehearsed the dialogue, planning to deliver it warmly, remembering her grandma's advice that honey gathered more flies than vinegar. "I'm Dr. Weathersby, and I'd like to see Dr. Cardozo." But a blast of even colder air shot into the car as the door opened. It sobered her. She understood she had no entitlement to ask for the presence of any doctor in that hospital, or in any other in the world, and that no matter how she phrased it, no matter who she claimed to be, there wasn't a grizzled, nightshift nurse on Earth who would drag an emergency room doctor into the waiting room for some exhausted blonde covering her obvious anger with a plastic smile.

She thought of simply waiting until Cardozo popped his head through the door, then accosting him, but Khai wondered if she'd even recognize him, for she had seen him only once, at a county-wide Grand Rounds. He was presenting the case of a young man with an appendicitis who had been sent home from the Evanston Medical Center with a diagnosis of indigestion and a treatment plan of TUMS. When the ambulance got him to Mitchie-Sterling two hours later, Cardozo diagnosed the problem and started running antibiotics for the ruptured appendix before checking on allergies. The teen had an anaphylactic reaction but was in surgery with a breathing tube before he suffocated from a throat swollen shut by Cardozo's ill-chosen medication. In the end, though, the child died just four days later, consumed by the original missed infection, not the botched ER treatment.

During the lecture, no mention was made of Cardozo's medication error, for administering the wrong drug was as common in hospitals as soiled bedsheets. The thrust of the discourse following Cardozo's presentation was that, while LMDs, local medical doctors, might be fairly skookum, particularly those on Mitchie-Sterling's medical staff, the pool of doctors in the county had been polluted by the emergence of walk-in clinics. Many in the audience turned to Khai and her colleagues, who had been ordered to the meeting by the director of the county medical society.

Slowly, Khai rethought her urge to march into the ER and, dejectedly, restarted the Lexus to drive off the hospital's grounds. Several times, she considered turning around but reminded herself she had no allies and no friends in the medical community, or any community. The only doctors she had spoken to were from the McKinley Clinic, desperate calls begging them to see her sick patients. It was not lost on her that not one of the doctors had ever said yes with a smile, sent a note of thanks, or even mailed a follow up letter. And now, there was Cardozo's diatribe to add to the catalogue. She steamed silently for a moment until her jaw tightened and she murmured, "I'll be damned if I let them treat me like a charlatan, some piker," but she quieted again and negotiated herself down to waiting until dawn to mount an attack.

As the Lexus entered the 740 North ramp, she prepared for the ever-growing stream of cars and trucks flowing toward Seattle, the road perpetually impassable even in the earliest morning hours. She was, though, immediately struck by how alone she was, facing the sparsest traffic she'd ever waded through on the interstate. In the boredom, her mind soon drifted back to the way Cardozo had dismissed her, and more grating, how he had ignored the needs of a very sick patient.

She thought of the thousands of patients who had come to her clinic and remembered sending only two to the ER at Mitchie-Sterling: the coach with life threatening hypertension; and a three-year-old girl whose leg had been essentially amputated when her father, who cut firewood for a living, drove a mowing tractor over a pile of hay in which the child had been playing. Khai had stemmed the bleeding, but there was near total vascular collapse from the blood already lost. She found a single, tiny vein in the other foot and started an IV, but the amount she could drip in was not going to be enough to save the child. As they did not start central lines in her clinic, she was left with no choice but to perform hypodermoclysis, the placement of a butterfly IV needle into the subcutaneous skin of the child's belly. She would attach a second bag of normal saline to that new line and maybe deliver a teaspoon of fluids every five minutes. While trauma was not the role for which hypodermoclysis was developed, there was nothing else Khai could do.

She guessed it would be half an hour, at best, before the ambulance arrived at the clinic, the child was loaded aboard, it made its way through the interminable traffic, and a proper line was started at the hospital. She estimated the amount of fluid she could deliver in that half hour was 350 milliliters, a third of a liter, 150 ml from the needle in her abdomen and 200 ml from the IV in her foot. Khai multiplied in her head: the toddler weighed thirty 30 pounds, 13.6 kilograms, and the average child had 80 milliliters of blood per kilo of body weight, or a little more than one liter of total blood volume. A third of a liter might keep her alive long enough to reach the ER.

Khai went along in the back of the ambulance—the wait in the clinic and the trip itself took fifty minutes, but the child was still alive, maintaining a barely acceptable blood pressure when they arrived at the ER. Khai gave the staff a report but was not permitted into the treatment area, so she called the clinic for a ride back.

With the doctor gone, Sharon had made the executive decision to close the office then tramped down to the basement for a nap on the moth-eaten couch. When Khai called, the receptionist woke Sharon and asked her to drive to the hospital. She refused. The receptionist called Dr. Weathersby, who ordered Sharon to the phone, then commanded her to come to the hospital immediately. But Sharon hung up and called the home office in Bellevue to file a workplace harassment complaint. The office manager sent a filing clerk from Bellevue to McKinley, but the woman lost her way, and it was hours before the clinic reopened.

Management docked Khai's pay for that day's miserable bottom line then threatened to dismiss her when she requested the clinic forgive the little girl's bill. The child survived and smiled at Khai when the father showed up two months later at the clinic offering cut firewood in payment for his bill. Khai hugged the little girl, who sat so proudly in her wheelchair, then told the family the bill was being covered by the same federal funds that addressed the $350,000 amassed at the hospital. When they left, Khai handed the receptionist her Visa card and told her to make it look like the family had paid for the clinic's portion of the bill. Sharon, though, reported the irregularity, and management accused Khai of a lack of professionalism for having become emotionally involved.

They also cautioned her about the negative feedback from the emergency room at Mitchie-Sterling Hospital. Essentially, that she had violated doctor-etiquette for having transported a dying child who required immediate surgery to the hospital without a call ahead of time to determine if the ER wanted to see the patient, or if the child should have been airlifted to Harborview, the regional trauma center. And now, just months later, Dr. Khai Weathersby had the impertinence to dispatch yet another dying patient who needed immediate surgery to the very same ER doctor.

At her cold apartment on Capitol Hill, Khai dressed in sweats and dropped into bed, but the harder she tried to sleep, the more her mind roiled with Sabrina Maddingly, with her helplessness, her beauty, and how few seconds away every soul crawling the Earth was from the end.

At 4:30, she got out of bed and called the hospital. Though she introduced herself as Dr. Khai Weathersby, Sabrina's attending physician, the nursing supervisor would say only, "The Maddingly woman is in intensive care." That was followed by a silence so potent, the only way Khai knew the line was still open was by the distant, but ever discordant, beeping of a dozen heart monitors.

"Was she operated on, is she stable?"

"Doctor, I don't see your name on the list of hospital staff. All I'm going to say is that she's in the ICU. Now I have work to do." There was a click. Though surely less deafening than Cardozo's or the ER receptionist's, it was, nonetheless, a thud of merit.

35

CHAPTER FIVE

An hour and a half after the Maddinglys took seats in the ER waiting room, Sabrina's head fell against Mike's shoulder. He thought she had fallen asleep, but a receptionist walked past them toward the restroom, stopped short, stared at Sabrina, then dragged the triage nurse over. Mike went alongside Sabrina's gurney through the inner emergency room doors into Treatment Room 4 but was forced into a corner as Dr. Peter Cardozo rammed his way to the bedside. Arms crossed over his chest, he peered down at Sabrina. "This the one from that quack up in Evanston?" The nurse flushed and nodded surreptitiously toward Mike. "I don't give a damn. It is what it is." He took Sabrina's wrist and felt her pulse. His eyes widened. "Get an IV started in a both arms then push saline. Cross and type five units, stat!"

As that nurse ran from the room, another took her place beside Cardozo, who nodded over his shoulder at Mike. "Get 'im outta here."

The woman froze for an instant, but Cardozo's face tensed malevolently, and he shouted, "Now, goddamnit."

She took Mike's arm and yanked him toward the waiting room. "I'm sorry, sir, but we need to let the doctor do his work." She forced a smile and pushed the wall switch, though as the broad doors opened a crack, she spun on her heels and sprinted back to the treatment room. Mike took another step to exit, but his chest clutched with a sense of dread, one that stopped him abruptly. He turned and looked back into the treatment area to see scrub-clad figures darting helter skelter through the halls, some screeching orders, others pulling medications from shelves, dumping them frenetically on carts—the final seconds of the annual Safeway give-away.

A nurse jerking the resuscitation cart from Bay 3 backed into the woman hauling an ultrasound machine from the broom closet. Vials of exotic remedies and plastic ketchup bottles of ultrasound gel arched across the hall to bounce against the walls.

As the doors pivoted closed, Mike stepped quickly into the waiting area, surveying the room for an empty seat. Not five seconds later, before he had taken a single step, a screech erupted from behind the doors, one that echoed off the waiting room walls. "I need that blood in here, NOW!"

Mike stood frozen, heart thumping out of his chest, until a nurse flew into the waiting room and jogged toward the receptionist's desk. When he heard her tremulous whisper, "Maddingly," his mind blanked, and, by instinct, he about-faced and dashed through the closing electric doors. Facing the madness again, he ducked out of the way into a treatment room, where he stopped to calm himself. After a few seconds, he spotted a stripe of light coming from the far wall through a six-by-eighteen-inch rectangular glass panel. He moved toward it and realized he was looking into Sabrina's room. It was hard to see through the glass, so he closed the door in his cubicle and turned off the lights.

He stood trembling, the hope in his heart dimming as the blur of blue-clad ghosts darted back and forth blocking the image of Sabrina's ashen body. Occasionally, there were snatches of a nurse, hands quaking more than Mike's, poking at Sabrina's left arm with an IV needle. As the seconds passed, and the woman could not find a vein, she began jabbing wildly, and it was just seconds before a large lump of blue erupted in Sabrina's forearm.

Cardozo looked down and growled, "Great, that's both arms you've blown." He punched his own fist and spit, "Jesus Christ. Prep her for a subclavian. Get me the ultrasound." Cardozo was now obliged to start a central line, a large bore IV placed just below the neck, one that would allow easy access to a sizeable vein. It was a second choice, after IVs in the arms, but would be adequate to pump volumes of fluid, saline and blood, into the patient who was bleeding to death before their eyes.

Two nurses cut away Sabrina's blouse and a third washed the area under her right collarbone with orange betadine solution. Another tore out to fetch a sterile subclavian IV kit. Mike could see Sabrina's eyes fluttering, though they soon closed, and her head sagged to the side. He watched helplessly as the muscles in her face went slack. She was unconscious, he knew, but an instant later, her eyelids began to pulsate rhythmically and soon her body was shuddering.

Several nurses looked up from the sterile drapes they were spreading. One finally straightened, turned to Cardozo, set her jaw, and spoke bluntly. Mike, though, could not hear what was said. Cardozo stared down at Sabrina and, while silent for a moment, finally shook his head angrily, his lips twisted in rage. There followed a string of barked orders that triggered an even more calescent frenzy over the comatose patient. Some of the technicians repositioned the sterile blue paper wraps just under the neck; others scrubbed the area with the betadine. Two new nurses entered the room wheeling IV poles; another hung bags of saline and unwound plastic tubes toward the patient. Cardozo slipped into surgeon's gloves, but Mike saw the man's hand ever so slightly brush a corner of the table that had not been covered in the sterile drapes. Cardozo looked down at the fingers of that glove, ignoring the blunder with an impatient shake of his head. The contaminated hand reached forward to pull a sterile shield off the instrument tray with which he wrapped the head of the ultrasound probe. The small tuft of the once-sterile cloth he'd touched with his once-sterile glove now sat directly over the head of the device, which he ran over the once-sterile, betadine-prepared skin just under Sabrina's collarbone.

Cardozo found the subclavian vein on the ultrasound screen, and, without looking up, felt for the introducer needle on the once-sterile tray. He placed it slowly against the skin. Eyes still glued to the ultrasound image, he quickly pushed the tip into the skin then gave the needle a hard thrust. When nothing happened, he shook his head and pulled it out for a second try. The needle, though, slipped from his quaking hand and rolled off the drapes onto the floor. He lifted his head and snarled for a new kit. As the crew stepped over and around a growing hillock of detritus—syringes, plastic IV tubing, and rubber gloves—yet a new nurse barged into the room clutching three vinyl bags of red-purple fluid. Cardozo looked up and barked, "What the fuck? I said five units."

A nurse standing by an IV pole looked away from him and grabbed one of the blood bags, her hands shaking nearly as badly as Cardozo's. She punctured the access port with the sharpened tip of an IV line and hung the bag from a metal pole. Another nurse took the patient end of the tubing, opened the valve, and let the line fill to the tip with blood from the transfusion bag. With that, the scene became deathly silent as the crew of eight or nine stuffed into the room waited breathlessly for Cardozo to find the neck vein with his introducer needle.

There was no movement in the room aside from the nurse who had hung the bag of blood and then turned to glare at Cardozo's face, the eyes over her mask fiery with temper. As her tremulous fist tightened more and more on the bag, ready to squeeze blood into their fading patient, it seemed as if she was really preparing to shoot venom into the doctor.

Cardozo, still hunched over Sabrina, poked and poked, the tip of his needle shredding the subcutaneous tissue. Stab as he might, the tip of his needle did not find the subclavian vein. He cursed under his breath and arched to stretch his back. With that signal, the nurse at the bag end of the blood assumed the doctor had completed placement of the IV. The wait finally over, it was time for her to morph into the central instrument of the team that would save this beautiful young woman. Complimenting herself silently over her professionalism for remaining sufficiently cool to wait three seconds for the nurse at the other end of the tubing to snap the line in place before squeezing, she performed her count, opened the petcock at her end, and gripped the plastic bag until her knuckles blanched as white as Sabrina's skin.

With that compression, a loose connection partway down the plastic line flew apart, the exhaust end of the tube whipping vehement jets of blood. As if in a Jackson Pollock painting, coppery, rust-smelling, liquid splashed over the staff and much of the room. The only item left untouched was the tube feeding the catheter that had yet to be started in Cardozo's fading patient.

The nurse holding the patient end of the tube was so stunned by the gush of free blood, it was seconds before she was able to scream for the other woman to stop squeezing. She tied a quick knot in the line, but most of the unit had coated the room, including several stand-by subclavian IV kits a nurse had readied. Wiping blood from his glasses, Cardozo's arms came up violently as if to shove the nurse closest to him, but he gathered himself and just bellowed, "Jesus Fucking Christ. Fuck! Goddamn you..." as irate as a Marine drill sergeant dressing down a trainee who had fired his rifle through the barracks' TV.

The nurse at the blood end reached out her arms to attack Cardozo, screeching, "Blasphemer!" but slid on a viscous puddle of blood. She clutched madly at the gurney to right herself, grabbing a fistful of Sabrina's hair, nearly lugging the comatose patient to the floor. Still desperately trying to regain her balance, she flailed like a first-time ice skater as she wove for the door. When her Nurse Mates shoes gained purchase, she ran through the waiting room, leaving behind a trail of blood worthy of a CSI season finale. She dashed into the November rain and to her car, where she lit a cigarette and sat bawling.

The doctor screamed after her, "Jesus fuckin' Christ! Moron!" A second nurse dissolved in a pious twit, twisting about like a Dervish. She finally stopped, faced Cardozo, and stomped her foot. "Doctor, if you continue to take the Lord's name in vain, I will walk right out of here."

Cardozo backed away from the table, fingers shaking harder than an old man with end-stage Parkinson's. Another nurse, her eyes wide with fright, turned slightly away from Cardozo and uncovered Sabrina's groin. She asked tremulously, "Doctor, do you want us to prep her for a femoral stick?"

Cardozo looked up and hissed to no one in particular, "Her blood pressure's so low, lost so much blood, all of her damn veins are collapsed flat. Not even gonna try the femoral vein." He thought for a moment. "Get the IO kit."

While that nurse dashed into the supply room, a nursing student followed her and asked, "What's IO mean?"

As the nurse pulled a tray from the storage rack, she spoke over her shoulder. "IO, that's interosseous. It's a needle drilled into the bone marrow of the shin bone, directly under the knee. Easy to do. Even Cardozo can get a line started that way."

Mike watched breathlessly as a nurse in the treatment room ripped the blanket from Sabrina's legs and began to prep the area below her knee, rubbing the skin with one betadine swab after another. It was standard procedure for an IO line, as any stray bacteria on the skin that got pushed into the bone along with the drill bit would lead to an infection that would likely last for the rest of Sabrina's life. Mike, though, had no idea there was such a thing as an IO, and he struggled to understand why they were preparing to operate on her knee. With what he could see through the small area of window that was clear of blood, it seemed the team had given up on the IV and were going to let whatever was left of Sabrina's life ebb away.

CHAPTER SIX

Mike shot blindly away from the window in his warren, drawn instinctively toward Sabrina. Sucking lungfuls of stale hospital air, he wrenched open his door only to be blocked by two sprinting bodies in OR gowns and masks. As the pair disappeared into Sabrina's room, Mike dropped back into his lair to watch through the window as a tall man in wire-rimmed glasses shoved Cardozo and the nurses aside. The new doctor bent over the patient and in one fluid motion snatched a clean central line kit from a trolley and had the needle out and unsheathed faster than Mike could follow. Within seconds, he was directing the path of the needle using the bedside ultrasound. Cardozo pushed his way back toward Sabrina and spoke from behind the man. "Thirty-something, white female, positive pregnancy test, empty uterus, likely ectopic on the left. Lost a lot of blood. Vascular collapse. Apparently blood on the ultrasound. Good luck. You're gonna need it."

The radiology tech, who had followed inches behind the new doctor, moved the portable x-ray machine into place to confirm the correct placement of the IV catheter. The doctor, however, shot his elbow forward and blocked her. "Not now. It's in there. No time for an x-ray."

The IV nurse stepped up to the IV pole, hung a fresh bag of blood, and raised her hands as if besieging the Lord at a revival meeting. Her lips twitched in what appeared to be prayer, but she was actually mumbling, "Fool me once, shame on you; fool me twice, shame on me." As it became clear from the doctor's body language that the IV had been successfully placed, the nurse brought her hands closer to the bag.

With no flow, the nurse who had accompanied the new doctor into the room snapped over her shoulder, "Let's go!"

Still there was no flow, and it was several seconds before the nurse at the IV pole cawed, "Dr. Gauthé, Are you ready for the blood?"

"Yes!"

"Are you sure?"

"Do it! NOW!"

There was a semi-squeeze then a delay. When nothing appeared to be spraying, the bag was emptied into Sabrina in a matter of seconds. In the turmoil, though, no one had gone down to the blood bank to gather the other two, now three, units of vital blood. There was but a single bag left in the treatment room.

The IV nurse sighed in relief, and her shoulders relaxed when the last drops of blood flowed out of the first bag. But the new doctor looked up at her and boomed, "Keep it coming, and Krystal, gimme a BP."

The nurse startled so, her shoulder thumped the IV pole. It teetered toward Sabrina's head, but the doctor caught and righted it with his thin, though muscular, arm. He looked up at the IV pole. The old, drained bag was still hanging. He barked, "Nurse, run—the—next—unit—of—blood!"

She turned to him, eyes down. "I can't find it, Dr. Gauthé...wait, there it is." She bent over and picked the bag from a puddle of red on the floor. "I couldn't see it because it blended in with..."

The doctor's groaned, "What in God's name?" silenced her, but as she lifted it wincingly from the linoleum tile, a flap of congealed blood stuck to the bag wagged as if a scolding tongue. All color drained from the woman's face, and she wobbled from the room. Krystal stepped over and grabbed the blood, hung it in a single, smooth motion, then squeezed the entire unit into Sabrina. She started a bag of saline before shifting to the bedside for a blood pressure. Pumping but a few strokes was sufficient to inflate the cuff high enough to clamp Sabrina's barely-inflated arteries. Krystal frowned and hissed, "Seventy over palp."

Three more bags of blood arrived. Two were infused quickly, along with normal saline, and Krystal stepped up for another blood pressure. She exhaled loudly, "Whew. Dodged the old bullet once again. One hundred over something. Good job, Doc."

Gauthé looked up and called out, "Where's Cardozo?"

A nurse standing at the door spoke softly. "He's in looking at a kid with a bad cough."

As the next bag of blood was hung, the doctor faced away from the staff toward the window between the rooms. Mike read the whisper on his lips: "Keystone Cops."

The doctor wrote for several more units of blood as standby then asked the charge nurse if the OB-GYN surgeon was ready up on the operating room floor.

"No, Dr. Gauthé, we're having trouble getting someone to come in. Apparently, the on-call OB's not answering her phone."

"What? She's onnnn calllll. That means answer the phone. What am I missing?"

"We got a bunch of calls about some doctor out in the community phoning OBs and ordering them to come in and see the patient. When she got Dr. Winningham on the phone, she said she'd come in, but we haven't heard from her, and there's no answer on her home phone, and her cell's going straight to her mailbox. I don't know what to do."

"Any OB residents up here this month?"

"No, but..."

From inside the treatment room, Krystal snapped, "Get more blood." Gauthé jumped back inside the room. Krystal monotoned, "BPs heading south again. Sixty-five over barely palp."

Gauthé ordered, "Get her up to surgery. I'll do it myself. Twenty-some years since I did a bleeding tubal, but I can fake it. How hard can it be?" He grinned and rolled his eyes.

This time, Mike heard the comment and saw the smirk. He flew from his darkened room into Treatment Bay 4. "What the hell's going on here? Where's the right doctor?"

Gauthé was shocked silent. The charge nurse bellowed, "Who are you? What are you doing back here?"

"That's my wife, damnit. And you're killing her. What is wrong with you people? Key Stone Cops, my ass. Do something!"

A clerk dashed to the phone. Seconds later, an ashen man in an over-large, green sports jacket and greasy ponytail hitched into the treatment room. The clerk pointed toward Mike and yelped, "That's him!" The guard grabbed Mike's arm and yanked him backward into the hall. Mike could not stop backpedaling and slipped on the trail of blood that tracked far into the hallway. He fell, smacking the back of his head on a corner of the nursing station desk. It took several seconds before the light from the intense flash faded, and he regained his bearings. He reached forward to grab the wasted man's trousers, to lift himself from the floor, but the security guard pulled back sharply, kicked at Mike's head, and lost his footing, landing on top of his prisoner. Mike pushed him off, sprang to his feet, and pivoted like a pulling guard to run back into Sabrina's room.

The gurney, though, was gone. He barked at a nurse on her knees peeling sheets of jellied red off the floor. "Where'd they take 'er?"

"You just turn around and leave this hospital, young man. You've caused enough trouble already. I'm about to call the police and have you thrown right into jail."

Mike turned and screamed at the charge nurse. The woman stood, extended her arms, palm down, then lowered her hands gently. "Please, sir, everything is going to be okay." Mike sucked in a deep breath to fuel the coming blast, but the woman softened her face and spoke with a smile. "Sabrina is fine. She woke up after the last transfusion, and she's just upstairs having the problem fixed. All she needs is to have the bleeders tied off, and we'll keep the tank full of blood. She'll do great. Sir, listen, this is what we live for, to reverse a terrible problem and see the patient go home to live a great life. Thank goodness you got her to us in time."

Mike's head dipped in contrition, a jolt of guilt lancing his chest. Had Dr. Weathersby called ahead and warned them of the Maddinglys, of the macho husband who had huffed and puffed, seeking to intimidate a young doctor in a lonely clinic miles away? Did everyone know how, in truth, he had delayed his wife's care? He forced his head up a few degrees and sighed, "Thank you for helping us."

"It's our privilege, Mr. Maddingly. Now, let's get one of the clerks to take you up to the surgery waiting area."

Mike nodded and stood silently, watching as a crew of housekeepers descended on Treatment Bay 4, hissing in a foreign patter, arms crossed across their chests, waiting for the IV nurse to swab every last red cell from the linoleum. When the nurse finally struggled to her feet, torrents of Pine Sol were poured into buckets, the deep gurgles of the magic disinfectant calming the women as they began their sullen mopping. The scent wafting into the hallway was so strong, Mike turned away, though got only a few steps before three uniforms burst from the elevator, the disheveled guard behind two unkempt, behemoth colleagues. "That's the bastard, that's him."

The charge nurse jumped to place herself between the stampeding bulls and Mike, but Mike had, by reflex, dropped into a near-crouch, fists and forearms tensed in front of his chest. The woman stiffened and held her ground as she raised palms in both directions, then just as quickly relaxed and smiled warmly. "Everything's okay, under control. Sorry for the misunderstanding." She turned to the security detail, and her voice hardened. "Thank you for coming so quickly, but you can leave now."

"Well, he don't do that, pardon my French, shit to one of the brotherhood. No way."

"Let's talk about in the morning. Everything's fine now."

With fixed sneers, both sides slowly backed several paces. The nurse took Mike by the arm and led him to the elevator.

CHAPTER SEVEN

K hai dropped onto the couch in her studio apartment, grabbed the remote, and stopped at the History Channel. The fare was but an infomercial for George Foreman's grill, the Champ carving a steak so blood-rare, juices sloshed across a white tablecloth. The audience cheered—Khai gagged. She snapped the TV off, grabbed her phone, and began to call the hospital, but stopped and muttered, "They can go to hell," as she flipped the phone onto the coffee table.

An instant later, though, she jumped to her feet, grabbed the clothes she'd thrown on the bed, and began a stagger to the Lexis. After several steps in the hallway, she stopped and realized that to appear at the hospital a homeless waif demanding to talk to an ER doctor would elicit the exact reaction her mien warranted. She went back into the apartment, jumped in the shower, pulled a comb through her hair, and gathered a bag of cosmetics, but decided to wait until she was on I-740 to do her makeup. The ride back to McKinley was as desolate as it had been an hour before, the boredom only giving her more time to ruminate about the past night. In the parking lot at Mitchie-Sterling, she grabbed the stethoscope off the passenger seat, draped it around her neck, and made her way to the elevators and up to the ICU.

A nurse on sentinel just inside the doors looked up with bloodshot eyes and focused on the stethoscope. She waited for Khai to speak. "Is the OB who operated on Dr. Maddingly still here?"

"No. Actually, I don't think she's due in. And I don't recognize you. Are you on the staff here?"

"I am not, but Dr. Maddingly is my patient. I have no intention of

46

writing orders in her chart or treating her, but I have a right and duty to see my patient." The woman was silent. Khai took a deep breath and spoke softly. "Probably best if I speak to her attending. Meanwhile, could you tell me which room my patient's in?"

The woman hesitated. "I'm sorry, doctor, but the hospital is closed to visitors at the time."

Khai smiled plastically, "Look, the hospital has 24-hour visiting rules. I'll find her myself."

As Khai turned to look at the site map, assuming Sabrina would be in the ICU overnight, the woman whispered into the desk phone. A grizzled charge nurse was waiting at Sabrina's door. Khai snapped, "I am Dr. Maddingly's primary care physician. I'd like to see her, please."

The nurse heeled around into Sabrina's room. Khai followed, but the woman turned back, a puffer fish growing shoulders and arms. She growled a few words over her shoulder to Dr. Gauthé, who shook his head and went on writing, pointedly refusing to face the nurse or the interloper. The woman addressed Khai. "The attending physician is very busy, as you can imagine."

Khai stiffened, "And what is the attending physician's name?"

"Ma'am, I think you should be leaving the intensive care unit now. It's long after visiting hours. As you know, you aren't on my staff."

"*My* staff? And you have no visiting hours." Khai pushed past the woman into the room, stopping in front of the man in bloody scrubs. "Excuse me, sir, but I am Doctor Khai Weathersby, and that's M.D. I am this patient's primary care physician. First, sir, may I have your name?"

He looked up bleary eyed. "You're her PCP?"

"Yes, I am."

"Sorry, nurse just said, 'some lady.'" He looked into Khai's eyes, and, after a pause, caught himself and spoke softly. "I'm Chris Gauthé, general surgeon. Lemme just finish these orders, and we'll talk." He managed an exhausted smile.

For the first time in hours, Khai's shoulders relaxed, but it was only for an instant, for the platoon of guards, which had grown to four huffing bulls, pushed their way into the room. The diminutive, scraggly combatant from the emergency room trailed, limping, behind the herd. When the men didn't see Mike, they turned to the charge nurse questioningly. She nodded, "It's that lady over there."

They stepped toward Khai, chests puffed. The tousled one pushed through his compatriots. "I'm still on patrol." He grabbed Khai's elbow and spit, "You need to come with me, lady, or you're going to jail."

Gauthé knocked the man's hand away. "Don't touch her again! You understand? She works with me, and as far as I'm concerned, you just assaulted a medical doctor."

"Yeah, well, the lady at the desk said someone broke into the ICU and said it was a woman with dirty blond hair. Not my fault. Just doin' my job."

"Yeah, well, if she told you to punch me, would you? Just doin' your job?"

"No, doc. You're a doctor."

"Well, I just told you, she is, too."

"How am I supposed to know that? I already got attacked right here in the hospital tonight. I'm here to tell ya, it ain't gonna happen again. That's why we're on special alert—Code B."

"Well, good. All of us should be on alert for people doing wrong here at Mitchie-Sterling." He turned to Khai. "Doctor, I can finish these notes later. Let's go chat."

They walked slowly to the surgical lounge. "Coffee, tea? Maybe some toast? Mitchie-Sterling Hospital's long on condiments, but a little short on civility and breeding."

She smiled. "Just doing their jobs." He shrugged mockingly, and she added with a smirk, "We must always walk a mile in the other gal's pumps."

Gauthé nodded "Very Christian of you at 4 A.M. after the night you've apparently had."

"My dad emailed me this article from some journal, that it's easier to practice when we," she made quotes with her fingers, "'reframe' the way we perceive how people treat us. He's also a doctor—happily retired, though. Says he now knows there is a God, because anything as good as retirement has to be heaven-sent."

"A little burned out?"

"Loved the work; despised the axe hanging over his head from the insurance company executives, hospital corporate staff, hospital CEOs, the doctor wannabes who didn't have the moxie or the you-know-whats to get into medical school."

"Looks like you met a few of them tonight."

"Ah, I'm used to it. But he loved the profession. He'd laugh that in every surgical lounge in the free world, I think he put it, '...a man can get himself white toast, peanut butter, ketchup, and in the Western world, cream cheese in little tin cups.' And I think I'll imbibe in the toast and, being the naughty soul I am, in two cream cheeses, and coffee — please God."

He laughed and put four slices of Wonder Bread into the toaster, poured the coffee, and sat. "Well, let me give you the lowdown on our patient. She went through a fairly long period of hypotension in the ER. Cardozo couldn't get an IV started. I don't like to talk out of school, but it got to be such a circus, one of the clerks, can you believe that, a clerk, she calls up to surgery and begs me to come down. Nurses must've been scared for anyone else to see what was transpiring, or should I say, expiring, on their little anthill. You won't tell 'em I said that, will you?"

"No way, but what was going on?"

"Look at me, stirring the pot. Such a bad boy, but it was like a Fellini movie. Helter skelter. Nurses darting from room to room, walls and ceiling in the patient's bay splattered with a unit of bank blood that was supposed to be circulating in their patient but wasn't because Cardozo couldn't establish a central line—ER 101. I can't believe I'm spreading this story."

Khai screwed up her face. "Yeah, I wanted to ask about him, but first, how's the patient doing?"

"Like I said, some protracted periods of marked hypotension..."

"How bad?"

"Seventy or so, maybe less, and that was after we got a subclavian in."

"Ouch."

"Yes, indeed. Anyway, I took her to surgery..."

"Why you? You said you're a general surgeon. Didn't that OB come in?"

"Nope. There was no choice. When I got into the pelvis, the products of conception had eaten through the left fallopian tube, up high, right below the ovary. Also, a lot of cysts. The tube was bizarre—doglegged hard just down from the fimbriae. I've never seen that before...suppose the OBs have. Need to look it up. There were all sorts of other irregularities down there—got a tiny look at a bifid uterus. Never seen that either. And there was a lot of blood in the pelvis and abdomen. Do you have any history on her?"

"Not much other than, somehow, she was exposed to Agent Orange via her father, who was in Viet Nam. Thought she couldn't get pregnant."

Gauthé laughed cynically. "Heard that before once or twice. You a female under 70, as far as I'm concerned, you're pregnant whether you deny intercourse, whether you're a virgin, whether you swear on your mother's grave you've never even shaken hands with a man. I don't listen to a word of it. Sorta like when they tell you they only have one drink every other night, or only smoke two or three cancer sticks a week."

"Amen. I also know she was paralyzed on the left, partially at least, because of a neural tube defect. She said it was the same etiology, Agent Orange."

"Gotta look that up, too. I hope she does okay. Saying my prayers, but the hypotension, and who knows what other defects she has going on..." He thought for a moment and sighed, "Like I said, praying for a break. On the other hand, she's quite stable, awake. We'll get you in to talk to her after the coffee, give the worker bees time to fly back to the hive."

"Thank you. I'd like that."

He put two more slices of Wonder Bread into the toaster and asked over his shoulder, "So, Dr. Weathersby, where'd you come from? How come I've never seen you before?"

Khai shot her eyes to Gauthé's ring finger. He noticed, and she noticed he noticed. There was nothing there, but, of course, he had just come from surgery where rings and bracelets, anything that couldn't be sterilized and might touch the patient, was verboten. She broke the silence with a bare smile. "Been here a year or so. Left the East Coast couple of years after my residency. Had to get away. And here I am, a 'Doc in a Box.'"

"Bad divorce?" Gauthé asked sheepishly, but when Khai looked away abruptly, he added, "I'm sorry. I shouldn't have done that."

"It's okay. Natural question these days." She turned back toward him and took a breath but stopped and sat quietly.

Gauthé cleared his throat and rose. "Well, let's let the toast cool off and go see how our Mrs. Maddingly's doing."

Mike was standing by the bedside holding Sabrina's hand. He looked up, a beaten man. When he recognized Khai, his face paled even further. He mumbled, "Oh, Dr. Weathersby, thank you for coming in. And, like I said before, I was out of line." His head sank a few more degrees.

"Don't be silly. It's all good. With the reputation we doctors have these days, I might have done the same thing. You're protective of your wife. Good for you." Khai tapped him on the shoulder then stepped to the other side of the bed. As she took Sabrina's left hand, Khai felt her own face lose color. She forced a smile to cover her alarm. Gauthé, though, noticed.

Sabrina's hand was cool and limp. Khai tried to recollect if she had touched Sabrina on her bad side during the physical exam. She could not remember, but she did recall Sabrina did use her left arm, though ever so slightly, to steady herself when she was on the exam table. Sabrina opened her eyes and gazed up at Khai. She slurred in a raspy whisper, "My throat...so sore. Nurse...water."

Khai squeezed Sabrina's hand gently, expecting a clasp in return. The skin, however, was disturbingly lifeless, with not the feeblest tightening of the fingers. She gripped a bit harder, then even more forcefully, to the point it should have caused discomfort, all the time watching Sabrina's face for the slightest flicker, one that did not emerge from the sagging, pallid face.

The surgeon nodded, "Well, let's all of us allow Mrs. Maddingly some time to rest. Dr. Weathersby, why don't we put our heads together and write some orders. Mr. Maddingly, I'm going to give your lovely wife a sleeper, so she's not going to be much of a conversationalist for the next six or so hours. And we should let the nurses get her settled into her new hotel suite. You might want to go home, catch some winks, start getting the house ready for when she comes home. Be a few days, maybe even five or six."

Mike nodded and sat with Sabrina until the nurse injected a few ccs into Sabrina's backside. Drs. Weathersby and Gauthé took Sabrina's chart and ducked back into the surgeons' lounge.

Khai began before they were seated. "Her hand was limp and cold. I don't think she even felt me touching her. Certainly didn't return my squeeze."

"Yeah, I saw that. Probably an intercurrent CVA. You know a lot more about this than I do. What do you suggest?"

Khai nodded. "Yeah, right. But I think the latest is a non-contrast CT scan of the brain; that is, for a stroke that's less than 24 hours old. Don't think she was nearly so weak in my office six hours ago."

"Well, one way or the other, if it's a stroke, it's acute. Happened somewhere along the line between leaving your office and right now. Cardozo said the ultrasound showed she was bleeding..."

"What?" Khai snapped, "I talked to the radiologist myself. Good guy. He specifically said there was no blood of note in the pelvis—said it twice."

"Dr. Weathersby, I believe you. But all I can tell you is what Cardozo told me. He was probably confused—pucker factor and all that. He may just have assumed there was already significant bleeding because her BP was so low. Not to worry, it'll all come out when we get a look at the ultrasound."

"Well," Khai exhaled, "I'm sure you're right." A moment later, though, her voice tightened. "But if she was walking around in the hospital before being seen by Cardozo, and was stable during surgery, BPs of a hundred and on a ventilator, that means the stroke's not on your watch, probably happened pre-op, in the ER."

Gauthé nodded. "Thanks for the vote of confidence." He picked up the phone and ordered the CT, then called the house operator who put him through to the neurologist on call. When that specialist picked up, Gauthé explained the situation stonily. There was no reply, so Gauthé ended the conversation with a tart, "I look forward to seeing you in ten minutes, Worth. Thank you."

He called Cardozo to ask for the blood pressure records and notes on how much blood had been introduced. Again, there was a long pause. "Look, Peter, I'm not, as you say, trying to bust your," he looked over at Khai and rolled his eyes, "your you know whats." I just need it for the emergency neuro consult on the Maddingly woman." There was a pause. "I know you're busy, early Thanksgiving morning and all. You must have gurneys overflowing into the parking lot." Gauthé listened for a moment and interrupted, "Whatever, Peter. I need those records in intelligible form, and stat."

Khai could hear the, "Not gonna happen," from across the room."

Gauthé put the phone down with a grunt. "That was Cardozo, as you might guess. Pretty gutsy after his performance, or lack thereof."

Khai had been determined not to whine about Cardozo that night, but she asked sharply, "What performance?" When Gauthé paused, she shook her head. "It's okay. You can tell me some other time. I don't need another punch in the gut tonight."

Gauthé shook his head. "Look, let's put it this way. Did you ever read Trinity, Leon Uris?"

"Probably, a hundred years ago."

"Well, he describes one of the characters as a 'toothache of a man.'

Let's leave it at that for the moment." As Khai smiled back, Gauthé's cell phone shrieked. "Hey, thanks for coming in. Let me know as soon as you've read the study." He ended the call and nodded at Khai. "She's down in CT as we speak."

Khai mumbled, "Let's say a prayer."

He smiled and scrutinized her in mock curiosity. "Are you religious? I mean, are you a Christian?" She stared at him blankly, and his eyes dropped. "I did it again, didn't I? You probably think I've been drinking, don't you?"

"To be honest, with what I've seen of this world, there is no God, no way, no how, despite my father's opinion. And he's not so sure anymore. I pray for her well-being, yes, but not to an old man in the sky striking down non-believers on this insignificant particle of soot in space."

"You mean you're already disillusioned by what you've seen in medical school and hospitals?"

"And other places. You ever traveled, been in the Peace Corps, the service?"

"No, escaped both, thank God. Way too busy. And volunteering's not very conducive to setting up a decent private practice. Those guys wind up working for the VA. Dead end. No thank you."

"Probably right about that," she mumbled and turned away.

Gauthé's face reddened, but he said nothing and made a couple of calls about his other patient. When his cell phone rang suddenly, he listened and shook his head sadly. "Thanks again for coming in." He looked up at Khai. "Yep, she's had an acute embolic event in the right hemisphere. I'm going down to the ICU and meet with the neurologist. You're welcome to tag along, but let me warn you, as if you didn't already know, the staff down there treats new ones like lepers—old ones, too."

"Thanks, but I think I'm going to drive home and get a couple of hours of sleep. They scheduled me for Thanksgiving Day because, they said, I was the only one without a family. How rude and uncaring! Problem is, they're right."

CHAPTER EIGHT

K hai tossed in bed for an hour before giving up. She took a seat at her computer and started scripting an email, surprised at how easily the words came.

Harvey Klat, M.D.
Medical Director
Mitchie-Sterling Hospital
McKinley, WA.

Dear Dr. Klat,

I am sorry to write to you about so unpleasant a subject, but I am sure you want to be kept informed about the goings on regarding your staff.

I am Khai Weathersby, M.D., board certified in internal medicine, and fairly new to the Northwest. I have chosen to work at the Evanston Walk-In Center until I feel more comfortable living here. I am totally devoted to the care and safety of my patients, and, in that regard, I am sure I am no different than you or any of the physicians under your aegis.

Last night, just before our scheduled closing at 2100 hours, a woman and her husband presented to my clinic. She complained of marked pelvic pain. My clinical diagnosis was ectopic pregnancy. As we had neither a laboratory to do a serum pregnancy test, nor ultrasound capability for confirmation, I sent the family to your hospital. I stayed in the office until past 1 A.M. to coordinate her care by phone. Your lab confirmed a positive pregnancy test, and the radiologist confirmed with me over the telephone that, while there was no free blood in the pelvis, he found no products of conception in the uterus. I felt sure the patient had an ectopic pregnancy that was unstable.

I asked the radiology tech to walk the patient and her husband to the ER and have them sit there until I found an OB to provide definitive care. I phoned the ER, and after several dropped calls, spoke with Dr. Cardozo. As soon as I identified myself, he launched into a profanity-punctuated diatribe denigrating my medical ability, my morality, and my parentage. He muttered a word describing me in terms of my genitalia, refused to see my patient, and terminated the call by slamming the phone down.

I called several OBs who refused to come in. Finally, Dr. Winningham agreed, but only after I assured her the patient had excellent insurance. I quietly accepted her threat that, "You better be right about the ectopic." She, however, never presented and would not answer her phone for the rest of the night.

It fell to Dr. Gauthé to start a central line in the ER after Dr. Cardozo was unable to do so for so long, it appears the patient suffered a CVA due to hypotension that commenced in the ER. Without an OB present, Dr. Gauthé had to take the patient to surgery and save her life. He scooped out four units of blood from her pelvis.

Sir, this is not right, and on so many levels, but for now, the only concern is that we almost lost a patient, a PhD professor at the U., whose husband is a high school teacher in Evanston, not that their titles matter. And over turf?

I trust you will investigate, and perhaps we can open a dialogue to smooth the way for our mutual patients.

Respectfully yours,

Khai Weathersby, M.D.

As Khai ruminated, she realized her email would never survive the gauntlet to the medical director. She thought about requesting a face-to-face meeting but knew she would be deflected to a secretary, her concerns fed to the medical director as so much Pablum. She would receive a perfunctory excuse from an assistant, and there the matter would die. Khai decided the best route to the medical director was to take a sheet of her personal letterhead and print out the note, put it into a sealed envelope - PERSONAL AND CONFIDENTIAL - and drop it off at Klat's office on her way back up to Evanston that morning.

As she was about to pull out of the hospital parking lot three hours later, Mike was driving back in. They stood outside their cars, Mike apologizing again, his shoulders so drooped, the irritation and frustration she'd held for him for twelve hours disappeared.

She walked with him into the hospital. Sabrina was being evaluated by a new neurologist. They were told to remain in the waiting area. Khai considered declaring she was Sabrina's primary care physician but decided against opening a new front in the war. She and Mike went to the cafeteria and sat over lukewarm coffee, talking. He asked what had caused the stroke, if it would resolve with time, or if it meant the total loss of her left arm and, now, her left leg as well.

Khai's gut clenched as she created an answer that hovered over blaming him, blaming herself, blaming Cardozo, and blaming the surgery. "You know, we can never pinpoint what causes these things. Never." She explained that Sabrina had been treated with tissue plasminogen activator, tPA, for the stroke. It was a blood thinner that had the ability to dissolve clots in the brain, but only if used very early in the stroke, before too much damage had been done.

"Mr. Maddingly, the last thing I want to sound like at this moment is a doctor, but there is no way to tell. I'm sorry. Sometimes, the symptoms resolve after anticoagulation therapy, sometimes not. You know, we sure don't like to use tPA right after surgery. There's no way to tie off all the tiny vessels that continue to bleed after any procedure, no matter who the surgeon is, and Dr. Gauthé's right up there. With tPA, bleeding can be a bigger problem than the blood clot. In Sabrina's case, the decision was made to try and dissolve the clot in her brain." She paused and looked at him cautiously. "I hope I can be frank."

"Strange first name for a woman, Frank, but these days, who knows?" She paused for a split second before her eyes rolled and her head shook. When she smiled, Mike's shoulders relaxed a bit. "I'm sorry, I've spent most of my adult life trying to make up for a lot of unhappiness in my child life. I do it by injecting humor into the bad. Well, Sabrina doesn't call it humor—no one does. Look, Sabrina is the only good thing that ever happened in my life." His eyes clouded. "Damn hard for me to say this, but I'm scared to death. Just trying to hide it."

"Don't be scared. And, to be honest, that's the first time I've smiled in about a year. Now, I want you to remember one thing. Ready?" He nodded. "'And this, too, shall pass.' That's my prescription. Say it three times a day for ten days. The both of you will come out the other end of this thing. You'll be teaching high school kids; don't know how you do it..."

"Drugs and alcohol. Kids keep me supplied. Did you know an 'A' buys a math teacher two grams of blow?"

Khai laughed this time. "You are incorrigible, aren't you? And Sabrina will be helping patients at the U. I want you to know Sabrina is being watched like a hawk. We can reverse the tPA, or we can do something surgical to protect her from excess bleeding. But if she has a greater deficit on the left when it's all over, you guys will learn to deal with it. I'm not trying to be dismissive, not one bit, but you will adapt. We all have to adapt." Khai, though, looked away when his eyes began to redden.

Mike took a deep breath, stood, and extended his hand. "Don't know where you came from, Doctor, but, apparently, it's a very good place. Thank you again. Okay, I'm gonna go try and see my wife, if they'll grant me the privilege."

"Second prescription: Like Ivar says, 'Stay clam'. These folks are in the driver's seat. Accept it. They ain't givin' up the twenty seconds of control they have over your life. You see, right now, you're in their house. Just smile and nod and say, 'Yes, ma'am, no ma'am, three bags full, ma'am;' and behind the façade, just remember that for every mean, nasty, snotty, arrogant word out of their mouths, another check mark goes into their bad karma box. Not all the sadness on Earth is from Karma, but I am absolutely sure each tick on the bad karma list has to be paid off eventually. And I'm late for work—bad karma."

CHAPTER NINE

It was 8:30. Sabrina was still asleep. Mike wound through the hospital trying to relocate the cafeteria. Down a corridor filled with the scent of broiling bacon, he came to set of doors he absentmindedly pulled open. The aroma transformed instantly to one that caused his chest to clutch—he was in the ER, standing frozen, swathed abruptly inside a veil of despair. A woman in scrubs marched up to him. "Can I help you?" He wondered if she recognized him, and if security was already on the way. He just shook his head and shuffled away. He glanced back before turning the corner to see her still filling the doorway, hands on hips.

In the cafeteria, gangs of the scrub-gowned knocked back runny eggs and cold bacon before jumping up to dash back upstairs. Mike tried the cheese omelet, but it was so loose, he muttered, "No wonder everyone around here is such a sourpuss." He bussed his tray to the plastic garbage cans and stood, reading signs, trying to decipher which bit of trash went into which recycle bin. A woman behind him tsooked and let her tray jab Mike's back. He turned and mimicked her saccharine smile then doglegged right to the moving conveyor, dropped his tray, and apologized to the worn little man on the other side of the belt. The man waved Mike away, and, in a soft foreign accent, whispered, "You leave it to me, sir." They reached across and grasped hands.

By the time Mike stumbled back to the ICU, Sabrina was sitting up in bed. She had tried to feed herself with her right hand, but, after the first spoonfuls of apple sauce, she became so fatigued, the nursing assistant took a seat and fed her.

Mike's jaw dropped. Sabrina looked up and whispered, "Better close your mouth. Flies'll get in."

The assistant froze before looking around the room. "No have fly in hopitill."

Mike walked to the bedside. He motioned to himself and then to the spoon. The woman looked up warily. "You husbin?"

"I husbin."

"You do. I see." She pointed to her eyes.

Mike sat and offered Sabrina a barely rounded teaspoonful. The woman shook her head. "You make too much big." She grabbed the spoon back and pointedly half-filled the next offering.

Sabrina took it and nodded warmly. "Much better." She smiled at the woman, "Thank you."

As Mike sat back down, Sabrina winked at him weakly. "You don't have to feed me, Honey."

"I'll never stop doing everything. Hey, I talked with Dr. Weathersby after you went to sleep. She says everything's going to be okay. Go ahead and try to move your left hand. Let's see." He pulled the sheet back, and she stared at the fingers. His face and shoulders tightened as if trying to generate a radio pulse, and when there was not a flicker of movement, he smiled uncertainly. "Well, we just need to give the tPA some time. You remember, that's what the neurologist said." As he bent forward and kissed her forehead, the hovering nursing assistant blushed and left the room.

Dr. Gauthé swept in on afternoon rounds at four. The surgical drain he'd placed in Sabrina's abdomen fed into a bag that hung under the bed. Fashioned of clear plastic, it collected the blood and angry fluids that seeped from the violated tissue at the surgery site. When the bag had been changed several hours before, Mike noted the fluid had been thin and only tinged with blood. Now, a far more viscous, redder effluent was edging up the sides of the bag. Reading the gradations of ccs on the face of the bag, Gauthé scratched a pen at a corner of Sabrina's chart, adding the amount listed from the old bag to what he read off the new one. He pulled up a chair and sat down.

"There's been a bit more bleeding. I'm not that surprised because of the blood thinner—you know, the tPA we're using to dissolve the clot in your brain. We just need to keep an eye on things. One of the best ways is to monitor the blood pressure and heart rate. If the pressure starts going down because too much blood has leaked out into the abdomen, we should see an increase in the pulse. That's the heart beating faster trying to keep the pressure up. So, for right now, let's get a blood pressure and see what's up."

It was 102 over 56, her pulse 98. Gauthé stood and thought for a minute. "BPs a little on the low side. Let's get a quick hemoglobin." Mike's head turned in question. Gauthé nodded. "Just a blood test to tell us how much hemoglobin is in the bloodstream. Hemoglobin's the compound inside the red cells that carries oxygen around the body. Easy to measure. At the moment, that's the most important thing we need to do—keep the oxygen supply going to all the tiny little corners of the body. Normal hemoglobin's roughly between 13 and 17. If it drops below 10, we get antsy. If the hemoglobin's low, that means, at least in our case here, that blood is leaking somewhere, and the bloodstream is pulling water in from our IVs and from the muscles, and anyplace it can find it, to try and keep the circulation full of something. For you, Dr. Maddingly, most of the extra water is coming from the fluids we're giving you via the IV. But IV fluids can't carry oxygen around the body. If we dilute the blood too much with IV fluids, even though we're keeping up with the volume loss, now there's too little oxygen to keep things working right; so, once again, the pulse increases to speed up what red blood cells are still left around to deliver oxygen faster. It's like if too many UPS guys go out with the flu, the ones still there have to drive like crazy to pick up the slack. Eventually, they will burn out, and people don't get their packages. Here, it's the heart we want to keep supplied. Don't forget, the heart's just a plain old muscle, no different than the ones in your arm. If you beat it enough, it's gonna get too tired to do any more meaningful work. In your arm, when you just can't lift another shovelful of snow from the driveway, you drop the shovel and go inside for cocoa. In the case of the heart, when the muscle gets that tired, it won't give up; it can't do that, but it'll contract so weakly, it won't even be able to supply itself with enough blood to keep the rate extra high to make up the difference. Then we got problems.

"Now, that certainly won't happen here. I'm just explaining why you may see us do certain things. We are very good at tweaking fluids. Very good. We add up the number of ccs of water you take in by mouth: drinking, in the hospital food—if you can call it that—from your IV, and then we add up the ccs coming out—in the urine bag under the bed, in the drainage bag from the surgery site—and we have a formula to calculate how much water you lose in sweat you don't know you're sweating, and even how much water you breathe out over an hour."

Mike turned his head again. "You lose water when you breathe?"

"Sure. Like if you huff on your glasses to clean them. That's water from the breath."

"But that's tiny."

"Add it up. Breathe twelve or fourteen times a minute, that's what, seven, eight hundred times an hour; that's nearly 20,000 times a day. That's equivalent to the fluid in a couple of units of blood, half a quart or so."

Mike raised his hand. "Dr. Gauthé, may I ask, right now it seems Sabrina is drifting onto the wrong side of the blood curve. Is there a problem just giving more donated blood? If it's a matter that the insurance won't pay for it, we will."

"Not an insurance problem. Not at all. It's just that there are cautions we need to follow. I mean, we won't let Dr. Maddingly run out of blood, no way, and we won't let her heart work so hard it begins to give up the ghost. No way. But there's also a concern with giving too many transfusions. It's really complicated, and I'm not saying that to be condescending. To be honest, I don't understand near all of it, but that's why we have hematologists. They're the ones who know all the rules—got 'em memorized, like you know that impossible calculus you teach."

"Oh, God, I hope you know more about blood than I do about differentiation. We want Sabrina to get better."

Gauthé looked at him askance then turned to Sabrina and laughed. "In your case, Dr. Maddingly, we don't want to add more and more tPA to the new blood to keep it from coagulating, and we try not to use too many units of blood—there are sometimes allergic reactions your body can have if we mix blood from a lot of different donors. So, it's a juggling act, but that's why we find the right people to keep the balls up in the air no matter how fast the wind's blowing. Surgery's the easy part. The thinking and coordinating care, that's the challenge.

"But for right now, we'll just forge ahead. No big changes. Go slow and keep reevaluating. I would like to ask that you not take anything by mouth for the time being. We'll check things over and over. I'll be honest: if we have to go back to surgery to tie off any little bleeders, we don't want anything in the stomach that can come partway up the esophagus during surgery and find its way into the lungs. Let me tell ya, that would be a pain in the old derrière."

Because there were two drainage bag changes by midnight, the nurse called Dr. Gauthé. He came in, totaled the numbers in Sabrina's chart, and when the nurse asked if he wanted another blood draw for hemoglobin, he growled, "Draw the blood. Have the lab call the result up to the OR. I'm taking her back to surgery right now. Get a stat team ready, and order five more units of packed red blood cells. Thank you, Liz."

She gave him a tap on the shoulder, bent forward, took Sabrina's hand, and whispered, "Honey, don't you worry even a bit. He's the best."

Gauthé found the belly full of uncoagulated blood. He mopped and mopped until he found a couple of vessels that appeared tied off but were slowly leaking. It was not much to see; there was no gushing, but with time, these two, small, innocuous arteries would have taken Sabrina's life.

While Sabrina was in surgery, Mike sat in the waiting area staring into space. An hour later, Gauthé came in and sat with him. "Sorry, it all happened so fast, but that's the way things go around here. Tied off two bleeders. No big deal, but there's not going to be any more tPA. So, next step is to do some imaging and see if the tPA worked and broke up the clot in the brain over the past twenty-four hours. Stick around, if you can. Need a note for school?"

"Nah. Principal's great, District is okay, too. Other teachers are already donating their sick days, so I don't lose all mine. Good people out here."

CHAPTER TEN

Gauthé called Khai several times over the first full day of Sabrina's hospital admission, and again at 7 the next morning. "Hope I didn't wake you, but I haven't been to sleep in three weeks, so why should you?"

"Nope, up and taking a shower..." She paused to let him think about it for a moment then went on. "I imagine you are calling at this hour not with news of having won the lottery."

"Very perceptive, Doctor." He described the most recent complication and sighed, "That's two strikes. The stroke and the bleed, and who knows what else when you consider all the possible congenital possibilities. We're not out of the woods. May be heading even deeper into the forest, I mean jungle."

"A truism of life, or at least medicine: things come in threes—or in Dr. Maddingly's case, looks like by the baker's dozen."

Gauthé mused, "There's got to be an easier way to make a living. I saw on TV in the surgeons' lounge that K-Mart's looking for greeters."

"Yeah, but I hear they're pretty particular. You bring any experience in that line of work? Got references?"

"Dr. Khai, you willing to write me one?"

"Oh, it's just too soon."

"Okay, then why don't you stop by the hospital on the way up to Evanston. See our patient, maybe grab a cup of coffee and sit with me?"

Khai paused for a bit but forced a smile as she answered. "Sure. See ya in an hour."

As Khai dressed, she asked herself why she'd agreed, grumbling impatiently, "You're not ready, girl; the scars are still way too scarlet." She reflected that she did not know a thing about him, only that he was a surgeon. She laughed; that might be a big deal from the patient's perspective, or with a shadchan, but it surely was not in her world; perhaps even a check in the bad box. She thought of the article she'd just read on the internet, the one about the professions most associated with psychopathology. CEOs, lawyers, and surgeons headed the list.

As she drove, though, she wondered why she had made the comment about the shower and, worse, just about bullied him to think about it. She pulled into the hospital parking lot and realized she had not heard a sound from the radio, her mind lost in a curious pleasantness. She tried not to smile when she saw him waiting for her outside the ICU.

Sabrina was asleep. Mike was at the bedside, holding her hand. He looked up at Khai with a weak smile. She touched his shoulder and again saw moist redness in his eyes before he turned away.

Gauthé held the chart and nodded in approval. "Your lovely wife is quite stable. Blood pressure's back up, pulse is slower, hemoglobin's cruising along—gettin' close to eleven. That's good."

Mike interrupted quietly. "Doctor Gauthé, I thought you said thirteen was bottom normal."

"Good memory. We'd actually like to see fourteen or better for a patient out in the community, but your wife's numbers, considering what she's been through, are just fine. We never shoot for perfect—it's the enemy of good. I wish more of my colleagues understood that. Sometimes it's smarter to stop treating, let Mother Nature intervene to polish things up for us. Look, if all my patients had a hemoglobin of eleven, I'd be outta work."

Khai nodded and was about to add a word but shrank back, abruptly aware that her presence at that hospital was at the pleasure of the attending physician. Gauthé sensed the tension and asked Mike if he had any questions. He demurred, so Gauthé nodded Khai toward the door.

In the cafeteria, he bought two coffees and walked to a corner table. Khai followed and noticed several women in scrubs looking up at him then glaring at her. Her head sagged; the shoulders followed. Realizing she was walking almost obsequiously, she growled under her breath, "Remember who you are, what you've seen, what you've done, girl." Her back snapped arrow-straight, and she pasted on a glower that would have shaken a company of errant army privates. She dropped into a seat facing out, the sneer deepening.

Gauthé asked with a wry smile, "You okay?"

"Friendly crowd."

"Yeah, like I said, the newbie syndrome. Ignore them. They're jealous."

"I'm sure."

"Really. Look at you and then look at them." He laughed uneasily and went on. "So, Dr. Weathersby, I hear you rattled a cage or two here in paradise. Good for you."

"What you mean?"

"You know, you didn't take crap from that moron, Cardozo."

"All I did was send a letter to the Medical Director. Don't tell me he's already going around bad-mouthing me for informing him about what's going on in his little kingdom."

"No, not him. He's a horny old bastard. I saw a man in his 60s the other day with a t-shirt that said, 'insufficient memory' and an arrow pointing toward his head. I wanted to pull it off his back and give it to Medical Director Klat.

"Nah, I'll bet one of the secretaries opened it before it got anywhere near Klat then passed it around the office, priority, and eventually, someone shot a copy down to the ER."

"That is so unprofessional."

"Honey, welcome to the metropolis of McKinley, Waahh. The gossip value and the esteem for the leaker is worth far more than the threat one of the administrators will raise an eyebrow, which they won't, because they're afraid of a harassment lawsuit if they try to discipline a filing clerk. You're from the big city, huh?"

"Boston, for a lotta years. And Mass General was big and bad, a zoo, but the boss's secretary didn't open mail from a doctor that was marked 'Personal and Confidential' and publish it to the staff. Holy mackerel."

He clucked, "Not to worry, it'll be forgotten in four days, just like everything else in the world."

"Dr. Gauthé, I don't want it forgotten. What happened with Cardozo was not right."

"Well, and by the way, my name is Chris." He stared into her eyes. "May I call you Khai?"

She hesitated for a breath then nodded. "Of course."

"Khai, look, this isn't the East Coast. Please don't be angry at me; I'm just the messenger, but these are stuffy, outwardly politically correct souls who bridle at anything out of the ordinary. Cardozo is an asshole, but he's a critical gear in the local money-generating engine. He makes referrals to his favorite specialists, those docs get busier, and richer, and the quality of your waiting room and your car convey the mantle of godliness in the medical community, at least in this one. When these guys get tired of seeing patients, that financial padding allows them to go to the dark side and become administrators. No more malpractice suits hanging over your head; no more threats of imprisonment for giving a suffering patient meds; no more interminable regulations that make you change your practice twice a day; no more electronic medical records eating away at your soul; hey, don't even have to take call. Hospitals pay their stooges real good. It's the perfect life, still a doctor, or at least you can convince yourself you are, still a big shot in the community. Old farts become executives, wait a few months, then join the bandwagon to squeeze the nurses and non-medical staff for pay freezes. Out of the other corner of their mouths, they push for raises for the guys in the trenches who put them, and keep them, there. And round and round the crooked wheel turns. Maybe not that simple, but shy of coming to work drunk, or smoking weed behind the dumpsters, Cardozo's untouchable. That's because the local medical community claims to police itself. Sucks, but what can you do?"

"Well, Chris, thanks, and I'm not really surprised, but I'm glad you told me. Goes onto the balance sheet for good and bad in suburban Washington. Which reminds me, I gotta get over to Evanston to work to make enough money to stay here where I probably don't wanna be. But thanks for the coffee."

"Can we do it again?"

She smiled back and sort of nodded.

CHAPTER ELEVEN

Sabrina woke at eleven and stared at Mike. A minute later, she shook her head as if trying to clear her head. As he squeezed her hand and bent forward to kiss her cheek, he inadvertently snagged one of the wires that formed the thick umbilical cord attached to his wife's body. A whooping alarm sounded in the room and at the nursing station, one that drew a tiny, hard-faced woman in blue scrubs. She checked the monitor, reconnected wires, pushed buttons, and huffed, "Please don't touch the equipment." And just that fast she spun on her heels and marched from the room.

Sabrina managed a frail smile and whispered, "Do I have to take you off my visitor's list?" She groaned, "I feel like I've been hit by a truck."

"If only it was that straightforward. Hey, but Dr. Gauthé says things are going according to plan, your numbers are getting better, and we're on the mend. That's good, huh?"

Sabrina sighed, "Wish I could believe him."

"Hey, that's not my Sabrina talking, is it? And this, too, shall pass. A doctor told me that."

"I don't know, Mike. I've never felt like this before. Never been so helpless, so totally dependent."

"Look, Sweet Pea, I'm on your six, every second of every day. Don't you ever forget that."

She nodded gently and whispered, "I know you are." They held hands for a few seconds until her head drooped, and she mumbled, "Mike, I'm sorry. I'm fading already. Mind if I close my eyes for a minute?" Her voice trailed off.

"I love you so mu..."

Mike leaned forward to kiss her cheek. The siren blared. He made it through the door before the flash of blue streaked by.

He came back an hour later. Sabrina was awake, though barely. He was not sure she recognized him as her lips formed disjointed words he could not understand. He sat holding her hand, and while her eyes opened occasionally, they only stared at the ceiling. After two hours with Sabrina motionless, he went back to the cafeteria. Barely able to finish a bowl of soup, he soon returned to the room. Sensing it was a bit warmer than when he'd left, he slipped off his sweater and dropped into the chair next to Sabrina. She was still asleep, arms and legs not having moved a millimeter. Her hand, though, was clammy, her brow moist. As it was snowing lightly outside, he assumed the heat had been turned up in the room. He walked to the wall thermostat. It was set at 70.

He went to the nursing station. The unit secretary looked up without a word. "Jees, my wife in 119 seems awfully warm."

"Oh, you can never tell by touch. Not to worry, we take our patient's temperature very often." She smiled weakly, dropped her head, and went back to work.

When the floor nurse came to do vitals, Sabrina was sweating freely. The nurse stopped and stared at her. As she ran a digital thermometer over Sabrina's forehead, her eyes grew wide, and she left the room without a word.

Dr. Gauthé strode in minutes later, still wearing his surgical hat and booties, the latter tinged with blood. "So, what's going on with Dr. Maddingly? A little warm, I hear." He did not, however, look at Mike before he called to the nurse. "Let's get a stat white count with diff."

He turned to Mike. "Looks like a bit of infection, but a collection of blood in the belly can cause a fever, too. No matter. I'm going to start her on an antibiotic just to be sure. We can take her off it if it turns out to be nothing." He wheeled around and went to the computer at the nursing station.

An hour later, a new doctor appeared. She introduced herself as, "...just the hospitalist." Mike had no idea what that meant but shrank back and stared out the window as the woman examined Sabrina.

The doctor pushed buttons, and the head of the bed rose. She opened Sabrina's gown from behind, letting it fall off her shoulders. Mike turned back and noticed a faint halo of rosiness surrounding the bulky bandage under

Sabrina's right clavicle, exactly where Cardozo had tried so many times to start an IV. The doctor sensed Mike's stare and turned halfway around to look at him crossly. Though Sabrina's breasts were exposed and easily visible to the visitor traffic passing the wide-open door, the doctor pointedly shifted her back to block Mike's view.

She listened to Sabrina with a stethoscope and mumbled to herself, "Got some junk in her lungs." She called for the nurse. "Get a chest film and send off some fresh urine for culture and sensitivity."

The nurse asked sheepishly, "Do you want me to send off some of the fluid from her surgical drain, too?"

"Yes. Of course."

Mike withdrew toward a corner as the portable x-ray machine was wheeled into the room, and even further when Sabrina was manhandled to get the film cassettes in place. She actually stirred and clawed at the bandage on her collarbone, but Mike came over and held her arm gently. He noticed that, despite Sabrina's agitation, the left arm showed not a flicker of movement.

Two hours later, though Mike had not moved from Sabrina's side nor spoken a word to the staff, he rose when Gauthé returned. The surgeon glanced at the chart. "White count is nearly 20,000. She's got an infection. Just trying to find out where. We're looking at the usual suspects—checking the lungs for pneumonia because she's not breathing very hard; I mean, the surgical incision hurts when she tries to take a deep breath or cough, so she's not blowing out the regular old bacteria that float around in the air."

Mike grimaced. "I thought the hospital was clean."

Gauthé paused, his lips twisting as if trying to hide a sarcastic smile. "No place on Earth's free of bacteria. Even the docile bugs you take in with every breath, if you don't breathe hard enough to get them out, they take up residence, hook onto the wall of the breathing tubes, start growing in pockets, and soon that turns into an infection, what we all know as pneumonia. The body pours water in to dilute the poisons the bacteria produce, and that water clogs the breathing tubes. The irritation causes coughing, as you might imagine, but Dr. Maddingly may be too weak to cough at the moment. It happens, and not infrequently. Since we can hear fluid sloshing around in your wife's lungs, I'm betting that's where the infection is growing."

Mike appeared confused, so Gauthé added, "That's all pneumonia is, an infection in the lungs. No different than an infection in your finger: swelling, pain, heat, and redness, the latter of which we would actually see if x-rays were in color. But we don't need to see the color because we can easily see a cloud of water around the infection on a plain old x-ray.

But we'll also get some urine from the bag under the bed to check for a urinary tract infection. Whenever you put something foreign in the body, like a urinary catheter, no matter how smooth it looks, bacteria are so small, they hide in the microscopic nooks and crannies and start growing. And we'll also check the surgical wound for an infection. Last thing is a lumbar puncture, but we'll wait on that until we rule out all the other places I just mentioned."

Mike spoke mechanically to hide his fright. "Lumbar puncture. What does it entail, Doctor?"

"We may need to see if there's an infection in the cerebral spinal fluid. That's the liquid the brain and spinal cord bathe in. But let's not talk about that until we rule out the easy stuff. And, anyway, we already have Dr. Maddingly started on a very good antibiotic. It's broad spectrum, which means it will kill most of the different bugs that ever show up in the Seattle area. When we find out exactly which bacteria we are dealing with, and where, we'll narrow the antibiotic down to something very specific. But for now, we're covered.

"So, let's just take it a step at a time. There'll be an answer soon. We'll let the hospitalist do her thing. She's great at finding bacteria. That's what they live for—hunting down bugs; a virtual army of Orkin men and women floating around the hospital squirting germ repellant on their hands and searching for pockets of pus in their patients. And I'll see you in the morning, but if you have any questions that can't wait until then, have the nurses get ahold of me."

Mike nodded and murmured his thanks then squeezed Sabrina's hand. He whispered, "Honey, they're on top of things. Don't fret one little bit. I love you so much."

She did not stir.

CHAPTER TWELVE

Norman Harp, Mitchie-Sterling's CEO, adjourned a top-secret conference of the institution's elite on the Sunday morning after Thanksgiving. Harp had reckoned the sensitivity of the gathering so critical, he had made the calls himself. The invitees were urged to tell their spouses the get-together involved the burgeoning power of the insurance industry to limit doctors' income. "Your wives should be particularly interested in that subject," Harp had laughed coldly with each surreptitious call he'd made late the evening before.

No one was ever sure where Harp bought his boutonnieres, but, even during the winter, each morning saw a fresh bud in his lapel. This Sunday was not an exception. He began his remarks in the most solemn tone, his lengthy, pointed nose just so many degrees atop the horizon. "In the past, our institution has provided the City of McKinley with quite satisfactory care. It was never our intention to replace the U as the medical investigational center of the Northwest. Our staff has always been totally dedicated to the proposition that the community is best served by following the fundamentals of medicine." He stopped for a sip of water from the crystal glass he carried from meeting to endless meeting.

While there had been perfunctory pre-summit grumbling, the attendees had assumed the real topic was going to be worth the sacrifice of the one day of the week they were not in the office or on call. Now, though, eyes were beginning to roll.

"Gentlemen and lady, please remain focused. As your CEO, it falls on me to deflect any flutter of disorder wafting in our direction. I want to nip in the bud challenges for which we might be seen accountable. Let me preface my remarks by saying much of our predicament these days is the result of a new breed of alleged doctors, lone wolves, who have slithered into town to man grubby walk-in clinics. They're hatching all over the county like nests of snakes. I have discovered their corporate leadership to be as questionable as the riffraff hired to churn out poorly arrived at diagnoses, followed by frankly dangerous treatments. We are all aware of the pediatric patient who lost his life because of the delay one of those so-called health professionals triggered, the quack who diagnosed a stomachache when the child was actually critical with an advanced appendicitis.

"Thankfully, the court settlement did not do us substantial harm. Regardless, sadly, despite that litigation, there still has been no legislative control of these charlatans. As a result, once again, we are faced with a new problem generated by one of these medical impostors. Several nights ago, one of the frauds over there in Evanston abandoned a woman suffering with an ectopic pregnancy. As I am not a doctor, I will leave a discussion of the gravity of that act to you professionals. Dr. Gauthé was closely involved so, sir, would you mind giving us a quick rundown of the most recent encounter with our," he raised his fingers to exaggerate quote marks, "'colleagues' to the east?'"

Chris Gauthé's shoulders tightened. "I'll tell you what I know of the matter, but I can only speak to what happened after I arrived on the scene in the ER, Norman. I think Peter Cardozo can give us a better idea of what led to her arrival on our campus. I'm not sure I understand why he's not one of God's chosen here today."

Harvey Klat, the hospital's medical director, raised a finger. "Cardozo's in the ER. Suffice it to say, we invited only the hospital's discriminating thought leaders to this meeting. I can summarize what Cardozo told me, and what I gleaned from a nastygram I got yesterday from the girl in Evanston.

"Long and short of it, a 34-year-old white female accompanied by her husband presents to the walk-in clinic in Evanston with debilitating abdominal pain. This is on Thanksgiving Eve, it's near closing, and they don't invite the patient in to stabilize her, if they even know how, if they even have the equipment to do so. Just send their train wrecks down here and let our doctors assume the malpractice risk of putting them back together.

"So, the female doctor tells the husband to transport the patient down here. No ambulance, nothing, just drive as fast as you can. She calls the ER and demands to speak to Cardozo. He's busy with two MIs at once and tells one of the nurses to tell the triage lady to tell the lady doctor he's not available. I guess the girl from Evanston becomes antagonistic, and Cardozo steps in, quite appropriately, to back up his staff. He grabs the phone from the triage gal. Lady doctor starts using profanity, threatens to sue him, so he hangs up, which was the professional thing to do.

"Meanwhile, the patient is actively bleeding from a rupturing ectopic, and everyone thinks it's an acute abdomen, because that's what the bogus doctor in Evanston has screamed over the phone to anyone who'd listen.

"Around 2 A.M., patient finds her way into the ER and is sitting there waiting for God knows what. Just sitting there. Our triage nurse is well-trained. She frequently looks out into the waiting area to make sure everything's copasetic. Sees a lady in the corner, white as a sheet, so they take her back, but she's lost so much blood, she's suffering from vascular collapse. Dr. Cardozo did the right thing. Swallows his ego and calls upstairs for a surgeon to do a cut down for a central line.

"Dr. Gauthé responds, manages to get a central line going quickly, and takes her to surgery—saves the woman's life. So, Chris, why don't you take it from here."

"Well, first, I think there's a bit more to the story prior to her presentation at our ER. The doctor in Evanston sent the patient and her husband down for a serum pregnancy test here at our lab, and for an ultrasound. SPT was positive, but the ultrasound didn't show any products of conception in the uterus. We do not know what the radiologist saw, other than what he supposedly told Cardozo, that there was a belly full of blood. Doctor in Evanston claims the radiologist specifically told her there was no blood at all. So, we do not know if there was free blood in the pelvic cavity when she came to our ER. It's a he said-she said right now. I haven't been able to find the films. Seems no one's seen them, and then there was the power outage. Isn't even clear if the radiologist dictated a report. No one in weekend-transcription remembers doing it. And now, with what's happened, we aren't going to be able to ask the rad himself."

As Gauthé paused, there was a sudden, deathly silence in the room. Harp, who had been distracted reading from his laptop, lifted his head at the silence and grumbled quickly, "Yes, Dr. Gauthé, please go on."

Gauthé's shoulders tightened, and he went cheerlessly back to his narrative. "Anyway, patient winds up in the ER after the ultrasound, eventually gets taken back, and like Dr. Klat said, it was a rough ride from there. One of the toughest central lines I've ever placed. By now, no question, she's bleeding out. No OBs around, so I took her to surgery with the hope of just stopping the hemorrhaging. My thinking was that we'd have an OB take her back to surgery in the morning, or when she was stabilized, at least not bleeding out, to, you know, neaten things up."

"Dr. Gauthé," Harp interrupted, "let's approach this with the attitude that, while you might not be an OB/GYN, you are a senior surgeon, supremely capable of entering the abdomen and controlling severe bleeding, no matter where it's coming from. As always, I want there to be no second-guessing on our part in regard to the care we provided. And I don't think there has been. So, please go on."

"Okay, lots of blood in the pelvis."

Harp raised his palm toward Gauthé. "So, even without the ultrasound, we know that there was bleeding. Yes?"

"There was bleeding, but that begs the question of when it started. But just let me finish what I did in surgery. Plugged things as quickly as I could, but there had been a long period of hypotension in the ER before the central line, and it looks like she suffered an intercurrent stroke."

Harp snapped, "Culpability?"

"Happens when eighty percent of your blood has gushed out of the vessels into a big pool in your pelvis. Uncertainty remains about when the bleeding started. If she arrived on our doorstep already half empty, no jury is going to pin it on us."

"So, how do we establish where she was when she walked into the ER?"

Gauthé hesitated. "Well, if the ultrasound doesn't show any free blood in the pelvis, it'll mean the bleeding started on our watch. To be up front, my guess is that because she was ambulating without difficulty when she arrived here, I mean walked into the hospital, then downstairs to the basement lab, the only one open that night, back upstairs and over to ultrasound, then all the way back to the emergency room, all on her own steam, and she sits there awake for who knows how long, that's not easy to do on half a tank. It means, at worst, she might have been leaking when she arrived here, but the gushing hadn't gotten going. The science of it lies in the radiology findings."

Harp's shoulders tightened. "Dr. Klat, why is there no radiology report?"

"Don't know."

"Dr. Gauthé?"

"I do not know if there ever was a report. Most of the rads will dictate the note before they leave the building. Like I said, I never saw the ultrasound, either, just got a verbal from Cardozo that led me to believe there was no fetus in the uterus, so with a positive pregnancy test, the products of conception had to be in the tube. I will say, in Cardozo's defense, he only mentioned it in passing that the rad said there was blood. When I arrived on the scene, all that mattered to him was that her blood pressure was tanking, and it was obvious blood was leaking—fast. The exact moment it started was not important for what he had to do."

Harp's voice rose. "I hope we are on good terms with the rent-a-rads this week. DeepSight Radiologists—a bunch of effete technicians. No loyalty to the institution. They're bleeding us dry, no pun intended. I love the latest: all of a sudden, they're demanding we pay them to overread every single x-ray we take here."

Chris Gauthé interrupted. "Norman, it's a rip off, no doubt, but the first time one of our docs misses something on a chest film or CT, the lawsuit's gonna cost more than hospital's worth. We have no choice. They have us over a barrel. And they're pretty good at what they do. And, given the circumstances, we need to tread very lightly."

Harp growled, "What circumstances?"

"Norman, are you not aware that the radiologist was killed out on 740 Thanksgiving morning?"

Harp paused for two seconds. "No, I was not informed. It's a different corporation."

"Drunk came across the highway and killed him, his wife, and one of their two kids. He was a good guy; everybody liked him."

"Well, I'm sorry to hear that, and my office will be sure to extend our sympathies, send flowers, but we need to remain focused. This is serious business. Lot of families depend on our corporation for their livelihoods." Without a pause he scowled. "Now, maybe there isn't even a formal report. I mean, if Dr. Gauthé's scenario is correct, the patient shows up with telephone orders for an imaging study from an unknown doctor not on our staff. Patient gets rushed through because the girl from Evanston is screaming bloody murder, has everyone rushing around like chickens with their heads cut off. I can picture it. Discipline breaks down, patient gets an ultrasound before she's even checked in, doesn't sign consent forms, on and on, no insurance info, radiologist doesn't even know her name, or the referring doctor's name. It's late at night, no one around to transcribe his findings. So, maybe, he says he'll come in in the morning and dictate the report. Maybe he says the hell with it, that he'll do it Monday. All he has to do is look at the film for fifteen seconds, if that. I mean they don't need to lay eyes on the actual patient. Correct?"

Klat held up his palm. "Norman, that's not necessarily the case. Some of the rads, actually most of them, are pretty decent docs. Most of them want to learn the medicine when there's an unusual case. He might even have done a physical exam to reassure himself about his reading. I don't know. We don't know, and we'll likely never know. But the rest is history. Best we can do is ask the tech if she remembers the patient. And I heard she's not handling this well."

Harp scoffed. "Not surprised. Weak sisters. In my experience, we won't be getting much from her. Our techs are not the sharpest knives in the drawers. Have their own little cliques—don't understand the concept of a corporation. If we ask her for a statement and tell her it's a legal document, you know very well what's going to happen—probably faint, get admitted for a few days, then file a harassment complaint the instant she's discharged, before she even goes home to feed the cat."

Dr. Sonya Laureano, the only woman on the board of directors, and the only woman who had ever been elected to the board in the hospital's nearly eight decades, had remained quiet during the proceedings. In most meetings, she said nothing until her colleagues' huffing and puffing wound down and Harp, sure he would get his way, called for a vote. Generally, Dr. Laureano would nod, apparently in agreement, when the CEO blathered on about his opinion, and then, with a warm smile, almost always side against the administration."

This time, though, without waiting to be recognized, she blurted, "Norman, hate to break it to you, but some of the staff have more loyalty to this hospital than a couple of dozen doctors we can all name in about thirty seconds. They work hard—get paid a few pennies over minimum wage." She stared at him poker-faced. "Just wanted to let you know."

"Sonya, of course you're correct. I'm sure they're wonderful, but I'm not willing to trust the future of this corporation to a clutch of technicians who barely made it out of high school." Before she could retort, he shot, "As for the radiologists, they make twenty times the minimum wage and are about as reliable."

Sonya Laureano spoke softly, "Thank you, Norman. Now, have we thought about calling the radiologists' medical director, whoever that might be this week, and ask him or her to get ahold of their head transcriptionist? Have her go through their work queue for the last few days, job by job."

Up came Harp's palm. "Waste of time. Never get ahold of one of the principals on a Sunday. They keep bankers' hours. He'd probably not want to call the fragile creature who runs the typing pool on her long weekend. It'll have to wait until morning." He smiled plastically, "So, Dr. Laureano, would you be so good as to get ahold of whoever's the CEO du jour and discuss the findings?"

She nodded. "First thing in the morning."

"Thank you. And where, exactly, is the patient, medically, at this juncture?" He pointed at Chris Gauthé.

The surgeon nodded. "We're pretty early in the process. What I can tell you is that she had a stroke in the hospital, and that she's developed an infection postoperatively, all of which looks, from the outside, like there's going to be hell to pay in terms of lawsuits. It turns out, however, she has an unusual congenital neural tube defect, supposedly from her father's exposure to Agent Orange in Viet Nam. Perhaps that has something to do with the stroke and the infection, but we don't know yet. And, importantly, she had very limited premorbid use of her left arm. Also, there was possibly weakness in the left leg, but I'm not sure about that because she was a runner, of sorts. And the left side is where the current stroke is manifesting itself. Right now, she's got no use of the left upper extremity at all, and very little of the left leg, but it's early."

Harp raised his palm toward Gauthé's face. "Dr. Gauthé, are you saying there's some wiggle room there?"

"Certainly doesn't hurt that her pre-stroke problems are pretty close to those after our intervention. I mean, the neurologist got a history of a young, healthy woman, thin, non-smoker, good diet, no birth control pills, no high blood pressure, no diabetes, no trauma; you have to wonder," he asked rhetorically, "why did she have a stroke?" You can argue there must be some serious underlying disease for which we can't be held responsible. And, you can contend that, at least, we saved her life."

Harp interrupted. "Is she going to live?"

"We'll do our best to get the infection under control. We're not sure where it's coming from yet. This is not your usual case. We need to wait and see when she wakes up how much more damage is present."

Harp locked Klat's eyes. "Okay, let's move on. Harvey, what do we know about the husband trespassing in the ER? Was his presence disruptive to the provision of our high standard of medical care? Are we going to be able to turn that to our advantage?"

Klat answered. "We don't know how or when he entered the treatment area the second time."

"Second time?"

"Yes, the first was when he accompanied his wife into the treatment bay. Cardozo ordered him out, and the nurse escorted him into the waiting room."

"Into, or just pointed him in the right direction?"

"The nurse assumed he had gone through the doors. No one knows for sure. Don't forget, it was pretty frantic down there, at least from what I understand."

Harp's jaw tightened. "Haven't they been trained not to assume? That's a step in the wrong direction. And, please, let's not sully our case with expressions like, 'pretty frantic.'" Gauthé nodded.

Harp hissed, "Go on, please."

"Well, out of the blue, there he is in the hallway."

"This the first or second time?"

"Probably the second, and how much he saw of our," air quotes, "'vigorous efforts,' is a mystery. We do know that once he was apprehended, he assaulted one of our security staff."

Harp again held up his palm to Klat's face then turned to Worth Weegun. "Doctor, you're our safety officer. What is the situation with this employee? I understand he was supposed to work last night but didn't show up."

"That's correct, Norman, but it's only been a couple of days."

"What's his excuse?"

Weegun smirked. "He reports that the patient's husband threw him to the ground in the parking lot. The attack, according to eyewitnesses, was unprovoked."

"There were witnesses in the parking lot?" He sighed, "Were they patients?"

"We don't know. Several of the other security guards state they observed the attack. They tried to subdue the man, but he ran back into the ER and continued raising hell."

"Does that mean there was a third incident?"

"No, only two as far as I know."

"How long has the poor man worked for us?"

"Two months."

"Is he sympathetic? I mean, in regard to a jury. This could be the injured worker who laid the golden egg."

Weegun hesitated. "Well, I haven't met him personally, but I guess he's had his struggles."

"Struggles." Harp's pupils narrowed. "How sensitive. Please don't tell me touched a patient?"

"No, it was with the law. Minor stuff. Was incarcerated at the county jail for a year."

Harp winced. "For what? A felony?"

"I don't know. We weren't allowed to ask—remember? Had to offer him the job based on his 'credentials,' and only then would we be allowed to look into his past."

"Well?"

"We didn't look into it. Slipped through the cracks."

Harp monotoned, "Now, we don't need to publicize his history. None of anybody's business. Man has a right to his privacy. He may still come in handy. And, the worse his injuries, the more sympathetic he appears. What's his complaint?"

"Says his back hurts."

"They all do, don't they? Go on."

"Asserts his legs are so weak; he can't stand to use the rest room. Also, claims he's seeing double. Filed an L&I claim."

Harp snapped, "I want to see his records."

"They're not here. He went to one of the walk-in clinics on Friday morning. Doctor gave him three weeks' time loss right off the bat. We offered light duty. Doctor refused. Dollars to donuts, this is going to be a time-loss nightmare. Lawyers, litigation. Mark my words."

Harp shook his head. "Heck of a lot cheaper than if the family wins a malpractice suit. Cajole him for as long as it takes to keep him on our side. You know these L&I people—turn on the employer first chance they get. Sniff a few hundred dollars...

"Okay, that's enough for today. We have some direction, but there's also a lot of work to do to fill in the blanks. Harvey, let's start collecting the woman's former medical records. Worth, let's meet with our loss control people and get on track with this injured worker. Don't want problems with him." Without taking a breath, he went on, "Dr. Laureano, you are going to contact the radiologists. Thank you. Please send our regrets, blah, blah, blah, and find out if a report was done. They'll be nicer to you than if it's a male trying to extract information.

"Devil's in the details, gentlemen and lady. I want to get all our ducks in row before we present this to the attorneys. We have some time, but not forever. We'll meet again after I've discussed your reports with the lawyers. And I don't need to remind you: absolute security is essential."

CHAPTER THIRTEEN

Early that Sunday evening, Mike drifted in and out of wakefulness in the corner lounge chair. Though in a near coma, he began to sense the presence of lay persons in the room, voices tentative and faint. He rubbed his eyes, but it was too dark to make out anything other than a pair of thin figures bent over Sabrina's bed, silhouettes that sprang upright with a start as Mike lifted from his recliner.

Mike howled, "Mom, Dad. What are you doing here? I told you not to worry."

Even in the bare light, Mike discerned in his father-in-law a face devoid of color or expression. His mother-in-law was crying quietly. They had traveled through the past night and most of that day from Wilkes Barre, Pennsylvania. As the three embraced, the woman's tears exploded, but her husband wiped them away softly with the back of his hand.

Lincoln Friday was tall and lanky, his face hardened by things about which he never spoke. Mike imagined the man's parents conferring the name Lincoln on the day of his birth, somehow presaging the square jaw and towering cheekbones. Yet that would have been unlikely, for neither had read on greater than a second-grade level, not much time on their hard scrabble Pennsylvania farm for history books about slavery and the Civil War.

Isabelle was also tall, and regal, with eyes as blue-green as the waters of Waikiki. Her hair remained light, tinged with the subtlest red, validating her western European ancestry. Mike was still taken with her comeliness.

Lincoln leaned forward and kissed Sabrina's moist forehead. He, too, began to cry. "Ya know Mike," he caught his breath, "when our little girl was born, there were problems. Doctors knew it right away. Most of them just shrugged—a few of them babbled, 'luck of the draw, I guess.' One of the smart ones sent us to a geneticist. Shoot, Mike, you've heard all this before. I should be quiet."

"Dad, I need to hear it, and so do her doctors. I don't think anyone here knows what's going on. Each new problem's like a bolt of lightning. Please, tell me."

"Okay. Maybe it'll help. Geneticist said she wasn't sure if it was congenital or from environmental things, but she started to ask questions about where Isabelle and I were born, raised, what month, on and on. Isabelle was worried we were getting an astrological reading. But she also asked a lot about things we'd been exposed to—me on the farm, Isabelle when she a nurse in the hospital back home. She wanted to know about all the different kinds of aviation fuel in the helicopters I flew, and she got excited about the JP-4. Had benzene in it, you know.

"But when she heard that I sprayed Agent Orange all over Viet Nam from my helicopter, she leaned forward and started taking lots more notes. That was the first I had heard of Agent Orange causing defects in the children of GIs. She told us the government denied it, but I guess there were a lot of articles about it in their genetics magazine. She warned us there might be problems later on. No one knew all the possibilities. I just wonder if this is all part of it."

Mike nodded. "That's what one of the doctors here thinks. We should have you meet her. Good lady. Put up with my crap and didn't abandon us. Let me give her office a call and see if we can make an appointment to talk to her."

Mike phoned the Evanston Medical Center. The receptionist would only put him through to Khai's nurse, Sharon, who cut him off quickly and grumbled, "We're slammed. I'll tell Weathersby when I get the chance."

The next morning, Sabrina's eyes fluttered and she appeared to be gazing about the room. As her three guests sprang from their chairs, Sabrina shied back, though her face slowly relaxed, and when she focused on Mike, her eyes filled with tears.

Mike laughed nervously. "Great romance. First thing wife does when she wakes up from oblivion and sees who she's married to, she bursts into tears." As Isabelle punched his arm, the corners of Sabrina's mouth curled up faintly.

Standing so fixedly over the bed, they did not realize another figure had walked up behind them. Mike, though, soon felt the warmth on his neck and turned abruptly. It was Khai Weathersby.

He brightened. "Mom, Dad, this is the doctor I told you about." He turned to Khai. "You didn't have to come here. I just left a message that we could go up to your office and do a doctor's visit, you know, pay for your time, and maybe you could explain things to Sabrina's folks." He rolled his eyes. "Oh, man, I'm sorry; this is Isabelle and Lincoln Friday."

Khai took their hands and smiled warmly. "Beautiful family. I'm not surprised, but I am mortified. You say you left a message? Who did you speak to, the receptionist?"

Mike hesitated and mumbled, "No."

Khai's face flattened. "Okay, I'll take care of that. Can't have a message service that's a sieve. Look, if you want to talk, let me know when Sabrina needs a break. We can sit up here or go to the cafeteria. I'm done for the day. Got plenty of time."

Mike turned his head curiously. "If you're not doctoring today, what are you doing up here in Metropolis?"

"Came to see you guys."

By the time they turned back to the bed, Sabrina was asleep. Lincoln kissed her forehead, and they left for the cafeteria. Mike pushed Isabelle and Lincoln on line first, and they nudged Khai ahead of them. Lincoln smiled. "Please, we're treating."

Mike laughed, "Good. I'll have the Surf and Turf, and the pecan pie. Nah, I'm not all that hungry. Just some coffee."

Khai turned back to Mike. "Mr. Maddingly, you need to start taking care of yourself. You've already lost a couple of pounds. You get sick, you'll be of no use to Sabrina. She's counting on you. We were taught in medical school not to badger people dying of cancer to eat. You're not dying of cancer. You need to stay strong."

"Okay," he chattered, "it's back to the Surf and Turf, and half a pecan pie," though he pulled a sliced turkey sandwich from the cooler.

They sat in the same corner she had with Gauthé. She was not sure if she was excited or scared, but quickly looked about and saw that she was invisible.

Mike faced Khai. "Doctor, The Fridays are quite special. Mrs. Friday's

83

family were, are, quite prominent in Pennsylvania. Her dad was a World War Two pilot. Never met him, but he was a wonderful man. And Isabell's mom is as stately as a queen, and three thousand times warmer. And I love Isabelle almost as much as Sabrina. She's a great lady."

"And you're a dream for a son-in-law." She leaned over and squeezed his hand, her eyes moistening.

"And Mr. Friday is quite something as well, not as good looking, though. For a start, he owns a very successful helicopter company near Philly."

Khai unconsciously bolted straighter in her chair. Lincoln noticed her hands clutch ever so subtly, as if grasping handles. When her cheeks flushed, Lincoln probed, "Doctor, you're familiar with helicopters, aren't you?"

A nervous rigidity overtook the table. Khai nodded. "Yes, sir, I am."

Lincoln smiled warmly. "Army?"

"You are a very perceptive man, sir. Yes, Blackhawks. Two all-expenses paid vacations in Kuwait and Iraq; Thirty-Third Mech. My father's old unit from Viet Nam. And you, sir?"

Lincoln straightened subtly. Isabelle and Mike stared anxiously. Khai was sure the hue of his eyes took on the faintest blush. "Two tours in Viet Nam. Hueys."

The silence was so painful, Mike could not help but blurt, "Mr. Friday won the Medal of Honor."

Khai froze, her face losing all color. She bolted to her feet, standing at near-attention, her eyes glassy. With the sudden hush around their table, she was sure the entire cafeteria was watching. She did not care. "It is an honor, sir."

He nodded slowly once, and she retook her seat, but her eyes clouded further as Lincoln spoke just beyond a whisper. "And an honor to meet you, ma'am. The profession is lucky to have you. And thank you for your service." He broke into a slight smile. "And thank goodness you had the I.Q. to get out of aviation. Especially as a rotor head. The fun of pushing buttons and pulling levers wears off pretty quick when it's for the rest of your life. Just another business with insufferable customers; most of them are mad at you most of the time, and not one, even the satisfied, pays his bill on time, if ever."

"Sort of like medicine," she laughed, "except you, Mr. Friday, actually accomplish something at the end of the day. Something you can see."

Lincoln rolled his eyes, and Mike cackled, "Well, Dr. Weathersby, just think, at the end of your day, you can take heart in laundry baskets full of soiled sheets."

Isabelle reached to her side and punched his shoulder lightly. "Dr. Weathersby, I apologize for Mike. He can't help it—congenital, I think."

Khai laughed. "Oh, I've known him for three whole days. Didn't take long to diagnose his syndrome. Wish everyone was suffering from it." As the mood at the table lightened, Khai straightened in her chair. "Okay, let's talk about Dr. Maddingly. Looks terrible right now, but this is what we see all the time. We call it a stormy postoperative course. But it isn't all that atypical. The stress of an infection, on top of the stress of surgery, on top of the stress of an early pregnancy, pardon my French, knocks the crap outta ya. Don't care who you are. We can control the infection, and pretty well, actually. After all, in fact, Sabrina is really quite a strong young woman. She has no real medical history since birth. Never been hospitalized, except for a routine appendectomy, doesn't take any medications, so she is a good candidate for a decent recovery."

Isabelle asked, "You say 'decent.' Does that mean the stroke is permanent? Will she get back some use of her arm?"

"I'm sorry. Wish I could tell you somebody knows. But no one does. As I told Mr. Maddingly, humans are incredibly adaptable. Did you know that last year a blind man summited Mt. Everest?"

Mike interrupted, "Yeah, I read about that on the internet. Guy got to the top, and all he did was complain about the view. 'Can't see a damn thing from up here.'"

"Mike, you're pushing it," Isabelle hissed, but shook her head and smiled.

"Yes, he is," added Khai. "So, I can't tell you anything except that we have to wait, and that Sabrina's getting excellent care. And let me warn you up front that there are going to be annoying little mistakes and problems along the way. When you see them, and you will, it'll scare the pants off you. But in the greater scheme of things, they're minor, and they must be part of the plan, because they are so common. And when all is said and done, the little glitches don't amount to a hill of beans.

"So, we'll wait and find where the infection is, then do a number on it." She rubbed her eyes. "Okay, I think I'll head back home." She took out a card and wrote her cell number on it. "You call me anytime. I'm serious. All of a sudden, we're family." She looked directly into Lincoln's eyes. "Again, sir, it is an honor. I can't wait to tell my dad. Hueys '68 and '69." Her eyes reddened again. "Maybe we'll talk about it sometime." They shook hands.

CHAPTER FOURTEEN

K hai's cell rang as she turned onto the highway toward Seattle. It was her clinic; the labs were back on a sick, older woman who had presented at closing two nights before. Khai groaned, took the next exit, then got back on toward the clinic. She smiled weakly recollecting the encounter. The woman sat on the exam table gasping for air, howling it was the acute onset of lung cancer. In fact, she was not short of breath at all, just having trouble drawing a breath deep enough to feel she was inhaling fully. It was a common complaint, and almost always associated with stress, as were the bulk of the problems Khai had encountered during her ten years in medicine. She urged the woman to draw air through her nose instead of her mouth. It worked.

The woman leaned forward and hugged Khai. "Oh, such a smart lady doctor. Good for you."

Khai could not miss the reek of stale, and fresh, urine wafting from the woman. She asked gently, "How's your bladder, Mrs. Cooper?"

"Why, now that you mention it, that's been a problem lately." She suddenly became very quiet, and her head drooped a bit. "Can I tell you something?"

"Of course. Anything."

"Well, I guess I can say this because you're a doctor and all...but you see, I have a problem with my private parts. I've got some red things, you know, down there. They hurt so bad when I pee. Oh, my, it is so painful. Do you know what it is?"

"Is this new?"

87

"Oh, yes. Just this week."

"Ever had anything like this before? Anything?"

"No, never."

"Well, I'm not trying to be nosey, but are you sexually active?"

"Oh, my goodness, no!"

"Of course not. But you know, Mrs. Cooper, what kind of doctor would I be if I didn't ask? Let's just take a quick look."

"Is that really necessary?"

"Be over in a second. I promise. The nurse'll get things ready."

When Khai asked Sharon to prep the patient for a vaginal exam, she sniped under her breath, "Woman comes in for shortness of breath, and all of a sudden, this one wants to do a pelvic!" Though Khai glared, Sharon rolled her eyes, grabbed a gown, and bristled into the room.

There were four dime-sized, angry red sores on the woman's labia. They must have hurt terribly when the woman urinated, the acidic liquid streaming over the lesions. Khai was sure it was a herpes infection. She asked again about any intimacy.

"Well, if you mean, did I have sex with that guy, the answer is no, no, no! Things don't work so good down there anymore. Don't think you could get a pencil inside."

"Well, did that guy touch you, or maybe, you know, kiss you all over the place?"

"Oh my God. Is this from him?"

"Well, did he kiss you down there?" The woman began to cry when Khai leaned forward and put a hand on her arm. "It's okay, Mrs. Cooper, everything's going to be fine. I promise. This is no big deal."

"Well, I suppose I have to tell you. He does that sometimes. I mean, when I let him in the door. He's right across the hall. Always knocking. Thinks I'm some kinda sex object."

"Nothing wrong with being close to someone."

"I guess so, but not if he gives you a disease."

"Well, he probably didn't know. Given what you've said, it's not the bad kind of rash." Khai started to explain that there were two different types of herpes infections that can infect the genitals: Herpes One, the kind that causes cold sores around the mouth, and Herpes Two, that is notorious for finding a home on the genitals.

"Mrs. Cooper, nearly everyone on Earth has Herpes Type One, so that type is no big deal. Maybe you were one of the lucky ones who didn't get it as a kid, but if he did, and he kissed you down there, well, you can just think of it as a few plain old cold sores."

"He didn't tell me he had cold sores. You think I'd let him do that to me if he did?"

"Well, Mrs. Cooper, even if you don't see the cold sores, even if he didn't see them, it can still be passed on. If the virus is hanging around his mouth, like it is in most people..."

"You mean I have the virus?"

"No, not that virus at all. Million different kinds of viruses. This one's just like getting a simple cold."

"He should have told me he was sick."

"He wasn't sick, probably. You see, herpes stays with you forever."

"Oh, my goodness, I can't hurt like this forever."

"Of course you won't. This will all be over in a few days. Don't worry a bit. Tell you what. Let's just send off a culture and figure out what's going on for sure. Send some urine off, too, and see if you've just got a mean old UTI."

"He gave me that, too?"

There was an accident on I-740, and Khai didn't get to the clinic in Evanston until past eleven. The woman had a UTI, probably from holding urine too long because it hurt so to pee. The results of the woman's viral cultures, though, were not there, and she called the lab, pestering them until they put the pathologist on the line. He hemmed and hawed that there was clearly an infection, and in both the skin scraping and the urine, but he wouldn't commit himself about the sores until the culture came back—two weeks, at best. Khai knew better than to ask the man to make an educated guess. She wanted to get home and sleep, not listen to the standard pathologist waffle about opening himself up to malpractice litigation if he actually made a confident, useful diagnosis. She grumbled a thank you, phoned the patient, and spent some trying to explain the need for two medications: an antibiotic for the UTI and an anti-viral for the rash. The dialogue became so confused, Khai offered to come to the woman's apartment and go over it in detail.

The woman bridled, "You goanna charge me for the house call?"

"Of course not, ma'am."

When Khai arrived, the woman's friend was standing in the door. His jaw set, he glared at Khai, finally barking, "Who the hell are you to tell her..." he jabbed his thumb over his shoulder, "that I gave her VD? I'm a Christian, ya know. Have been ever since I got outta the joint. Ain't ashamed of it no more, either. Did my time. Lotta years ago. Just 'cause I'm an ex-con don't mean I go 'round infectin' the ladies."

By the time the dialogue with the angry lovers had reached a stalemate, it was past one. Khai called in the prescriptions from her cell phone then drove back to the clinic to gather charts to work on at home.

An envelope on top of the pile was from the Office of the Medical Director, Mitchie-Sterling Hospital, McKinley, Washington.

Dear Dr. Weathersby,

I am in receipt of your letter regarding a conversation that took place with a member of my staff on Thanksgiving Eve. My secretary has spoken with the party involved. He categorically denies using either the tone of voice or the deprecating language you have alleged. He does allow that he was busy with two patients suffering myocardial infarctions and did not have time to discuss the disposition of a patient who was unknown to him. I'm sure you can understand that.

I was particularly sad to hear that word of the purported incident was widespread before I had an opportunity to respond to you. Doctor, we are a collegial and professional medical community. Allegations of this sort undermine the integrity of health care delivery in the McKinley community.

I note that you have not joined our county or state professional medical societies. If you choose to seek membership, you will have to present testimonials from member colleagues. I am not sure the recent episode is the best way to achieve the respect needed for sponsorship.

Very truly yours,

Harvey A. Klat, M.D.
Medical Director

Khai read the letter twice, her teeth grinding harder with each word. She grabbed her phone to look for Gauthé's number and cocked a finger to punch the call button but stopped abruptly. "I don't need to be begging some full-of-himself surgeon to handle my problems. Put the phone down."

As her finger retreated, the cell rang. She looked at the screen. "Oh, shit, the call went through anyway. How the hell is that possible?" She thought briefly about ignoring it but hit TALK almost as a reflex.

Before she could excuse herself claiming a butt-call, he answered cheerily. "Khai, hey, how are ya? Just wondering what you're doing."

Her jaw tightened. "Just fine. Enjoying another day doing God's work here on Earth."

"You don't sound fine."

"It's okay."

"Where are you?"

"Ah..."

He interrupted, "Hey, had a cancellation. I'm done for the day. I know you're not up at the clinic..."

"How do you know that?"

"The receptionist used some other name when I asked who was in the hot seat today."

Khai was silent again as she contemplated hanging up on her only possible ally within the surrounding two to three thousand square miles. "Well, Swami Chris, I am up in Evanston, but just about to get the heck out of here."

"Perfect. How 'bout I meet you at Sergio's, down by the Port. Two hours. Late, late lunch, or early dinner. Ever been there?"

"Yes, it's a lovely setting." She looked at her jeans and Harvard sweatshirt and shrugged. "Not dressed properly."

He laughed. "This is Seattle, man. All you need is a credit card."

"Okay, two hours."

"Perfect. We can watch the sunset."

CHAPTER FIFTEEN

Lincoln and Isabelle Friday returned from a walk around the hospital. Mike was asleep in the corner recliner. The hospitalist was standing over Sabrina's bed, her head buried in a cell phone, fingers tapping furiously. She did not realize the family had entered the room and was standing right behind her. A nurse pushed past them dragging a stainless-steel cart piled with tubes and syringes. She stopped and spoke formally to the family. "You may want to leave the room while we do the LP. Shouldn't take too long. Why don't you try back in a half hour?"

The hospitalist looked up and turned toward them. Her hair had not been washed since the first time she had come to see Sabrina. As the mood in the room darkened, Mike startled from his uneasy sleep, rose groggily, and stepped forward. His nose wrinkled at the fishy odor wafting from the woman. He asked tautly, "What's going on?"

Barely looking at him, she monotoned, "We're going to do an LP."

"I thought that was the last step, when you couldn't find the infection anywhere else."

"That's correct. We have not found the infection anywhere else. Nurse said while you were gone Sabrina woke up and thought she was in a hotel. That means she's confused. And I sense a bit of a stiffness in her neck when I try to flex it forward. We need to look at the CSF."

Mike growled, "I forget what that is."

"CSF, cerebral spinal fluid."

Mike raised his eyes to the ceiling and mumbled, "That means a brain infection."

"No. It only means we're looking for an infection in the meninges, the envelope that seals the brain and the spinal cord away from the rest of the body. We catch it now, and it won't get into the brain."

Mike mumbled, "But what about that redness around the tape where they couldn't start an IV, you know, right below her collarbone?"

The woman pulled the gown down slightly and looked at what was now just a Band-Aid. Oh, that's just redness from pulling off the dressing over and over. I don't know, maybe your wife is allergic to tape."

"Shouldn't you check it for an infection?"

The hospitalist sighed, "If we culture it, it will come back full of bacteria. All the usual bugs on everybody's skin. I am certainly not opening a healing wound. And even if it was the source of the infection, that no longer matters if it has gotten into the meninges. Sir, we are going to do the lumbar puncture. We must find out if there is an infection near the brain."

Mike barked, "You wait. Don't do anything until I speak with Dr. Gauthé."

"We don't have time to wait. Your wife has a fever, she's confused, hard to wake up, and she has a stiff neck. That's all the indication I need to do an LP."

Mike took the surgeon's card from his pocket and pressed the keys on his cell phone. Gauthé answered on the first ring. His voice was clipped. "I was unaware of that. Let me speak with the hospitalist." He and the woman went back and forth in a patter, little of which resembled English. The conversation became totally unintelligible as the woman's frustration deepened.

She handed the phone back to Mike, who spoke with the man curtly but eventually nodded and ended the call. He asked the doctor to wait until the family talked over the alternatives, and her face tightened as if to say there were no alternatives, but she held her piece.

The family retreated toward the elevators. Mike's voice was unsteady as he reported Gauthé's words. "He says not to worry and that that doctor does these procedures several times a day. Mom, do you believe him?"

Isabelle mumbled, "I don't know if I do, but I don't think we have a choice. From what I remember, the only way to see if there's an infection in the CSF is to do the lumbar puncture. Actually, I remember seeing a lot of these. Even helped on a few. Most of the time the patient's awake, and it's no big deal.

They have the person lie on their side and pull their knees up to their chest, to help spread the spinal bones apart. The patient may blink when they put in the needle with the Novocain, but that's about it. They wait a minute, to let the skin get numb, then put in a thin needle and go into the spinal cord, well, not into the cord itself, but into the fluid around it. Pull off a little CSF and send it to the lab to see if there're any white blood cells in it. If yes, that's means an infection. But, Mike, don't worry, the needle's so thin, there really isn't any damage. And then a Band-Aid, and it's all over that fast. On old guys, it can be a task—lot of arthritis in the spine to get the needle past. Sabrina'll be okay. Let's just back off and let them do what they need to."

Mike started to chafe and was about to recount the episode in the ER, but squeezed his eyes shut and nodded reluctantly. The three left quietly, heads down, for the cafeteria. They barely touched their coffee.

When they returned, a nurse was hanging new bags from the IV pole. Isabelle asked, "Why the change?"

"It's a different antibiotic. Much better at treating meningitis."

Mike took an aggressive step toward her. "Meningitis, what the hell?"

Lincoln put his hand on his son-in-law's shoulder. "Let's define the problem before we get too excited." He whispered to Mike, "And then we'll beat the crap out of 'em."

Mike's shoulders barely relaxed, but he forced a smile. "Mom, do you know what's going on?"

"I think so but let me go chat with the charge nurse."

She came back in two minutes. "Sabrina apparently has an infection in her CSF. Again, that's the cerebral spinal fluid. Apparently, the CSF they drew off was cloudy, which is not normal, and under the microscope they saw lots of white blood cells, which is what made it cloudy. There shouldn't be any more than one or two under normal conditions. Like I said before, white blood cells usually mean the body is fighting an infection, especially if there's a fever and a lot of sleeping. So, that's what they think Sabrina's got."

Mike growled, "They think?"

"Mike, it's okay. Remember what Dr. Weathersby said. They have to try and grow some of the bacteria on a culture plate to know exactly what's in there. In the meantime, Sabrina's getting antibiotics that cover almost everything that commonly gets into the CSF."

"That's what they said last time."

"Mike, look, we need to be patient. They're doing everything they can to help. We have to trust them."

"Trust them?" The crimson in his face deepened. Both Lincoln and Isabelle tensed. "You should've seen the botch job in the ER. I didn't want to tell you about it, but Dr. Gauthé called them Keystone Cops. These people are untrustworthy. They need to send Sabrina to the U."

Isabelle stared at him for a moment then sighed. "I wish you hadn't told us, but we'll address that later. Mike, it seems they're following protocol to the letter. Moving her now would be a disaster."

"They should have known she had an infection a long time ago, when she was getting worse instead of better."

Lincoln's hand touched his son-in-law's shoulder. "Mike, come on, we need to calm down and think straight. Let's try not to get ahead of ourselves. I saw people a lot worse off than Sabrina, in hospitals that would curl your toes, and they did fine. The doctor said she was strong, and we know she is."

Mike drew in a deep breath to fight back but nodded. "I'm sure you're right, Dad. I'm just so damn tired and scared. I'm sorry."

Isabelle spoke in a whisper. "Don't be. You have the right, and duty, to question every move they make, but for right now, I think they're on top of things."

They sat until the next dose of IV antibiotics had been injected into the IV. At eleven, the hospitalist came in. Isabelle smiled at her. "Are you still working?"

"Sure looks like it. One of my group's kids has a sore throat. He owes me big time. Let's just put it this way: both you and I are here against our will." She laughed briefly.

Isabelle tapped her arm softly. "Thank you for taking care of Sabrina."

"It's my privilege. And we're going to do everything we need to get your daughter stabilized. Now, look, Ms. Maddingly probably won't show any improvement for the first twenty-four hours, probably longer. You might want to go home and get some rest."

CHAPTER SIXTEEN

The late fall days are very short in Seattle. As Chris Gauthé had alluded, the sun was just dropping over the Olympics when Khai walked into the restaurant. He helped her out of her coat then settled her in a chair in a private niche along the grand array of bay windows. They sat just feet from Puget Sound and a roaring log fire.

"Whata you know. A clear afternoon. See what you've brought to the Great Northwest. Could it be an omen of times to come?"

Khai winced faintly but forced a smile and began to answer. The waitress, though, had already slid to a halt at their table, poked her head between them, and asked if they wanted to start with drinks.

Chris turned to Khai. "This is my treat. Should we get a bottle of really good wine?"

"You know, I never drink and drive. I think I'll stick to coffee."

"Aw, come on. One glass of wine isn't drinking and driving. Tell you what, we'll get half a bottle, and you can take a sip or two. The colors out there are too beautiful to waste on a clear brain."

The wine was there before they had a chance to speak. Gauthé poured a single swallow into both glasses and lifted his. She hesitated but with no choice, glasses clinked. "To your coming success on the West Coast."

She sipped two tablespoons of wine, and with her lips barely away from the glass, he reached over and poured a bit more than the last offering. She smiled and put the glass down.

Chris laughed softly and nodded. "You're a very strong person, aren't you, Khai Weathersby?"

"I hope just sensible."

He thought for a moment. "And formidable. And guarded. And, yet, you are incredibly warm and good with patients. How do you compartmentalize your life so well?"

"A girl needs to watch out for herself these days, ya know."

"That's true, but not with everybody. Too much skepticism ain't healthy."

"True, but the rub is figuring out who you can trust."

"Well, most people trust their surgeon." When she didn't answer, he shook his head. "You know, there's ups and downs in everybody's life. Relationships come and go. Just part of the sinus curve of the journey. I mean, once you're plopped down on this Earth, you don't have all that much choice in the matter." He took a gulp of his wine. Only way to live a perfect life is not to get born in the first place."

Khai screwed up her face. "Huh?" She pointed at his glass. "This stuff fortified, like Thunderbird?"

"No, I'm being serious. I mean, people fall in love, whether they admit it or not. It's natural. God makes it happen. Not sure why she does. So damn painful when it doesn't work. Makes you wonder if life's worth it. It's why I didn't want to have kids. Didn't want them to bear that kind of loss. Kills me when I think about them suffering."

"So, you have kids?"

He took a deeper gulp of the wine. "I do. Three. Light of my life. They take more time than work, which is fine, and as it should be. I love it. But not such a great a situation with their mother."

"Divorce sucks. I'm sorry."

"Uh huh. It does indeed. You? Kids?"

"Nope."

Chris stared into her eyes. "You want to talk about it?" Khai's face turned away slightly. She hesitated then drew a breath to speak, but Gauthé's cell phone rang. He slumped in his chair and took a gulp of wine as he answered. He mouthed, "Maddingly."

When the call ended, he shook his head. "Husband called me an hour or so ago. Hospitalist wanted to do an LP but he was refusing. Must have got him straightened out because looks like it she's got a flaming meningeal infection. Just calling to let me know."

Khai sighed. "What a mess. Every day something new, and worse. You know, I talked with the family this morning. It was hard. Came away with my legs shaking."

"Another dysfunctional tribe, huh? Saw the father limping. Left hand pretty shriveled. Probably all of 'em 5PT."

"5PT?"

"Yeah, piss poor protoplasm poorly put together?"

She laughed cheerlessly. "Quite the contrary. Wonderful family. Patient's father won the Medal of Honor in Viet Nam. Somethin' else. First recipient I ever met."

He nodded. "I guess that's pretty high, but I thought you had to get killed to get that."

Khai hesitated, her head shaking almost imperceptibly. "Not really, Chris. Lot of them are given posthumously, though. You're thinking of the Purple Heart, and that's either wounded or killed in action. And what you saw on the father are likely war wounds, so he probably also has a Purple Heart—maybe two. But Medal of Honor's completely different. The highest award you can get. It means he did something extraordinary, really extraordinary, far beyond what anyone else did. The process the military goes through before they commend a soldier to the President and Congress for the Medal is more grueling than becoming a saint. Everyone has to approve it. That means politics are involved. Disgusting that the fate of a troop that went through so much sits in the hands of the bums in Washington. Whole thing takes years and years."

"Ya know, Khai, I have to admit I never really learned much about that sort of thing. I was in medical school, or maybe it was residency, during the first of the Bushs' wars in the Middle East. Like I told you, I fought my own war to stay out of the army. Prayed about it a lot. God was pretty clear. He made me see the Middle East was just the latest in the endless wars man creates out of greed. Not for me." He poured himself another half a glass and downed it in a single swig. "Who was it, the Mayans or the Aztecs? Can never keep them straight. One of 'em used to do human sacrifices every day. Cut open the chest of some kid who was still alive, and very much awake, then yanked out the heart. Barbaric sons of bitches, huh? We're much more civilized. We send our kids off to wars to get shot or blown up in sacrifice to the horny old bastards in Washington, same old bums you're talkin' about who use heroes as political fodder. And let's not forget the business conglomerates that are really calling the shots."

Khai thought for a moment. "Ah, so you don't drink the Kool-Aid, do you? Can't argue. The wars are B.S., but the troops are the best the country has to offer."

With the half decanter nearly gone, the waitress rushed over and offered a refill, but Gauthé picked up his menu. "Hey, Khai, Do you like fish?"

"Of course."

"Great. Let's do the salmon." He looked up at the waitress. "Two Northwest Duets." He turned to Khai. "That's silver salmon, Alaskan, mind you, and shrimp from the coast right near here. It's the best. How 'bout a glass of white wine?" When Khai demurred, he nodded to the waitress, "I'll have a glass of the Cayuse Vineyard's God Only Knows. Great stuff. Ah, go ahead, make it another half carafe. It'll burn off before we leave." He turned back to Khai and grinned, "Or, maybe you can be the designated driver."

When she didn't answer, he took two swallows of wine. In a few seconds his eyes brightened, his face blushed, and his tongue thickened. He spoke pleadingly. "Khai, please, I feel like I'm walking on eggshells. Can you tell me what I did wrong? I just thought you might like a night out."

"No, Chris, it's not you. Actually, I'm flattered, and the evening is lovely, but it's just too soon for me to be acting like I'm on a date. Please understand."

"Of course. Thank you for telling me. But like I said, there isn't one of us who hasn't gone through it. Do you know a single soul whose first marriage worked?"

Her eyes reddened, and she answered coldly, "Well, mine did."

His head snapped back an inch or two. "Whew, I'm sorry. I guess I don't understand."

"No, I'm sorry, Chris. Didn't mean to do that." Eventually, she stammered, "I'm hurting, Chris, but it's my problem, not yours, or anyone else's." She thought for a moment. "Why I have to take it out on you and every soul I touch is beyond me. I know it's wrong, but I can't help it."

He thought for a moment. "I don't know, maybe it's a defense mechanism, I mean to shut everyone out when life turns rotten. Doesn't take long to learn that even though we crave someone to do something, fix it, hold us, make it all better, there ain't no such thing. We're all alone in the end. Gotta face up to it. And then there's the other side of the coin," he laughed bitterly, "no matter what they say, everyone's thinking to themselves, 'Yeah, yeah, too bad for you. Just glad it's not me.' Isn't that what they drill into our heads in med school and residency?"

"Didn't do such a good job on me, huh?"

"Thank goodness. That's why you're special. Why you still have the gift." He paused. "Why I like being with you." She looked back at him. "But you know what's funny, what they forget to tell you in residency, is that before long, it's going to be your turn. Everyone gets a shot at grief. Let's see how you like the cold-faced, impatient nurse doing vitals on your dying mom; how 'bout the arrogant specialist popping his head in the door to tell you, 'Your labs are still fakakta, but I'll come around tomorrow and check again.'"

"How do you know that word?"

"Went to medical school, remember. Half the class, maybe more, were Jews."

Khai winced. "Doesn't sound like that was one of the highlights."

"It was oaky. We did our thing; they did theirs."

Khai nodded, but without expression, then muttered, "I guess we're thrown into this mess without a lot to say about who we're plopped next to, huh? Can be pretty unpleasant, no one just like you to talk to."

Sensing the sarcasm, he mumbled, "Sounds like I'm a bum, huh. But, gimme a break; I grew up in Eastern Washington. Never saw a black until one poor kid in my high school. Father was an engineer at Hanford. Kid was smarter than the rest of us. They flew his cousin out from Chicago to go to the prom. As for the Jews, two whole families in town. One guy was a lawyer, other owned the Five and Dime. Kept to themselves."

"What did your father do?"

"Ornithologist at Washington State, but he did most of his work in the field. Where we lived was pretty rural. Mother was a teacher. Four-room schoolhouse. When she died of breast cancer young, I was devastated."

"Father hard to talk to?"

"Yeah, our conversations were for the birds." He paused, waiting for a laugh, but Khai just rolled her eyes. "You're cute when you do that." She rolled them even higher, and Chris laughed. "Really cute, but seriously, I found a friend who listens to me no matter what. Very comforting."

Her lips twisted doubtingly. "Sounds a bit like you're thumping. Like I told you, when you've seen some things, that's hardly a refuge. It's a trap, no different than a drug." She reached over, swiped his wine glass, emptied it in one gulp, then chuckled sourly. "What did you call it—God help us?"

He laughed. "You mean my friend or the wine? It's God Only Knows. Sure you don't want to talk about it?"

"You know, Chris, that's about all I have in me tonight. Maybe sometime. Maybe."

"I was going to invite you to be the designated driver and take me home, and maybe coffee, but I think I won't be a wise guy...but only for tonight."

"Perceptive. And how 'bout the kids?"

Chris tightened. "Oh, I keep an apartment in Soundview, so I can be close to my hospitals when I'm on call."

"And I keep an apartment in Seattle and can barely pay my electric. I'm in the wrong specialty."

"No, you're not."

CHAPTER SEVENTEEN

The culture of Sabrina's CSF grew Pseudomonas aeruginosa, a very common bacterium, but one that rarely caused meningitis, especially in a previously healthy, younger person. It was the same bug finally cultured from the wound of her central line under the right collar bone. Usually, it was seen only in the immuno-compromised, those patients so sick they couldn't mount a white blood cell defense against invading bacteria.

The hospitalist summoned an infectious disease specialist to examine Sabrina. When done, he sat with the family and explained, "Even though her total white count is high, it's hard to know if Sabrina's has a neutropenia. That's just a fancy word for an insufficient number of specific white blood cells we call neutrophils. And neutrophils is a just a fancy word for one of the many types of white blood cells that protect us from infection. Each type of white cell has its own mission. Some kill bacteria, some eliminate viruses, and some control fungal infections, and some even *cause* allergies. And there are those that have evolved to just clean up the debris after an injury—it goes on and on. It's like the military. Everyone wears nearly the same uniform, and from the distance, it's hard to tell them apart. When you get close, though, you can see some drive tanks, some fly, some cook in the mess hall, some work in offices.

"Of course, there's overlap, but basically, the job of neutrophils is to kill bacteria that get into the body, as opposed to, say, kill viruses, or fungus. Particularly when we see a Pseudomonas bacterial infection, other than hot tub rash or in the ear canal, swimmer's ear, you always wonder if there are enough neutrophils around, or if there are enough, are they working properly.

"You see, Pseudomonas is everywhere. It's on the ground, on plants, on medical equipment, and no matter what you try, it's impossible to get rid of all of it. So, we're exposed to it daily. Usually, the neutrophils kill it in no time. That's their job.

"Getting a Pseudomonas meningitis is quite unusual, and generally when it happens, we see more than one breakdown in the body. First, there has to be a way for the bacteria to get from the skin into the bloodstream, then a problem with the neutrophils themselves, and the hard part, the bacteria have to find way to get into central nervous system, that is the brain and spinal cord. Not terribly hard to get into the bloodstream. Every time you brush your teeth, the micro trauma from the bristles cuts the gums, and all sorts of bacteria, even the nasty ones, shower the bloodstream. The white blood cells, though, are constantly on patrol. They recognize the bacterial invaders, kill them very quickly, and we do fine most of the time.

"Sometimes, if you get a big enough slug of bacteria into the blood, they might overwhelm the guards and squeeze out of the bloodstream into the body itself through normal holes in the capillaries. Gives them a chance to set up house in the organs. That's dangerous, but even then, most of the time white blood cells follow the bacteria into the tissues and end the infection very quickly. In modern times, of course, we add antibiotics, which keep things under control until Mother Nature gets the white blood cell assembly line revved up to finish the job. Usually turns out fine.

"The big problem is when bacteria squeeze out of capillaries into the central nervous system. Not supposed to happen because there's this thing called the blood-brain barrier. The capillaries of the brain and spinal cord are different from those in the rest of the body. They are very tightly sealed and pretty much leakproof to toxins, bacteria, and even some medicines.

"So, unless there's a tear or some sort of defect in the meninges, that's the name of the barrier, it's like a plastic tube, the central nervous system is protected from bad stuff in the bloodstream. In Sabrina's case, and I'm not sure about this, but the neural tube defect may have compromised the blood-brain barrier, that is, provided a hole in the plastic tube that has allowed bacteria into the cerebral spinal fluid bathing the brain. We just don't know for sure."

Mike raised his hand, and the doctor stopped. "I thought we could see the neural tube defect on the MRI. Can't we tell from that?"

"Good question, but we're talking only about a microscopic hole for the tiny bacteria to get through. Problem is, the MRI reveals just the big picture. We'd need to take out all the blood vessels in the defect and look at them under a microscope to see if that's where the leak is coming from. For obvious reasons, we cannot do that. Good news is, it doesn't matter for the immediate problem. There's an infection in the CSF, we know that for sure, and we are going to treat it with the proper antibiotic, Ceftazidime. If Sabrina was president, that's what she'd be treated with, and for 21 days, just like everyone else with this type of infection."

Isabelle asked, "Doctor, what's going to happen over those three weeks? I mean, she's on the critical list now. Do you think she'll wake up, be talking, maybe get out of bed?"

"Can't tell you for sure, but my guess is that she will be groggy and maybe even a bit confused for a few days, but by the time it's over, she'll be chomping at the bit to get the heck out of this place. I feel she'll do fine in terms of the infection. The stroke is another story, and far from my field of expertise."

Isabelle went on. "Do you think we should stay with her by the bedside for the whole time? Will that help her wake up sooner?"

"May I be honest?" Isabelle nodded. "I don't know about your family, but most, mine on top of the list, well, it's like the old saying: house guests are like fish—begin to stink after three days."

Sabrina's fever began a downward drift over the next couple of days. Then her white count stopped climbing and, by the third day, began to decrease, a sign her body didn't need to produce as many white cells to fight an infection that was coming under control with the antibiotics.

The neurologist had suggested that if Sabrina was confused as to person, place, time, and situation when she awoke, it was the family's job to reorient her. And, indeed, on the fourth day, when she began to stir, her first intelligible words were a barely audible, "I don't like this hotel. I want to move."

Mike froze. He asked, "Sweetheart, do you know what year it is?"

She whispered, "1991."

"Sweetheart, who's president of the United Sates?"

In the softest whisper, "George Bush."

Isabelle, Lincoln, and Mike glanced at each, their faces tense. Isabelle took a step forward and asked, "Sweetheart, do you know who I am?"

Sabrina studied her mother's face then turned away and closed her eyes.

She was asleep before Isabelle's hands started shaking.

The next morning, Sabrina awoke again and looked around the room uncertainly. Her eyes reddened as she gasped faintly, "Mom?"

Mike jumped up and lifted her hand to his lips. "Honey, everything's going to be okay. We're all here."

Lincoln lifted from his chair, but Isabelle put her arm out to stop him. She shook her head subtly and undertoned, "Just let the two of them..."

Sabrina pulled Mike's hand to her cheek. "What's happened?"

"You were preg..." He hesitated and went on a bit louder as if to erase his slip. "You were pretty sick. Do you know where you are?"

She answered in a throaty, though frail, whisper. "Hospital? Smells like a hospital."

"That's right. You're in the hospital. Do you remember how you got here?"

"No."

"Do you remember that you had an operation? I mean, first, we went to the doctor in Evanston. Do you remember that?"

"No."

Isabelle whispered, "Mike, why don't we just let Sabrina rest for a bit. Plenty of time for questions tomorrow."

Sabrina's hand became soft, and Mike put it back on the bed. Her eyes drifted closed, and, in seconds, she was asleep, silently rigid.

Early that evening, she opened her eyes and stared at Mike. "Hey, you okay?" she whispered. "You look like you're lost in the woods." Lincoln and Isabelle walked to the bedside. Sabrina struggled to focus on them. "Mom, Poppy, are you really here? I must be dreaming."

Isabelle forced her voice to remain strong. "Yes, Sweetheart. We're here. All of us. And we won't be leaving you. Not for a minute. Oh, God, I love you."

Mike bent forward and kissed Sabrina's forehead. She whispered to him, "My throat is so raw."

"That's from the breathing tube. They said you'll be over that in a couple of days. Please don't worry. And you don't have to talk."

She reached out her right hand toward Lincoln. "Poppy, I love you."

He kissed her. "Sabrina, Pumpkin Pie, you have the best husband in the world."

Sabrina smiled. "So do you, Mom." She shook her head as if clearing cobwebs. "I don't remember anything. Maybe something about putting a turkey in the oven. There was a lot of yelling. And a crash, and the rest of it's a blur."

Mike's chest tightened. He drew a breath to ask Sabrina to move her left hand but stopped himself and went to the other side of the bed. He waited until she turned her head toward her parents before stroking the left hand. She seemed not to sense she was being touched. He squeezed the fingers gently, and when she did not acknowledge that, he tightened his grip. Still, she seemed not aware of Mike's test.

A day later, when she woke and tried to lift herself from the bed, a nurse walking past the door rushed in and stopped her. "Let's go slow, Honey. You lay back and let me help you." She raised the head of the bed forty-five degrees and after two minutes, nearly straight up. "Let's leave you like this for a bit, then we'll have you sit on the edge of the bed. See how you do." Minutes later, she called another nurse to help, and the two pivoted Sabrina's legs over the side of the bed one at a time. Sabrina did fine until she turned her shoulders to drag her left arm into position to steady herself. It, though, hung dependently, a tube of sand; she toppled to that side. The nurse smiled. "I guess we're not quite ready to sit up for too long, huh? No problem, Honey, we'll try again tomorrow. Got all the time in the world." As she was eased back down, her eyes closed, and she was asleep before her head touched the pillow.

The family retired to the cafeteria, but Mike had forgotten his cell phone and rushed back up. Sabrina had awoken and was wringing her left arm with her right hand. Her cheeks were wet with tears.

Mike stood by the bed stunned. "Sweetheart, please don't worry. The neurologist said it was still so early."

"Mike, it hurts so bad. I can't feel anything but pins and needles. It's worse than when your arm goes to sleep and you try to move it. It hurts. I can't live like this."

"Did you tell the nurse?"

"She never stays long enough to do anything but change the IV."

Mike bolted into the hallway. He stopped in front of the first woman in scrubs. "My wife is in terrible pain. You need to do something."

"Excuse me, sir, but let's calm down. First, who is your wife?"

"Sabrina Maddingly in 517."

The woman pulled a chart from behind the counter. "Looks like your wife doesn't have orders for IV pain meds. Doctor only wrote for hydrocodone by mouth. Let me get her nurse."

Sabrina's nurse was busy in the room adjacent to Sabrina's. The patient in there had just expired; a priest was standing by the bedside chanting a psalm as the family sobbed. When the nurse ducked out of the room to gather a breath, Mike descended. "My wife is in a lot of pain. You need to do something."

"Mr. Maddingly, look, I'm a little busy at the moment, as I am sure you can see. I'll be in there just as soon as I can."

Mike started to grunt something about Sabrina being the living patient but held his tongue. He went back inside, knelt by Sabrina, and put his hand on her cheek."

A new nurse came into the room with a single Vicodin in a tiny paper cup. She gave it to Sabrina and offered a sip of water. "Take about twenty minutes, maybe less," the last words spoken over her shoulder as she strode quickly back into the corridor.

When Isabelle and Lincoln returned, they stared at Sabrina's tense face. Mike explained that the nurse had promised she'd be feeling better in just minutes, but glanced at his watch and snorted. "Damnit, that's half an hour. Are you any better, Honey?"

Sabrina moaned, "Not much. I can't take this."

Mike shot into the hallway. He placed himself at the door of the next room. The nurse was working over the deceased, pulling cardiac monitor patches from beneath pendulous breasts. The patient was nude, on her back, frog-legged, the tube of a urinary catheter poking from her vulva.

Mike quickly averted his eyes and turned away. A swell of wooziness descended over him, and he wobbled to the desk, uttering weakly to the clerk, "Excuse me, my wife in 517 is still in pain."

A woman looked up. "Who, sir?"

"Dr. Maddingly, in 517. You gave her a pain pill half an hour ago, and she's worse."

She pulled the chart and spoke edgily, "Yes, she got Vicodin. That should've worked. You can go back in the room. I'll alert the nurse."

When the nurse returned to the room, she looked directly into

Sabrina's eyes. "Are you still hurting, Dear?" When Sabrina broke into sobs, she added, "Doctor only wrote for Vicodin. Let me get ahold of her."

But the hospitalist was in the middle of a procedure, and Dr. Gauthé was in surgery. The nurse returned quickly. "Let's give you another Vicodin. That'll hold you. You'll see."

But it did not and, twenty minutes later, Mike was back at the desk. "She's still in awful pain."

"She's already had what the doctor prescribed. We need to wait."

"Are you're saying you won't help her?"

"I'm saying that we don't medicate patients with strong narcotics until the doctor says so. And, sir, please understand, your wife is disoriented and may only be imagining the pain. We can't tell. And we don't use strong painkillers unless we're sure. Last thing we want to do is get your wife dependent on opioids here in the hospital, and then addicted on the outside. Next thing you know, we're to blame."

"She's not comatose. She's not confused. I know her. She's tough as nails. She wouldn't say she was in pain unless she was. This isn't right."

As the clerk's eyes dropped back to her paperwork, Mike spun on his heels and ran to the stairwell, flying up several flights to Administration on the top floor. He sucked in a resonant breath to fuel the explosion but stopped and marshaled a sham smile. The corners of his mouth, though, curled down, his eyes as tense as a raging grizzly's.

He asked the receptionist, "May I speak with the CEO, please?"

"In regard to what, sir?"

As he culled an answer, it suddenly all seemed so silly that he had come to the top executive to complain that his wife was in pain. This was a hospital, a house of pain. Everyone who passed through Mitchie-Sterling's grand doors was in extremis, five-hundred suffering or dead souls in the rooms just feet below.

"Well, ma'am, my wife is in the ICU, and she is in terrible pain. I just want someone to get ahold of a doctor to help her."

The woman rose and smiled artificially as she spoke. "I'm sorry. Mr. Harp's in a meeting. And I'm sure they are doing everything they can to make your wife comfortable."

At that moment, Mike caught the image of a figure just approaching the edge of a dividing wall, the red and white lapel carnation locking Mike's attention. At that instant, the receptionist slid backward toward the divider, flapping a frenzied hand behind her butt. The man stopped abruptly, about-faced and retreated to his office, slamming the door in punctuation.

Mike spoke softly to the woman. "I won't forget that."

"Are you threatening me?"

Mike turned silently and climbed back down the stairs to the ICU.

CHAPTER EIGHTEEN

By the sixth day of antibiotics, Sabrina was able to transfer to a wheelchair to use the bathroom, albeit buoyed by two nurses. That evening, she began to take a little solid food, but just tiny bites, pleading that she wasn't hungry. The nurse pushed the food, but Chris Gauthé arrived on rounds and halted the force feedings. He explained to the family, but loud enough for the nurse to hear, that when a patient was very sick and refused to eat, it was better to leave them alone. He nodded to the family, "She'll eat when she's ready."

Isabelle and Lincoln sat at the bedside and talked about her childhood, about their childhoods, and then about the weather. The next night, Sabrina ate a few ounces of mac and cheese for dinner. An hour later, she asked for more. Lincoln and Isabelle leaned back in their soft chairs and talked about going home.

Sabrina fought not to mention the pain in her arm, no longer agonizing, but sufficient to draw the muscles in her face taut several times an hour. The neurologist suggested the terrible burning was analogous to phantom limb pain, and he started her on morphine but warned it was only for the short term. He also treated Sabrina with gabapentin, a medication that stabilized pain nerves, preventing them from firing so easily. The downside was that it made her sleepy. He also added an antidepressant, duloxetine, purportedly for its calming effect on the norepinephrine sensitive nerves in the spinal cord, the ones that carry pain impulses to the brain.

The other arm of his decision, to add an antidepressant, was that duloxetine was designed to address Sabrina's hopelessness, helplessness, and her loss of appetite, all signs of a major depressive episode. The duloxetine he prescribed had a host of side effects, one of which was insomnia, which he hoped would balance the gabapentin. He sat down with Mike and explained it was a juggling act, but that none of the drugs had the potential to do lasting damage and could be discontinued at any point.

Mike went back to work half-time the next day. He kept himself away from the hospital while the physical therapist was in the room, for during the initial session, he sat next to Sabrina and coached, "Sweetheart, you can do it. Just concentrate on one finger at a time and move it a millimeter. I know you can do it. Just takes concentration."

The therapist ignored him at first but finally barked, "Mike, let me see you move your left ear up just a millimeter. Concentrate. I know you can do it."

For two weeks, Sabrina did PT twice a day, yet there was no change in the left arm or leg. She had begun turning away from that side of her body, as if it was unsightly. Mike could easily see the muscular deterioration on top of the pre-stroke wasting. He said nothing but also stopped looking at her arm.

When he arrived late each afternoon, she would force a smile and ask in a monotone, "So, how was your day?" but her eyes became unfocused after a second or two, drifting to a point beyond him. At the end of the third week, she barely kissed him back as he left for the evening. When he arrived the next afternoon with roses, he found her sobbing into a pillow. Though he asked if it was the pain or something else, she turned away without answering.

Mike stopped by the clinic in Evanston late the next day on his way to the hospital. He signed in as a patient, complaining of a cough. Khai laughed when she walked into the treatment room and saw him sitting sheepishly on her rolling stool.

He looked up and grinned, "I didn't want to waste the table paper. I have to admit the truth: I just wanted to talk to you about Sabrina. And, also, I didn't want to take your time for free. If you worked half as hard for your M.D. as Sabrina did for her PhD, you better get paid for your labor."

"That's very thoughtful of you, but it doesn't matter. It all works out in the end."

Mike smiled skeptically, "Not sure all your colleagues heartily agree."

She dropped down on the end of the exam table. "Some do, some don't, but how can I help today?"

"Dr. Weathersby, I'd like, straight up, to ask you what's going on with Sabrina. Is she ever going to recover from the stroke? She's not doing well at the moment. Seems so depressed. I've never seen her like this."

"I know. I've checked on her several times. She barely spoke to me." She paused for a moment and looked him in the eye. "Mike, I can't read the crystal ball. All I can do is regurgitate the statistics. From a doctor's perspective, all of medicine is statistics—probability that there will be a certain outcome. And that works out well over a career. From a patient's perspective, it's the opposite. You two are living in a binary world—all or none. I mean, if the odds of having a good outcome from an operation are ninety-nine to one, that's pretty safe, right?" Mike nodded. "But I have to warn you that if you're the patient, statistics are superfluous, meaningless. There's still one in a hundred that doesn't do well, and to that family, the other ninety-nine percent of outcomes count for nothing. That's why no doctor should ever pretend to know the future, no matter how sure about the outcome.

"But here goes. First, before we talk about mechanical recovery, more than a third of patients with a stroke suffer significant mood disorder. That's our word for depression, and it is more painful than having your arm cut off. Worse than cancer.

"Regarding how people do after strokes, here are the raw numbers: ten percent of those who survive will recover nearly completely. Twenty-five percent recover with only minor problems. Forty-some percent have significant impairments, and ten percent wind up in long-term care situations. Ten or so percent pass away.

Khai saw Mike's chest clutch. "Let's not get excited. That ten percent are generally the elderly with multiple diseases. In Sabrina's case, I would imagine, even if her new impairment is mild to moderate, it is still superimposed over a fairly serious chronic problem, the neural tube defect. Will she get a flicker of movement back? I bet she will. Will she be able to use the arm and hand as she has in the past? I personally don't think she will. Will she learn to compensate? That, I'm positive she will. Will this change your life? Of course it will, but just how is up to you, both of you. She will go back to work and will probably be an even better psychologist for it.

"And for the moment, and perhaps forever, none of it matters. She will slowly recover her vigor. Her strong personality will push through. It can't be stopped. You will strengthen your relationship. I know you will because I know who you are. You two deserve each other."

"Hey, thanks a lot."

"You know darn well what I mean. You're one in a million. You both are."

"That's kind of you. I guess I need to stop thinking so much. What will be will be."

"Yes, it will. I also know she's being treated with an antidepressant. I imagine that doesn't thrill you, either of you."

"Doctor said it was for the lack of norepi-something."

"Norepinephrine. That's true. But it's not working, which is not unusual. Stroke patients are especially difficult to treat—in terms of depression, I mean. Depression is notoriously hard to treat, even in those without strokes or without other underlying problems. We usually have to try three different antidepressants before we find the right one. And even then, the one that finally seems to work is only seventy-five percent effective, so we have to start adding additional medicines."

Mike's shoulders drooped. He spoke just above a whisper. "We don't want that. That's for the elderly. Is there some treatment to just cure it? Hit it hard once and erase the heart of the problem? Something drastic to do here in the hospital, get it over with."

"Mike, if I may, we don't cure, erase, much of anything. We manage illness, treat the symptoms so you live a more comfortable life until it's your time. We try not to do any collateral damage, well, as little as possible, along the way.

"Depression is cyclic—comes and goes. The best we can do is stretch out the time between episodes, and when one rolls around, which it will, blunt the lows. Not talking about bipolar—that's a whole 'nother kettle of fish. Just regular old, garden variety, clinical depression, one of the commonest diseases on Earth. It's everywhere, in every country, every society, every walk of life: presidents, kings, astronauts, great quarterbacks, truck drivers, and doctors, especially doctors. On the other hand, Mike, we're talking about Sabrina here, not the rest of the world. I'll get word to the psychiatrist who's seeing her. Give 'im a little nudge."

CHAPTER NINETEEN

On a grey Saturday afternoon, Chris Gauthé and Khai met for coffee at a Starbucks in Seattle. He told her he had just done an emergency splenectomy in the other hospital at which he had privileges, the University of Washington. His face was drained, and he hadn't shaven. As he templed his fingers and let his eyes close, Khai quickly looked at his face, but her eye caught his left ring finger. She wasn't sure if she saw the faintest impression under where a wedding ring might usually sit but also noticed a similar hollow on the thumb. Maybe the dents were just from the way he held his surgical instruments, or so she sought to convince herself.

He looked up. "Been following the Maddinglys?"

Khai answered glumly. "Some. At least her infection's better, but the stroke looks like it hasn't budged. I can't get it out of my head that I pushed on her adnexa too hard. Started the bleeding, brought the situation to a head long before it should have become a matter of life and death. You know what they'll say at trial. 'But for your improper, aggressive physical exam, Dr. Weathersby, there would not have been a need for an emergency central line, and all that happened in the ER, blah, blah, blah.'"

Chris shook his head. "And when I'm on the stand, your defense attorney will point at me and bark, 'Now, Doctor, let's talk about those two botched surgeries: one in the ER and then when you performed a procedure for which you had no formal training. What about that, Dr. Gauthé, blah, blah, blah?' Truth be told, none of us are out of the woods on this one."

Khai smiled easily. "What was the name of the wine, God Only

Knows?"

Chris laughed. "Good memory."

"It was a nice night."

"Thank you. Yes, it was." He reached across and touched her hand so softly, she was not sure he had. Though she did not move, her face reddened. Chris smiled and went on. "And on an even more entertaining note, it appears our Mr. Maddingly made quite an impression at the hospital, all the way from the monkeys on the security force, to the nursing staff, to the CEO's secretary."

"I'm sorry, Chris, I wish I could say he's just a loose cannon, and he got what he deserved, but something's off in that hospital. I didn't tell you, but I got a letter back from your illustrious Medical Director Klat. Didn't scan it into my phone, or I'd show you. Didn't want to push the wrong button, open it, and have to look at it again. But still hard to get it off my mind."

"Well, if you'd like to show it to me, I'll figure out a way to talk to him. Smooth things over."

"No, Chris, that's the point. I don't need help; he does. Got the facts completely upside down. Threatened to blackball me in the local medical community."

"Did you expect the impotent old bastard to invite you to lunch at the McKinley Golf and Country Club? No sweat off his back. He'd write it off to the hospital. Wouldn't cost him a penny farthing—he's president of that board, too."

"He blamed me for leaking the story all over the hospital."

"He probably believes it. Do you think his secretary 'fessed up? How 'bout Cardozo? You're kidding yourself if you think you'll get a fair hearing at the zoo. Remember, it's a fiefdom. All the parts work together to make sure the money keeps coming in and gets distributed according to the formula everyone has agreed on. Do you know how impossible it is to get a gaggle of doctors to agree on something as simple as, say, a healthy blood pressure? The facts are in. Everybody knows what's a good blood pressure, but these chimpanzees'll find some way to get their egos and their wallets involved in a fight to the death." He thought for a moment. "Funny, though, somehow the hospital found a formula of spoils-distribution that got most of the staff to shut their mouths. The chances of them allowing a newbie to waltz in and upset the apple cart—ain't gonna happen, young lady. You know we all think of ourselves as practitioners of the noble profession. When we have the annual softball game against the local lawyers, we call it the Healers versus the Stealers. But it ain't so, not by a long shot. You just haven't been around long enough to see."

"Yes. I have."

"Just wait. You've only found the easily observable flaws, the low-hanging fruit. Give it another ten years."

"Maybe I won't be able to."

"And you aren't going to be blackballed. I won't allow it. You're a great doctor. Don't worry, I'll corral enough backers to get you into the local medical society. You'll be the president in two years."

"What if I don't want to join?"

"Well, hope you enjoy making a fifth of what you're worth, because that's all you're going to see at a walk-in clinic."

"Maybe I'll just go back to the East Coast. Not sure it's all that great out here."

"Better in Boston? How 'bout the Bronx? Philly? Those are dead and dying cities—mostly the former. Maybe someday you'll fall madly in love again..." She screwed up her face, "Could happen. Have a family. You want to raise your kids in Baltimore?"

She laughed. "Oh, it's so comforting to peer into the future with Swami Chris."

"Look, Khai, it's a profession, this doctoring thing. There are traditions. And a lot of good people sweat blood to build that hospital into what it is, or what it could be. Tell me another walk of life where there aren't a hundred jerks in every direction you turn. Personally, I've learned to just get along. I ignore them, go to the OR, carve up my victims, and hope for the best. Gets me enough of a cash flow to buy coffee for a very special lady."

"Thanks, but it's hard to be called a stinking liar to your face and turn the other cheek. Oops. I mean it's okay to turn the other cheek, but it's hard as hell to forget what he said." She paused for a moment. "You know how the blacks say, 'He dissed me'? Well, now I know what they're talking about. Even in the Army, that would never happen. Superior'd be out of a job and a career in six minutes, he tried something so unprofessional."

Chris thought for a moment. "You know, we never talked about it, but I'm getting the impression you were in the service. Am I right?"

"I was."

"And there I was, generating all that hot air bellowing about how I worked my fingers to the bone to stay out. Truth is, sometimes, when I'm taking stock of myself, I think about it."

"Not too late."

"Yes, it is. Got a family."

Her face became suddenly serious. "It's the first time you've said that."

"Family, I don't know. I've got kids. I told you that. Not going to go into the Navy and get on a ship and be gone from them for six months every year. No way."

"And your wife?"

"You mean their mother?"

Khai's lips tightened. "Chris. I want you to tell me the truth. Are you divorced, at least separated?"

"It's not final, if that's what you mean."

"Well, do you still live in the house with her?"

"Under the same roof some of the time, but not," he made quote marks with his fingers, "with her. If you know what I mean."

Khai nodded, "That's a little uncomfortable."

"It is."

"No, I mean for me."

"It's not as though we've done a thing but talked a few times. I'm not dead. I haven't asked you up to my place, or if I could see yours."

"But you wanted to."

"Well, duh!"

She remained poker-faced for as long as she could before her lips curled up ever so slightly.

CHAPTER TWENTY

Sabrina remained in the hospital's Intensive Care Step Down Unit for eight more days. A bevy of internists, neurologists, and psychiatrists confabulated daily in a corner of her room, some with arms folded across their chests, others with fingers templed, touching their lips, weighing treatment options for Sabrina, especially for her worsening depression. There was even talk of electro-shock therapy, but with her recent history of meningitis and stroke, no one wanted to write the orders for any sort of brain procedure, even if they knew well it had been done successfully many times despite those confounding factors. Then again, what daring psychiatrist wanted to hop on the train wreck that was Sabrina Maddingly, especially when that train's next stop was clearly a multi-million-dollar malpractice case?

Eventually, though, she turned the corner and drifted toward clinical stability, getting neither better nor worse, but with little hope of the former. She was moved across the street to a skilled nursing facility, where she spent her days in bed staring at the acoustic ceiling tiles. She was simply not going to move, and that became a risk factor for one deadly problem after another. Would the blood in her legs stagnate to the point that a clot formed, a deep vein thrombosis, one that would grow like a tumor? Would a piece break free and be pushed along the blood stream to the lungs, to lodge there as a fatal pulmonary embolus? Would sores form on her legs from the constant friction against the bed sheets, become infected, and enter the bloodstream to take up residence in organs miles from her legs? Would she develop a bladder infection from having lost the gumption and strength to lift herself to use the bedpan and wash out the bacteria in her urinary tract? She was sufficiently compromised that a simple UTI might easily transmute over a single day into a roaring upper tract kidney infection, pyelonephritis, soon to spread throughout the body and threaten her life.

But the most ominous complication of her lassitude was the probability that she would develop pneumonia. The nursing home was an ideal culture medium for microbes so resistant to antibiotics, the CDC had not yet imagined such strains. It would not be long before those bacteria found their way through the ventilation system or were carried into her room on a nurse's uniform.

The respiratory therapists, having faced this scenario a thousand times, descended each morning at nine to browbeat Sabrina into a regimen of deep breathing exercises and coughing. She, though, just pretended to comply, giving up after the second or third breath, complaining that the pain in her surgical incision, and her left arm, and her left leg, and her lower back, was just too overwhelming to comply with their directions.

After each abbreviated session, they left quietly, heads hung, for they knew it was only time before a squad of nomadic bacteria would be drawn into her lungs. With such weak exhalations, they would not be swept back out before the tide of the next breath pushed them even deeper. A few hours later, the microbes would do what they had evolved so beautifully to do over the past several billion years—attach themselves to vulnerable tissue, in this case, the walls of Sabrina's throat. There, they would grow for a day or so, dollops eventually breaking off to drip further into the bronchi. Finally, they would trickle by gravity all the way into the bronchioles, the tiny breathing tubes deepest in the lung. As they multiplied in the delicious warmth and humidity, the body would mount a defense, dispatching white cells to kill them. Part of that process was the release of chemical messengers to draw water from all over the body into the lungs to dilute the poisons from the dying bugs. That fluid, along with the dead bacteria and exhausted white cells, became phlegm, a medium easier to cough out than just the dead cells. But that fluid also blocked the flow of oxygen from the lungs into the blood, a situation, in the worst cases, little different than drowning. The sputum simply had to be brought up and coughed out.

Still, though, Sabrina would not cooperate, and as the staff predicted, and feared, three days later, Sabrina was suffering from a flaming pneumonia. Once again, she drifted in and out of consciousness.

Mike stopped at the Evanston Clinic. He began to talk to Khai in the waiting room, but she pulled him back to an exam room.

"I know," she nodded. "I visited last night. You were out taking a walk, they said. And, also, just like at the hospital, I don't have privileges there. If they think I'm interfering...well, you know the story. I told them I was just a friend and that I'd be only a second."

Mike mumbled, "Thank you for sticking with us. You know, on the one hand, it's overwhelming, but on the other, I'm getting used to waking up to the crisis de jour. Like you warned, each calamity seems to pass on to the next up within a few days. The latest catch is the doctor who comes to the home to see patients. He's really old. I asked the staff, and they said that's all he does—nursing home care. Is that safe? I mean, who's watching him?"

"Mike, I don't know if anyone is watching any of us. If he screws up, hurts someone, then it's in the open, and he gets sued, or the Department of Health investigates."

"Can't the nurses keep their eyes on him and head off mistakes?"

"Nurses at the home are basically LPNs and nurse assistants. They're not all that trained up on cutting edge medicine, and that's not their job. They provide comfort and safety; that's why they're there. Most do a good job, a very good job, but I doubt they know if this guy's up to date. On the other hand, his age may not be a factor for what he's being asked to do. Surgeons, sure, shouldn't be allowed to go on after 65, though some do. And if an old dude wanted to operate on Sabrina, or me, I'd have a lot to say. But basic internal medicine is not rocket science. Guy needs to be able to handle diabetes, high blood pressure, respiratory infections, straightforward kidney problems, that kind of stuff just long enough to get the patient across the street to a specialist. Look, Sabrina's only minutes away from the ER. Ooooops. Sorry."

Mike snorted. "Yeah, but Sabrina's got pneumonia. Shouldn't she have been transferred to the hospital?"

"Well, let's look at it in terms of the things critical for life—the ABCs: airway, breathing, and circulation. First, nothing is obstructing the movement of air in and out of the lungs, like a piece of food stuck in the bronchus would. So, A, airway, isn't a problem. Then B, breathing. No doubt there's water deep down blocking some of the oxygen from getting into her blood, but she's getting enough through, maybe not to run a half-marathon, but quite sufficient for her present bodily needs. We know that because she has that little clip on her index finger. You remember that. It tells us exactly what percent of her blood that is supposed to be carrying oxygen around the body is, in fact, carrying oxygen. Yes, she's on supplementary oxygen through nasal prongs, but her saturation's right up near a hundred percent. Better than mine. Wouldn't be better if we admitted her across the street, so that's A and B off the table. In terms of C, circulation, basically heart function, she's maintaining her pulse rate and blood pressure very well on her own without medication, which we know because the nurses check it every couple of hours.

"Those are the things you admit people to the hospital for, when the ABCs may become compromised. On the less immediately critical things, we also know she's on the right antibiotic, which was the one chosen by a pulmonologist at the hospital after they took a sputum sample and cultured it. They know exactly which bug is causing the infection, and the good news is, it's plain old, garden variety, pneumococcus. We got lucky. That family of bacteria isn't resistant to our usual antibiotics, at least most pneumococcal infections aren't, yet.

"So, I guess the question is, what can be done at the hospital that the nursing home can't do? Believe me, Sabrina's much more comfortable and peaceful at the home. LPNs over there are just fine. It's a good facility. Far as I'm concerned, they're the ones doing God's work. Certainly ain't us doctors. And the respiratory therapists are the same folks from the hospital. See what I mean? Three or four thousand dollars a day versus the same, maybe better overall care that she's getting for three or four hundred a day at the nursing facility."

When Mike nodded, Khai went on. "Anyway, back to the specifics. Sabrina's got pneumococcal pneumonia. The pneumonia, itself is not as concerning as the fact that some of the infection has leaked into her bloodstream. That's why she's not fully alert. But, like I said, she's on the correct antibiotic that will cover the infection no matter what organs are involved. We just need to wait. Takes days before we kill enough of the bacteria for the body to take over and get even twenty-five percent back to normal. Hang on for three more days—you'll see. That's because there's pockets of enemy hiding all over the place. But they'll get the word. Get coughed out or die by the hand of the antibiotic.

"Promise me you won't get upset when she improves a bit, then goes back downhill for a day. Two steps forward, one and a half back. Remember, and this, too, shall pass. Patience, patience, patience."

Mike sighed, "Dr. Weathersby, I've kept you too long. But there's one more question. Promise me you won't take offense."

"I don't think I will, but..."

"Well, it's about the depression. Sabrina's slipped into another world. I've never seen her like this. The psychiatrist who's sort of running things keeps adding drugs, but anyone can tell they're not working. Comes by late every day, stands in the door, and asks Sabrina how she's doing. Before she even finishes her sentence, he writes in the chart and says, 'We're going to be trying something new.' That's it. If you open your mouth to ask a question, he mumbles, 'We have to be patient. Let's wait and see,' does an about-face, and walks off."

Khai thought for a moment then answered. "I don't know him, to be honest. But I'll ask around for a psychiatrist who's respected in town. And, again, the guy seeing Sabrina may be fine. Treatment for depression is as slow as frozen molasses. But we'll get to the bottom of it."

"Dr. Weathersby, look, I've already stressed you beyond words. You've got to be ruing the day, night, we showed up on your doorstep."

"Mike, listen to me, please. In case you didn't know it, you and Sabrina are the best this society has to offer. Nature is capricious, and that means challenges are part of my job. You might say glitches *are* the job. You have a problem; we'll work to fix it. I will do my due diligence on the depression, but you need to be strong and not give up. To some degree, that psychiatrist is right; we will see."

"Okay, thank you, again, but how do we jibe all your work with the fact that you aren't getting paid? I know, I sound like a broken record, but it just isn't right."

"Just stop by in two days. We'll talk again."

CHAPTER TWENTY-ONE

Chris Gauthé also had surgical privileges at the University of Washington Medical Center. He was perfecting a cutting-edge procedure for laparoscopic cholecystectomy, gall bladder removal, using a laser. He had designed the entire operation to be done through two trivial nicks in the abdomen and one very small incision. The innovative technique had the potential to reduce the operative time from one hour to sixteen minutes, and the recovery time to a few days. "Lasik surgery of the tummy," he laughed. The U had provided him with a wall full of surgical trays, the instruments laid out to his personal tastes, and a special staff of operating room technicians available at his beck and call. He'd even convinced the administration to train them at hospital expense. His final coup was to bring Krystal Kaywood, his personal scrub nurse from Mitchie-Sterling Hospital, with him. He arranged for her to receive a stipend from the U on top of her full salary from Mitchie-Sterling, the U even agreeing to pay for her to attend classes to master the physics of the laser. She became so good at programming, she created code that extinguished the beam if it slipped a single Angstrom Unit off target. The bioengineering company bought the fail-safe code for a hundred thousand dollars. Though Gauthé's contract stated explicitly that any external income generated by the new procedure belonged exclusively to the University of Washington, the hospital split the payment with her.

Krystal was the daughter of Arlington Spielman, Professor Emeritus of General Surgery at the U and retired president of the Washington State Medical Association. She had two brothers, one an M.D., the other a lawyer. Krystal, by far the brightest of the three, had been pushed by her science teachers in high school to enter the U in pre-med. Arlie, though, nagged that girls went into nursing—end of argument. He softened the thump by badgering her with notions of rising to charge nurse in a surgical suite, then to the director of surgical nursing. How fitting, he loved to muse, for Krystal's mother had been a surgical nursing supervisor at the U when Arlie'd met her. Years later, he sat after dinner in their Mercer Island living room, nursing a third scotch, beaming at his little girl, joyful with the prospect of his life coming full circle.

It was not long after Dr. Gauthé entered the FDA's approval process that his team commenced operating on dogs, dozens and dozens of them, to perfect the technique. This was at a special, secret, animal lab in the Cascade foothills. Krystal would stand beside him in the operating theater, anticipating her surgeon's every brainwave, ready with the next surgical instrument long before Chris's fingers twitched for it.

As they got better, able to knock off a gall bladder from start to finish—from the application of anesthesia to the dog back up on its feet peeing in his cage in less than 20 minutes—they started doing three cases a week after regular surgery until they could do them in their sleep. As the final testing on animals neared, they stayed later and later, doing two procedures per night. It was, though, okay, for it was summer, and Krystal's two-year-old was with her parents in Friday Harbor, on San Juan Island. Her husband's softball team had advanced to the Washington State finals. They practiced every night, and when it got dark, they retired to a local watering hole to drink beer until midnight.

With a week to go before the final FDA evaluation, they did three dogs in a row after a day with an appendectomy, a colectomy reversal, and a mastectomy. As the clock in the operating room approached 7 P.M., Chris looked across the table at Krystal and locked her eyes. He smiled lasciviously as he let his stare drop to the soft outline of her breasts in the surgical gown. She glanced away, face reddening. Before his eyes returned to the TV monitor that gave him a picture of the tip of the laser, he inadvertently brushed the edge of his surgical gown against the toggle switch that disarmed Krystal's fail-safe circuitry. As he pulled the instrument's trigger, thinking it would not fire until precisely on target, a pulsing tube of tissue under the laser's cutting tip vaporized. Krystal gasped. Gauthé had severed a major artery. It took him several seconds to understand what had happened, and after an unnerving silence, he called harshly for instruments, reverting to traditional, open surgery. By the time they finished, it was 9 P.M. Everyone was exhausted; wisps of Krystal's moist, silver-blond hair stuck to her forehead. Chris waited until the staff had cleaned the room and left the lab before asking Krystal if she wanted to get a bite and go over last-minute refinements of their technique. He did not mention his blunder.

Still shaken, she thought twice but nodded, though asked if she could first freshen up in the tiny room reserved for overnight staff. He tossed her the key, and she left, alone, but as she came out of the shower, Chris ducked his head into the room. He turned away quickly, though. "Oh, hey, sorry. I was just checking to see if you were ready. I tried to call, but there was no answer."

"Hey, Chris, that's dirty pool."

Still facing out the door, he stammered, "I know, but I couldn't help it, Krystal. You mad? You make me crazy. You hate me?"

She wrapped herself in an unsubstantial, hospital towel and spoke softly, "You can turn around and look, but not too much." She lowered the towel below her breasts.

Gauthé stared at the floor and shook his head as if chastising himself. "Krystal, really, I was out of line. It was like I was drawn here by some crazy force outside me. I mean, I'm a doctor. It's not like I've never seen a beautiful woman. You...you know what I mean. It's just the thought of you up here, out of your scrubs. You gotta forgive me. Please. It won't happen again."

She was silent, but he sensed her warmth as she came a foot closer to the door. He looked up and took an anxious step into the tiny room. When she did not turn away, his hands came up so very slightly and brushed her breasts. He leaned forward and softly kissed her left nipple. She sighed.

Chris whispered, "I don't want to hurt you, Krystal." She said nothing, and he spun around to take a step for the door. She reached forward and grabbed his shirt.

CHAPTER TWENTY-TWO

Several nights later, Khai stopped by Sabrina's nursing facility on her way home. Chris Gauthé rolled into the parking lot seconds after she entered the building. He waited outside in the shadows until he saw Khai write in the visitor's book, then walk toward the patient rooms. He followed cautiously into the facility, signed a false name, and asked for directions to Sabrina Maddingly's room.

Khai and Mike were standing on opposite sides of the bed as Chris poked his head in and paused, as if surprised to see Khai. "Dr. Weathersby," he smiled and nodded formally, "nice to see you again."

Khai had taken Sabrina's cold left hand gently, but with Gauthé's arrival, she unconsciously gripped it more firmly and looked down nervously to see if she had hurt Sabrina. The woman didn't stir, seemingly unaware of the people in her room. When her head did lift a fraction, the three leaned forward expectantly, but she just coughed weakly and settled back down onto the sheets.

Gauthé stood silently for a moment before asking, "You folks want to come out into the conference room and chat?"

Mike looked up but paused before speaking softly. "You know, I think I'm a little talked out. The doctor who comes around sat with me for an hour. Just left. Turns out he's a good guy. Tell me if this is right. He said everything's intertwined. When one organ goes bad, the next one down the line's forced to pick up the slack. Some can do it for a while, sort of as a temporary backup, but sooner or later that one gets pushed too hard doing things it wasn't designed to do, and the next organ up has to do three jobs at once. But he said not to worry, that it was his job to choose medicine that neutralized the toxins before they poisoned all the structures down the line. He said he couldn't cure Sabrina with the medicines, but he could buy time to let the organs rest and heal themselves." Mike's eyes reddened as he went on in barely a whisper. "So, I'm fine. Just going to sit here and watch my precious wife get better. Thanks, though."

Khai, her eyes clouding as well, came to his side of the bed and squeezed his arm. "Lucky woman. Everything's gonna be just fine. You'll see. And, your description of what a doctor tries to do was spot on. Took me a long time to figure that out. Good for you." She squeezed his arm again and left the room with Chris.

The two sat in the worn, padded chairs of the family room. Chris got up to turn off Wheel of Fortune. He dropped back into the seat, and they stared at the blank screen until he blurted, "You up for a quick bite? Nothing fancy. Something local?"

"Okay, but no alcohol, Chris. Gotta be up early tomorrow. Doing some research for the Maddinglys. Actually, I'd like to talk to you about it."

At the Burger King, they stepped up to the counter to order Whoppers, but Khai gagged, "So, this is where we finally wind up."

They turned to each other laughing as they ordered coffee. Chris asked, "Did the husband tell you that her depression is getting worse? It's not my specialty. Clearly, what we're doing isn't working, but I can't very well have the guy who's already on the job fired. Could be, no treatment will work."

"That's what I wanted to talk to you about. Maybe I can get involved surreptitiously. No one'll know who arranged for the consult. Touchy, though."

Gauthé shook his head. "Nah, husband can just say he wants a second opinion. No doc likes to hear that, but too bad about you. Patient comes first, not the tender feelings of a guy who's not making any progress."

"Guess we're on the same page."

"Feels good doesn't it."

"Yeah, yeah, yeah. So, Saint Chris, do you know any decent shrinks? Mike's afraid she's suicidal. I think we need to get right on it."

"I know one. Think she even has privileges at Mitchie-Sterling. I've not had the pleasure of engaging her professionally, but maybe I should." He stopped short and stared at the ceiling. "Look, I'll be honest. My wife was seeing her. It really made a difference, but then she just up and quit. Had some cockamamie excuse—too humiliating or something. The usual." He shook his head. "I shouldn't be talking out of school. I'm sorry."

"It's okay. It will never leave my lips. So, maybe, you can give me her name. And, if it isn't too much trouble, give her a call to let her know who I am, that it's all on the up and up."

"Be happy to. He took his cell phone and looked up the woman's office number. He dialed to leave a message, but there was a recording and Chris ended the call. "She's out of the office for a couple of days, but I'll get with her for sure." He drank the rest of his coffee in a single gulp. "Well, I'm gonna head down the road to my place in Soundview." He paused and peered into her eyes. "I know I shouldn't ask, but would you like to stop by for a glass of wine? I mean, we've got the psych issue under control. Sabrina can hold on for two days. She may not even be awake by then. Don't worry, this gal'll know everything there is to know about treating resistant depression."

"I don't know, Chris."

"Oh, she's real good from what I hear."

"No, I mean about your place."

"Oh, that. I can be trusted."

"Can you?"

"Cross my heart, hope to die, stick a finger in my eye."

Khai rolled her eyes. "Ah, such profound and scholarly words from the city's most distinguished surgeon, Christopher P. Gauthé." She shook her head and smiled subtly. "Okay, but just for a few minutes. I'll do anything to avoid walking into my place. It's a lifeless prison cell."

Gauthé's apartment was neat, but as icy as Khai's. She excused herself for a moment, and as she closed the door of the bathroom, she saw a dark speck on the floor in the shadow of the sink cabinet. She thought it was an insect and took a step away, but when she touched it with the tip of her shoe, it didn't bite back. She bent forward to look more closely and picked it off the floor. It was a tiny hair clip. Three strands of long blond hair were tangled in it. Khai looked closely; the roots were nearly as light as the rest of the strand. She replaced it on the floor and went back out.

Chris had a glass of wine in his hand and tipped it toward her. She shook her head no. "Well, at least sit and keep me company." He lowered himself onto the couch. She hesitated for a moment then dropped into the recliner.

She forced a smile and spoke softly. "Tell me about your kids. You have a picture?"

He nodded at a shelf and the picture of his family. His wife's hair was ebony; the two children were nearly as dark. He sighed, "The light of my life, those two. Their mother's Brazilian, not a bad person, not at all. It's the cultural differences. That's what's blown us apart. I should've known. So many people warned us—my parents, her parents. But what did they know? Unworldly peasants. I just hate what's happening. This is hurting the kids so much, hurting all of us. I've never felt so alone."

Khai nodded and mumbled, "I know the feeling." She looked down for a bit and finally mumbled, "So, you don't date? No one hovering? Hard to believe."

Chris's shook his head. "As celibate as a dormouse."

"Dormouse? Those things breed worse than rabbits."

He laughed. "You know what I mean." He stopped to rub his eyes. "Hey, look, Khai, I'm beat. I think I'm gonna turn in." He paused, "May I pose something? Just promise you won't go postal."

"Let me guess. No, no, surprise me. Pose away."

"Look, there's the couch here, and then there's the bed. If you want to stay, you take the bed, I'll camp out on the couch. I'll give you sweats. Lock the door from the inside. You can run the washer. Be all spiffy and spotless in the A.M."

"That's really tempting, Chris, but I need to pick some stuff up at my place to take up to the clinic in the morning. It was thoughtful of you though. Thanks."

He stepped forward and put his palm against her cheek. She started to pull away but stopped and leaned into his hand. Her eyes closed. His other hand brushed her breasts. She did not move for a moment but then slowly pulled away. "Maybe next time."

PART TWO

CHAPTER TWENTY-THREE

Sabrina awoke the next day, and by the end of the week, she was barely coughing. With her impending discharge, Medicare arranged for a no-frills electric wheelchair, a ramp into the house, and accommodations in several of the rooms, especially the bathroom.

An occupational therapist was waiting in front of the Maddingly's home as they arrived from the hospital. She let Mike transfer Sabrina from the car to the new wheelchair. When he nearly dropped her, the OT, perhaps a hundred pounds, slipped between the two, helped Sabrina back into the car, then used her arms and legs as levers to ease Sabrina into the chair.

She gave them a tour of their own home; Sabrina was most excited to roll into the kitchen. The woman, though, urged Sabrina not to use the stove. Confined to the wheelchair, it was deemed too difficult for her to lift hot pots and pans with one hand, especially onto the counters, all of which were, at best, at eye level with her in the chair.

A helper minded Sabrina during the day while Mike was at work. At three-thirty he'd rush out of school to go shopping, then dash home to relieve the elderly woman and start the cleaning, laundry, and cooking. Each week, he used sick days to drive Sabrina to her endless doctors' appointments.

By now, she was on three antidepressants, a slurry that blunted the overpowering despair, but also muffled her personality. Mike went back to see Khai. She recommended, given the slow, but seemingly incremental improvement, they hold off changing psychiatrists. "Mike, like we talked about, everything in psych happens in four-week increments, and we're generally happy for even a suggestion of progress. We need to look at the effectiveness of our treatment in months, not days. Then, maybe, we'll have the option of tailoring the medications to limit the side effects."

That night before dinner, Mike wheeled Sabrina to her place in front of the fireplace. He suddenly mounted a chair to lift a bottle of Bordeaux toward the heavens. "I hereby declare Season Eight of the Cocktail Hour." He had rigged a sports drink bottle with a long straw for Sabrina to draw in the wine. He measured one glass carefully, but after a week, she began insisting on a refill, though after the second glass, her words slurred, her head weaved, and she sat staring at Mike with a foolish grin.

He said nothing for another week but finally asked, "Sweetie, don't you think one is enough?"

"Well, you've had two."

"I'm twice your size, and remember what the doctor said, two for men and one for women. Not healthy for you to drink that much."

"Healthy? What the hell do I care about healthy?"

"Sweetheart, you know that's the alcohol talking. And..."

"And it's the truth, and you know it. So, you want to dictate the last bit of control they left me over my life? No way. If I want thirty drinks, I'll have them, even if I have to crawl to the liquor store."

Mike poured her half a glass of the Bordeaux, but she did not acknowledge him when he set the drink down by her side. She did, though, take the straw greedily and pulled the claret so hard her cheeks hallowed. With just a trace left, she took a final tug, one so deep, she broke into a paroxysm of coughing. Mike jumped to her side. He lifted his palm to lightly smack her back, but she arched away from him violently, her right hand lifting to cover her face. Even her left arm twitched. He stopped short, mouth agape.

"Sabrina, my God, what's happening to us? You think I'd hit you? Tell me. Tell me, damnit!"

She began weeping softly. As he warily put his hand on her shoulder, her head dropped, and she began to sob frantically. Soon, she was shrieking. "Don't let them do any more to me. What do they want from me? I'm already dead. They killed me. I just want it to be over. Why are you making it go on and on?"

Mike lifted her from the chair and carried her into the bedroom. They lay together, Mike holding her so closely, he was afraid he would hurt her. She quieted but panted, "Tighter, Mike, don't let me die alone."

The next morning, Sabrina rolled over in bed and held him, whispering, "Mike, forgive me for what I said. It was the alcohol talking. I never want to leave you, ever. I love living with you. You are my rock."

When she began to weep quietly, he kissed the top of her head. "And I'll never leave you. Every time you look back, that's me sailing right behind, every minute of every day, for the rest of our lives." He paused for a moment and whispered, "Hold on for a minute, Sweetheart." He lifted the phone and called for a substitute.

When the visiting nurse arrived, Mike drove to the Evanston clinic and waited for Khai. Ignoring the staff, Khai led him to the furnished sitting room in the basement. He gushed the whole story. "I'm not trying to be the doctor, but..."

"Tell me what you're thinking."

"I thought she was getting better, but a couple of drinks last night, and I'm afraid she's going to hurt herself. I've been doing some reading, you know, about that shock therapy. When they first mentioned it, I thought, like, not over my dead body. But she's on all this medication, and she's getting worse. I don't think we can wait anymore."

Khai muttered, "I think it might be time to see the psychiatrist Dr. Gauthé knows. What do you think?"

"Anything. I'm grasping at straws. She's too depressed to get dressed, and don't ask her to leave the house. She's talking about dying. I'm really scared."

"You go home and take care of Sabrina. Stay with her. I'll get things arranged and let you know as soon as I speak with the psychiatrist. Don't worry, we'll get it done. Just hang in there a little longer."

Khai called Chris later that morning. He didn't answer his cell, so she called his answering service. They said he was in surgery, but Khai knew he was off on Tuesdays and always spent the day cycling during the summer or skiing in winter. She left a message; he did not call back. She tried again at three, promising herself it was for the last time, and tried again at nine.

He finally answered, though his speech was muddled, as if he had been asleep." "Hello."

"Hey, it's Khai. Been trying to get ahold of you."

"Oh, hi," he slurred. "Been in surgery all day. Colostomy that went bad. Sometimes I wonder why I didn't go into dermatology."

She laughed, "You'd spend your life treating fourteen-year-old girls with pimples."

"Better than being bathed in feces day after endless day." He asked coolly, "What's up?"

"You okay."

"Yeah, fine. Just tired."

"Wow, your voice sounds like you're exhausted. I'm sorry to bother you..." She waited a moment for the perfunctory, 'Don't be silly, you're never a bother,' but he remained silent. She tensed and asked, "Just wondering if you have that number for the shrink we want to send Sabrina Maddingly to?"

"Oh, damn. I forgot. Sorry. I'll call right away." He also gave Khai the number, but had to repeat it twice, tripping on the threes.

CHAPTER TWENTY-FOUR

Mike called the psychiatrist's office minutes later. The earliest appointment was three weeks hence. He called Khai, who phoned the office. They denied having heard from Gauthé. When Khai introduced herself and told her about Sabrina, Dr. Claire Darling carved an appointment for them the next morning.

Mike noticed the woman's head shake faintly as she read down the list of antidepressants. And she caught, out of the corner of her eye, that he had seen her reaction. For the next few minutes, she occasionally shook her head subtly when benign subjects surfaced.

After listening to Sabrina's story, she leaned forward. "Okay, well, first, I don't know a soul who wouldn't be depressed with what you've gone through. But that's immaterial." She smiled and winked. "You may have heard that before. You have undoubtedly communicated that to your patients a thousand times." Sabrina smiled. "The bottom line is that your depression is severe, and whatever the cause is, it doesn't matter. There is nothing volitional that you can do about it at this point. You are a mental health professional, and intellectually, you know all of this. So, we have to advance the level of treatment. What are your feelings about that?"

"Right now, I have no feelings. You and I both know..."

Her voice trailed off, and the psychiatrist turned to Mike. "Mr. Maddingly, please don't be offended, but could you excuse us for a few minutes? You know, so we ladies can have a few words together. Pretend we're going to the powder room."

Mike looked at Sabrina, who nodded blandly.

Sabrina spoke first. "How did you know?"

"Just the way you would know with your patients. So, Dr. Maddingly, what are you most scared of? Let's get it all out on the table."

"You know, it isn't even the physical disability. I adjusted to my arm as a kid. But now, Michael is my responsibility. I don't want to curse him with my stuff. And for a full lifetime? I won't do that. It would be better for me to die. Let him have a normal life. He'll get over it. He is the gentlest man, so caring. I can't keep hurting him like this. It's killing him. I'm killing him. I need to have the courage to do the right thing and stop this."

"He is a special man. I can already tell. He has the sweetest face." She paused and looked into Sabrina's eyes. "Dr. Maddingly, on the other hand, you're sitting here talking with me, so, you must believe all is not lost. If it was, you wouldn't have shown up today. You know our field as well as I do. What can I do to help you climb this hill?"

"Hill? You mean Mt. Everest?"

"Why do you say that?"

"You know, when my patients talked about hopelessness, I wrote it down like a good little clinician. It was just a word, a puff of air, nothing more than a symptom of depression. Everybody knows that. But when you feel it, when there's only futility and a dark tunnel with a black, concrete wall at the end..." She stopped speaking, her head dropping to stare at her left hand. Dr. Darling leaned forward but said nothing. After a minute of utter silence in the room, Sabrina finally whispered, "Never felt this hopeless before, ever. Never knew anyone could. Never knew how much it could hurt." She looked up into Darling's eyes. "I've never seen a patient dragging this much mental and physical baggage. Even if my mood improves, that doesn't do a thing for the stroke, and how my frailty and helplessness are essentially ruining Mike's life."

Dr. Darling spoke dispassionately. "So, it's not the depression but the sequelae of the stroke? Is that the catch?"

"Catch?"

Darling stopped and let her eyes drift to the ceiling. "You know, every mental health professional has been taught not to rag patients about how small their problems are. That disaffirms what the patient is experiencing. 'You think you got it bad, well, let me tell you about Joe Blow...'" Her voice hardened. "But you're not the usual patient, so, even though I shouldn't tell you about a few people you might have heard of, I'm going to anyway. Knowing about these folks isn't going to cure you, but maybe they'll give you some perspective, buy some time to get you to reconsider your options. Stop me when you've had enough."

"Okay, roll out your menagerie of defectives."

"Let's start at the bottom of the pile and move up. How about Senator Robert Dole? Lost use of his right arm to a German machine gun in World War Two. A politician who couldn't shake hands, but he rose to Republican leader of the Senate in the 1980s. Ran for vice-president. Heard of Ray Charles? How about Little Stevie Wonder? FDR? Have you heard of Steven Hawking? They did okay, huh? I'm sure each of them considered doing away with themselves. I know that Senator Dole did back in the hospital in Europe. But, you see, the gift of life is something over which they did have volitional control, and they turned things around and managed to change the world while they were crying in their beer. And you and me, all we want to do is change a few lives along the way. Not that high a mountain."

Sabrina nodded. "Dr. Darling, intellectually, I get the point, but that's selfish of me, because what is most important is Mike's survival, not mine."

Dr. Darling smiled cynically. "That's very brave and noble, but it smacks of melodrama." Sabrina face hardened, but she said nothing, and Darling went on. "I'm speaking with you professional to professional for a moment, if you will allow me..." Sabrina's face loosened. "Good. For me observing from the outside, but with thirty years under my belt, what you face is an uphill road. Then, again, from my vantage point, it looks pretty well paved, curvy for sure, but it gets to the top. So, how far are you willing to go to start the journey?"

"I'm not sure what you mean."

"Well, we have a pretty big armamentarium these days. I'm going to be perfectly blunt. Your tool belt is talk therapy. You know more about, for instance, cognitive behavioral therapy in your little finger than I do in my whole body. And, for a panoply of the outpatient mental health issues we treat, you and I, CBT is a great option, better than meds. But you see, I have prescriptive power. So, I've made myself very familiar with a lot of meds and procedures not available to a psychologist."

Sabrina grew pale. "Procedures? What are you thinking?"

"You tell me."

"You mean the 800-pound gorilla over there in the corner?"

"Hold on, hear me out. Personally, I do not believe that you've tried all the medication possibilities, but each doctor has a favorite algorithm, and it's not my place to second-guess the guy down the block.

"On the other hand, even if I my choice of antidepressants is diff...hold on, let's get Mr. Maddingly back in here. We're going to talk about choosing options. I imagine you'll want him in on the process. That okay with you?"

Mike was nearly as pale as Sabrina when he took his seat. Dr. Darling leaned forward in her chair. "Mr. Maddingly, it's time for all of us to discuss the next step. My recommendation is that we make this a group effort. Are you on board?

"Whatever's best for Sabrina."

"I explained to Dr. Maddingly that there are all sorts of medicine combinations we haven't tried yet. On the other hand, most of the time, changing antidepressants around, especially when you're already on usually effective meds, seldom makes a quantum change in results. So, there is essentially no chance that I will pull a new drug out of my hat and all of Dr. Maddingly's problems will suddenly vaporize. In fact, no chance. There's no silver bullet. Doctoring doesn't work that way.

"Professionally, and personally, I think we need to break the vicious cycle, stop the depression as fast as we can, get things under control, and then we can reintroduce antidepressants, one by one, until we find the best combination. And, by the way, I do think it will eventually take more than a single, and perhaps even three, medications, to keep things copasetic over the long haul.

"So, bottom line, I'm recommending we don't rely on meds for right now but go straight to Electroconvulsive Therapy, ECT."

Dr. Darling faced more toward Mike than Sabrina, not surprised when his face tensed crossly. She smiled ever so subtly and nodded. "I understand, sir, but it's not at all what you think. It works in a large percentage of patients, and the side effects are quite mild and manageable. Heck of a lot more manageable than living with severe depression for the rest of your life. But we'll go through the possible hitches in detail, make sure we're all on the same page."

Mike sheepishly raised his hand. "Dr. Darling, are you saying Sabrina will have this depression for the rest of her life, no matter what?"

"To be honest, very likely so. Typically, depression is episodic, starts when you're young, teenager, often earlier; you know, kids who suddenly start to fail at school, become behavior problems. Typical early episode, you go downhill for a few months, plateau, or I should say bottom out for two or three, then resurface over the next few. Usual cycle is, say, eight or nine months. Goes away for a while, but, if you've got the gene and the right life circumstances, or, sometimes just the gene itself, it comes back in the vast majority of patients, usually a little worse each time."

"But this is her first time."

"May be. On the other hand, there could have been what we call sub-clinical depression in the past, you know, the teen blues. Sabrina?" She nodded subtly. "Well, we'll certainly be talking about that, and a lot, but for right now, there is a significant problem that the stroke and the terminated pregnancy unveiled. All that counts is that we're faced, today, with a serious depression, and whether it's the first occurrence or not, left untreated, the episodes become more frequent as you age, and the low points get lower. So, we don't like to let even a single depressive episode go on too long. What I'm saying is that we need to intervene sooner rather than later." She waited until Mike looked away from Sabrina toward her. "What are your thoughts?"

He sighed, "Shock therapy? I thought that went out with *One Flew Over the Cuckoo's Nest.*"

"Actually, in the film, after the ECT, Nicholson was feeling a lot better, so much so, that Nurse Ratchet had even less control over him. That's when she sent him for a lobotomy. That's what did him in, the surgery. On the other hand, I hear you. Seems very primitive, but it's not at all archaic; really quite sophisticated and safe. Let me tell you why this is my primary choice. First, we only use ECT when the situation is a relative emergency, basically when there is imminent danger to the life or well-being of the patient. Dr. Maddingly, let me put it bluntly: I think you are suicidal. And I think you are a candidate for admission to a mental health service—voluntarily or otherwise. I would like to admit you to Mitchie-Sterling's Mental Health facility. It's right across the street from the hospital."

Mike protested, "That's too far for you to drive."

"Nah, I'm up that way several times a week. I cover for one of my partners at a clinic near Evansville. Her husband's being treated for prostate cancer. Ride's not a big deal. And I've had privileges at Mitchie-Sterling for decades. Good facility." Mike rolled his eyes. "Not to worry, Mr. Maddingly, we're a very separate arm of the hospital.

"We treat three times a week for the first week and go on for as long as it takes to make a difference, usually once or twice a week for two or three weeks. That's my guess for you, Dr. Maddingly.

"The horror stories from the 50s and 60s are old news. These days, we sedate the patient lightly and give a muscle relaxer, so you don't feel a thing, and there's darn near no muscle movement at all. No pulled muscles, no soreness. That's all in the past. It's no more dangerous than undergoing brief general anesthesia.

"I will be honest and tell you there is a greater risk for side effects after a patient's had a stroke. ECT could, in theory, cause another blood clot, but we know what caused the first stroke, the first clot. That was during a very perilous medical problem, the loss of a large amount of blood, when anybody could suffer a clot, whether they're susceptible to clotting or not. In this case, I believe that has little to do with the chances of a second stroke.

"The most common side effects are confusion and memory loss after the procedure. Confusion is only right after the procedure. Sometimes there is loss of memory, Dr. Maddingly, you know, retrograde memory loss, that can go back weeks or even, rarely, months. Usually, the memory of the blank period starts to come back after a month or so. Infrequently, some retrograde memories don't come back."

Mike interrupted. "You mean Sabrina might forget the whole episode of the tubal and the hospital?"

"Possibly."

"How about not being able to recall things about psychology?"

"What you're asking about is losing memories from years before treatment. It is very unusual using the modern machines and techniques, but even if it does happen, the long-term memory loss always comes back. It's the short-term memory loss that occasionally does not return."

Sabrina shrugged. "That may not be such a bad thing."

Mike nodded. "Dr. Darling, I don't mean to cut you off, but that's a lot to think about. Most of all, that you want to put my wife in a mental hospital." He sagged and spoke softly. "On the other hand, the last time I argued with a good doctor, it almost cost Sabrina her life, so I'm going to leave it up to her."

They both turned to Sabrina. She spoke quickly. "I'm not going to fight either, but I do not want my employer notified. Can the admission be kept from them?"

"Well, I can't lie if I'm asked by someone who has a right to ask, but your employer is not one of those people. You are on medical leave of absence for how much longer?"

"It's open ended, but I told them I wanted to wait six more weeks before I tried to come back part-time."

"That gives us enough leeway to get you feeling better without having to apply for further LOA, and all the questions these nosey human resources people ask. Your insurance company will know the diagnosis, but they had better not share it with your employer. And there is no foreseeable way they would report it to anyone. You two would be able to retire after the lawsuit if the insurance company or one of the doctors let any of this get out. Don't forget, every time somebody accesses your medical records, documentation is made of the inquiry. Snoopy people, like those from human resources, are usually far from computer savvy enough to cover their tracks. That's not a concern.

"And, Mr. Maddingly, when we do the treatments, it's okay not to be there. I mean, why don't you come a few hours later? Much better for Dr. Maddingly and for you."

CHAPTER TWENTY-FIVE

Sabrina was admitted to the mental health facility across from the hospital that day. Mike drove to school and told them he'd be back in the morning. The next afternoon, though, was an in-service, and he skipped out of a meeting to see Sabrina. As he pulled into the parking lot, a figure cloaked in all black jumped from behind a parked car. An ebony cape pulled high onto the apparition's head did little to obscure a Scream Mask. The creature thrust a sign to the front of Mike's windshield, it's menacing letters blood red.

MITCHIE-STERLING DEATH HOUSE SNUFFS THE LIVES OF OUR LOVED ONES

Mike drove past, avoiding the man's eyes, and took a spot as close to the front entrance as he could. As the hospital doors opened automatically, he sensed eyes boring into his back. Stopping mid-stride, he looked over his shoulder to find the bizarre, black-clad soul staring at him twenty yards away. Edgy that he needed to be with Sabrina, Mike took a few more steps inside, but could not help himself, and slowly paced back toward the apparition. The figure stiffened, and the sign came up as if a shield. Mike called out, "Excuse me, but can I ask what's going on, what's happened?"

142

The being stood stock-still. "You an undercover cop?" The voice was so raspy, it was nearly unintelligible, but when Mike decoded the question, he asked cautiously, "Do I look like a cop?"

"Yeah, you do."

"Well, I'm not. I'm here to see my wife." He gestured toward the second floor.

"You a lawyer trying to get me to bad-mouth the hospital? Sue me for slander?"

"No. I just had a problem with the hospital myself. They harmed my wife—bad."

"How can I be sure you ain't a plant?"

"Look, man..." Mike answered quietly but shook his head and turned back to the entrance. He paced barely three steps into the foyer before his chest clutched. He wheeled around impatiently. "I'm telling you the truth." He fumbled through the papers in his hand and pulled free a thin packet. "Look at this. This is her discharge summary. You know what that is?" He paused for a second. "Come take a look."

The man walked forward slowly and craned his neck at the document. Mike snapped. "Tell me if I'm a cop." The man adjusted his mask to better align his eyes with the holes. Mike sighed "Come on, man."

"Okay, I'll talk to you."

Mike nodded. "Come sit in my car. And don't worry," he added caustically, "it isn't bugged."

The man slipped into the passenger seat and pulled free the skeleton mask. He was in his late 30s, dark and deeply handsome, though his neck was marred by a jagged scar that tracked from under his right jaw, over a deformed Adam's Apple, then coursed down under the collar of his OD tee-shirt.

When Mike's eyes locked on the wound, the man hissed, "Don't worry about it."

Mike grunted, "Okay, but what's up, man."

"Fuckin' hospital. I'm protestin' what they did to my wife. Took 'er in for bronchitis. Waited over four hours to see a doctor. Wasn't even a doctor— PA or something. Spent five minutes with her and sent her home with some pills, amoxicillin, same thing they give my little girl for an earache. I get snappy with the guy, tell him she needs something stronger, but he says if I want to see a real doctor, it's going to be an hour, maybe two. Meanwhile, babysitter's

143

watching Brie, my little girl. Got no time to argue with the asshole. Cocksuckers. Went home. Had to go to work in the morning, construction on the hospital annex, of all things. Boss didn't let me off, so, at noon, I snuck away from the job site to call my wife. She had tried to call me, but we ain't allowed to have the phone on during work. Some bullshit about detonating explosives. We ain't got no explosives on this job. Fuckers."

Mike growled, "Shit, I thought I had it bad. Go on, man."

"Anyway, I got no answer. Tried again at two. Foreman's lookin' for me. Chews my ass. Fuckin' Air Farce asshole. Hates me 'cause I was on the ground, a grunt, and got Purple Heart tags on my rig." Mike's eyes dropped to the man's neck. "Yeah, Afghanistan." The man's eyes reddened. "So, when I couldn't get ahold of her at four, when we were packing up, I left early. Boss caught me. Told him to shove it up his ass. Fucker fired me on the spot.

"When I got home, she was like blue, hardly could talk, she was having so much trouble breathing. I drove her back to the emergency room. They put her in for pneumonia. Told 'em I lost my job. No more insurance. Nurse said that even if I lost my insurance, the hospital had to take care of my wife because they had already started." His face tensed, but he remained quiet for a moment before blurting, "She was dead in two days."

The next silence lasted for many seconds until, through gasps, he choked that he had wanted to sue the hospital. "But they twisted the story into a fuckin' fairy tale 'bout the man who was too lazy to bring his wife back to the hospital right away when she got worse. Said she did it to herself by smoking. That's bullshit. She smoked with her friends when she was 19, all her girlfriends did, you know what I mean. But not one cancer stick since—fifteen years. She hated it. They lied and lied to protect their sorry asses. I fuckin' hate 'em. Now they're going to sue me for slander. At least that's what they've threatened. Cops said they'd throw my ass in the city lockup if I set one foot on any sidewalk near the hospital."

"Are you allowed to be over here?"

"Don't know, and I don't give a shit. My lawyer's a good guy. Understands these bastards, says they're too scared to make a big stink over an unhappy customer whose wife died in their hospital under crappy circumstances. Anyway, what can they do to me? They already killed my little girl's mom. Killed me inside, too."

Mike felt a cloak of despair wash over him. It was if he, himself, was telling the story to a stranger, and he sensed the same nauseating feeling that had blanketed him the night he watched through the window as his wife's life ebbed. His chest clutched remembering the rock-hard wall through which he had been powerless to crash and halt the madness.

Mike spoke softly. "Sorry, man. I hate to hear that." He paused and went on. "Hey, I gotta go in and see my wife. Not doing very well. I guess you know the feeling."

"Okay. But thanks for listening. I'm Scott Bialek. You?"

"Mike Maddingly. Hey, Scott, listen, I'm going to be heading home in a couple of hours. Can I buy you a beer? I mean, I'd like to hear more. It seems so similar to my story. You can be sure it's on the up and up. I promise I don't want anything from you. I promise."

Scott thought for a minute. "You seem real. Meet you right here. I'll be dressed like normal—jeans, blue hoodie."

CHAPTER TWENTY-SIX

S abrina was sitting up in bed. Mike smiled, "You look much better already."

She slurred, "I feel okay. How long am I going to be here?" She gazed down at her left arm, and Mike sensed she was trying to will a flicker of life into it. There was, though, nothing. Seeing him watching her arm, she added, "Was hoping to kill two birds with one stone."

Mike's smile diminished subtly, but he quickly forced up the corners of his mouth. "How was the treatment?"

Sabrina shook her head. "I'm not sure. They gave me an IV, apparently," she gazed at the back of her right hand, "but that's all I know for sure."

"Do you remember, like yesterday, when you were admitted?"

Her lips pursed. "Not really."

"How 'bout the psychiatrist, you know, Dr. Darling?"

"Who's he?"

Mike forced himself to breathe slowly. "She's your new doctor." His voice tightened. "Try to remember, Sweetheart."

"It's all a blur. But I'd sure like to get out of here. This place is a bummer, so drab."

He asked hesitatingly, "You looking forward to coming home?"

"God, yes." She closed her eyes and pursed her lips again. "A thought just flew through my mind. Darn. It's gone. Just that quick. Like trying to remember some part of a dream. Harder you try, more blank it goes."

At that moment, Dr. Darling knocked softly at the door and took a hesitant step into the room. Mike looked up and smiled—Sabrina stared. He put his hand on Sabrina's arm and asked gently, "Sweetheart, you remember Dr. Darling. She's your doctor here."

Sabrina looked up again. A faint smile came to her. "Yeah, I do. That's the face that flashed through my mind."

Dr. Darling smiled broadly and sat on the far corner of the bed. "That's great. You're doing better than most after the first treatment."

Mike asked, "How did it go?"

Darling nodded. "Just fine. Easy as pie. We only placed the cords on one side. Fewer adverse effects, and maybe just as helpful. Let me ask you, Dr. Maddingly, do you have any nausea?"

"No."

"Headache, jaw pain, or muscle aches?"

"No. I feel pretty good. Yeah, it's coming back. Well, a little."

"Good. You know, we used a very low current. First time and all. Hardly any movement of the muscles, which is usual and what we want, so you don't pull tendons and the like. But what I noticed was that your left arm moved somewhat. That means there are still some working connections between the brain and the arm. Good reason to keep up with the PT."

Mike sighed. "Insurance is saying that we've used up the physical therapy benefits. I don't know if that means here in the hospital, or at home, too."

"Yeah, I saw that. It's both but let me work on it. There's light at the end of the tunnel. I can make a statement to them based on objective findings of movement of the left arm. Hard for them to fight too hard when you can show improvement. I mean, they'll fight like caged animals, but we'll get 'em under control. Use one of those immobilizing dart guns."

Mike laughed. "Like they do on wild elephants?"

"More like what they use on snakes."

Dr. Darling and Mike were looking at each other but turned toward Sabrina when she giggled.

An hour later, Scott followed Mike to the Big Ugly Bear, a grill he and Sabrina had visited several times with their new friends from the school district. In the parking lot, Scott sighed, "Used to come here with Justine."

Mike grimaced, "Sorry, man. Come on, we'll go somewhere else."

"Nah, no matter where we go, it'll be the same. We both grew up in McKinley. It's okay. I'm gettin' better. Like they say, time heals, and all that sort of shit. I donno know, though."

Mike ordered two beers, and Scott pulled a crumpled five-dollar bill from long-unwashed jeans. Mike pushed his hand down. "Nah, I got it. I'm workin'. At least for now."

The beers came, and both chugged two-thirds before wiping away the foam with their sweatshirt sleeves. They laughed and high-fived.

Scott turned his face away from Mike slightly. "Hey, man, can I ask about your wife? I mean, is she gonna be okay?"

"She had a pretty bad stroke. Can't move her left side. Slurs when she talks. Bunch of other things. She'll make it, but future's pretty grim. Doesn't look like the movement's coming back to her left side." Mike paused, waiting for Scott speak, but when he didn't, Mike asked quietly, "By the way, who's taking care of, did you say...Brie?"

"Good memory. Yeah, my mom. But she ain't got nothin'. Social Security don't kick in for another two years. My old man died a few years ago. I'm doin' security work at night. Gives me time with my little girl. Take her to pre-school and then do my picketing around here. Waste of time. I know, but, what the hell, I met you."

"Thanks, man. I shouldn't say this, but it seems better knowing I'm not alone."

Scott nodded. "Yeah, me too."

"Hey, Scott, man, if you don't mind, could you tell me more about how the hospital screwed you?" When Scott didn't look up, Mike added, "I mean if you don't mind."

Scott exhaled. "No problem," but said no more.

Mike waited before asking, "Man, are you sure you can't sue? I mean, if your wife was so sick that..." He stopped suddenly. "Hey, look. I been thinking about it for the past two hours. Now, I'm no lawyer, but it seems to me there was obviously the potential for what happened, because it happened, and yet they let her go home? Aren't they supposed to, what is it they say, rule out all the bad possibilities? I mean, what's that about? Are they telling you that if she took some pills at home for the next 24 hours, everything would be just fine? That doesn't seem right."

"Yeah, you got a point, but it isn't that simple. We had to get a certificate of, what the hell was it? Oh, yeah, certificate of merit before my lawyer could file a case."

Mike interrupted. "I'm sorry, man, I don't know what that is."

"See, from what I understand, in this state, your lawyer has to get a statement from a so-called expert that the doctors screwed up. Can't file a malpractice lawsuit without it."

"Did you get that?"

"In the end, no. Couldn't afford it. No job. Spent all our savings burying my wife, and that was after burying my dad." He became very quiet again, and his head drooped."

"We don't need to go on."

Scott grabbed his beer and guzzled the last third. "No, man, no problem. Part of it's on me. My lawyer, Mr. Jennings, good guy. He wanted to help, but there had to be five grand up front to get some doctor in Texas to go through the files. Where the hell am I going to get that kind of money? Got a kid at home, wife wasn't working for three years. I made just enough to get by, but we both wanted her to stay home with the baby. My wife was a healthy young gal. Stronger than me. Carries the baby and the groceries up three flights day after day. Doesn't even breathe hard." He laughed dolefully. "Then, all of a sudden, she dies from a curable disease. You need a doctor to say on paper something's wrong with that picture?"

Mike raised his eyes. "Didn't your lawyer put up the money? I thought they did that. Collect at the other end."

"He's a good guy, but he can't be payin' my bills. They gotta have somethin' up front. Lawsuit can cost forty, fifty thousand before it gets to trial. He's got to know if it's worth it before he puts out all that money. And that doesn't count his time, just what he has to pay for copying records and paying experts and court fees. Can't stake every pissed off dude who walks through his door.

"He even called the doctor, the expert, in Texas. Told him about the case. Asked him if he would just talk about it for a few hundred bucks. Guy said okay, but when he heard it was nearly a day between us going to the ER the first time and going back, he said he'd heard enough. No case. Mr. Jennings said he was sorry then paid the doctor down in Texas out of his own pocket. Never heard of that before. His hands were tied. I don't blame 'im.'"

"Scott, I need to get going. Grade some papers. Haven't been all that good about keeping up. You know how it is."

"Well, like I said, thanks for listening. Glad I met you. Lemme know if I can help, I mean with the dirt I was able to dig up on those scum. God, I hate 'em."

They exchanged telephone numbers and hugged.

CHAPTER TWENTY-SEVEN

Norman Harp reassembled the members of his select team on a wintery Sunday morning weeks after the first meeting. His introductory remark was a muttered, "I was hoping to have this little challenge in the hands of our attorneys by now, but I got a report from security of some funny business. First, let me ask the medical director, where are we with the woman who had the stroke?"

Klat smirked, "Which one?"

With Harp's glare, Klat's head dropped a few millimeters. "She's woken up, discharged, but I understand she's been admitted across the street to the psych facility. Severe depression, from what I understand. Even suggesting ECT—that bad."

Harp snorted, "Nutcase, eh? Not surprised. Seems to go with the territory, doesn't it?" When no one nodded, he grumbled, "But they aren't going to try and pin that on us, are they? You don't all of a sudden wake up one day in your mid-thirties crazy. She must have a psych history. Was that part of the records you went over for the discharge summary, Harvey?"

"There was no mention of mental health issues. As I'm sure you're aware, depression is a very common complication of stroke."

"I see, but..."

Klat interrupted, "Also, something I need to tell you, Norman. Husband's mad as a wet hen. Says he tried to get you to help when his wife was at her lowest. Says Claire gave him the bum's rush, that you heard the whole thing and retreated into your office, slammed the door. Guy says you saw the whole thing."

Harp shook his head, dismissing Klat's stare. "Claire, you mean the girl that sits outside my office?"

"Yep, that Claire."

"Sorry, not in my job description to play nursemaid to every worried husband. Be reasonable. That's why we pay a staff." When Klat's stare became a frown, Harp asked pointedly, "Then tell me, is she going to die?"

"Looks like she'll survive, but with deficits."

Harp thought for a moment. "Well, if I remember correctly, she had all sorts of problems when she landed on our doorstep, and that's how we're going to structure our approach. I want all of her old medical records. We have a right to them."

Klat raised his palm. "Not until she sues us, we don't."

Harp snapped, "Must be one of our doctors seeing her at the loony bin, right?"

"Well, it's Claire Darling. She has privileges here from way back. Hasn't been terribly active for years, though."

"Good, have this Dr. Darling order every medical note this woman ever had written about her. Just make sure she's on board and willing to give us copies."

"Norman, I don't think she will. I mean, order records for non-medical purposes. She's pretty straitlaced. Does a lot of pro bono work; a dinosaur, plays by the rules she learned in medical school. Those were different days."

"Well, approach her. Say something like one of our docs wants to look into her past, you know, to see if there's any other underlying problems. Us working selflessly on behalf the patient. Might remind her that she's not been active on our staff, and we'd like to draw her back into the fold.

"Now, our legal representation advises that if this woman has been treated for a congenital problem since birth, that'll be enough to get the thing dismissed by the county medical panel. That's if we have the horses, i.e., her medical chart. It'll never see the inside of a courtroom.

"But let's be smart. We'll put together so much evidence, none of the local ambulance chasers'll even look at the case. Now, where's that ultrasound report? What does it say?"

"We're still not sure."

"Are you telling me, Harvey, that we still haven't found a routine radiology report?"

"DeepSight Radiologists haven't gotten back to us. I don't need to remind you about the contract negotiations. There're some tender feelings at the moment. And they're radiologists; don't move all that fast unless reading films a million miles an hour to beef up the number of x-rays they can bill."

"Can we just have a different radiologist read the ultrasound? Tell them we'll pay for a second reading."

"There are no films."

"Well, interview the ultrasound tech who did the study. Let's find out what she saw. I'm sure she's recovered from the shock, poor thing. Is she back to work?"

"Never missed a day."

"Admirable. Surely, she can read a basic ultrasound. Takes 'em forever to be trained to become techs. Is she one of those whose training we paid for?"

"She is."

"Well, remind her where she works, who pays her salary, and her contractual arrangement with us to pay off her school loan as long as she remains in our employ. Find out if she saw the blood down there, which I'm sure even she couldn't have missed. Get a sworn statement before the other side says we waited too long and that she couldn't possibly remember an incidental finding on a study in the middle of the night. Get her on paper now, and if she's a weak sister, let me know, and I'll have a talk with her department head."

Harp turned away curtly from Klat. He pointed at Dr. Weegun. "Worth, as our safety officer, what about the L&I guy? What have we learned about the man? First, are we taking good care of him, supplementing his time loss from the state with enough to bring him up to his usual salary?"

Weegun shook his head. "Norman, we need to be careful. That's a slippery slope. We don't do that—even for professional staff. Just encourages people to stay away from work forever. And then the next one'll want the same treatment."

Harp's eyes tightened. "Look, if we don't keep him on our side, he's going to cost us more in negative testimony than if the entire clinic was out on L&I. Simply a smart business decision."

"I'll see how the wretched man's feeling."

Klat raised a finger. "Norman, you know, I talked to one of the security guards. Left me kind of uncomfortable. He swears he and, he says, five other guards, saw the husband beating the tar out of the employee who's claiming injury. Says the husband had our man on the ground, pummeling him, smashing his head into the linoleum right outside the treatment room while Cardozo was trying to save the patient's life. I asked him why no one intervened. He hemmed and hawed that they didn't want to commit an assault on hospital grounds before they were on the clock. I asked around. The staff there that night, no one wants to talk. Best I could find out, the only security person in the ER at the time was our injured guy."

Harp glared sternly. "Is that in writing?"

Klat's palms came up defensively. "No, Norman, just from my conversations down there." Harp's face tightened. "And look, Norman, I'm just reporting." He paused for a moment before adding a bit more calmly, "Also asked him why all five of them were claiming to have witnessed the incident when there's only two on duty at any one time. More hemming and hawing. Says it was change of shift. But that's at 3 A.M, and the incident was hours before. I checked the timecards. Holiday eve, only one guard was on the clock at the time. To be honest, the whole thing sounds like a crock of you know what."

"Okay, but, bottom line, the main guy who was assaulted..." He watched Klat's face, "He was assaulted—yes?"

"Remains to be seen."

Harp rolled his eyes. "I imagine the employee was seen in our ER that night. So, let's get his records. See what signs of trauma they recorded. Must have been some. Also, get his records from the meatball medicine walk-in clinic where he's going for his L&I claim. They're granting him time loss—we have a legal right to those records. After all, his treatment's on our dime. This part of the story may not be worth pursuing, but we need him on our side, or at least neutral, and for as long as we can.

"Okay, that's all. Let's get back to work. And, Harvey, we really need to get on the ultrasound report and the woman's old records."

CHAPTER TWENTY-EIGHT

O n a Saturday morning, a few days after Sabrina was admitted to the psych facility, Chris called Khai. "Whata you heard from the Maddinglys? How's she doing?"

"Funny that you ask. Mike came by yesterday. They're doing ECT. Two treatments so far, and he actually smiled. Pretty much the first time I ever saw him do that, and..."

Chris interrupted. "ECT? Saw it in medical school once. Almost passed out. I'm sorry, please go on."

"Mike said she rolled over in bed and held him this morning. He was pretty emotional. He's a good man."

"He is. Crummy deal, but it always is when you get people who do everything right, and still they get screwed."

Khai paused. "And haven't heard from you in a while. What's new?"

"SOS. Same old stuff. Started doing the laser cholecystectomies. A little different than on dogs, but we're getting real good. Down to twenty minutes. And that's going through every step twice, three times if there's anything unusual. I even have a little tape recorder in my pocket. Sound activated, so as I'm operating and see something strange, a little twist in the plan, I can verbally remind myself after surgery, come up with a filler for that pothole."

Khai asked lightly, "I'd love to see one of the procedures. Don't mean scrub in, just stand in a corner and watch the master at work. I won't say anything to activate the recorder."

Chris' voice tightened. "Yeah...ah, let me see what the rules are down at the U—HIPPA and all that. They're a pain in the rear at the great Mecca. But let me ask, and I'll let..."

Chris stopped, and Khai could hear his voice break as he pulled the phone away to see who was calling. He was quiet for a second then said matter-of-factly, "Well, kiddo, need to get back to the salt mines. Call you later." The instant he heard the first syllable of Khai's answer, he interjected abruptly, "See ya," and aimed his finger at the key to swap lines. He, though, started to talk before the switch had taken place, and Khai heard him gush, "Hey, kiddo, how you do..." And with that, Khai's line went silent.

It was Krystal. "Hey, I was just about to hang up. You must busy at the hospital."

"Nah. Just getting coffee at Starbucks. Was trying to fish out my wallet when the phone went off. You?"

"Bob's got the baby. They're going to his mom's. I'm going shopping. What about you?"

Chris' chest clutched. "Nothin'. You wanna shop here in Soundview? Heard about a sale goin' on at the condos on 155th. You know the place? Pretty good stuff, from what they say."

"Yeah, been there a few times. Top notch goods. Twenty minutes?"

"I don't know. All of a sudden, I may not be able to stand up and leave the place for the next twenty minutes. Kind of embarrassing, if you know what I mean."

"Stop it, you. You're making it hard for me to keep my hands off myself—if you know what I mean."

Krystal got to the condo first and let herself in. She jumped into the shower and when done, took Chris's robe off the hook and lay back on the couch. He came in a moment later, face flushed. She sat up, let the robe open a trace, and smiled. "Hey."

He dropped down beside her, shaking his head, "If it isn't one thing, it's the oth..." He trailed off, but after a few seconds, he turned to her silently and put his hands on the edges of the robe to tug it further open. It was not long before both were nude, and three minutes later, done. She stroked his cheek then leaned forward to kiss him, but without a word, he pulled his head back and stood, beginning to dress.

She slipped into the robe and leaned back to stare at the ceiling for a while before speaking very softly. "You know, Chris, I'm not sure this is healthy—for either of us. I mean, I love it with you, but each time the guilt gets worse. It's like a switch. I can't stand waiting to see you. It's all consuming, and then I climax, and an instant later my mind darkens. And then I run out, call my husband, make some excuse, and when I get home, I can't look him in the eye— kids either. It makes me feel like a fraud, like I don't deserve to love them anymore. Don't you feel that, even a little?"

He sat back down a foot from her. She reached out and put her hand on his arm. He flinched faintly and started to speak but abruptly stopped and stared straight ahead. Finally, he turned back to her. "Are you saying you don't want to see me anymore?"

"I'm just saying I'm not sure the remorse is worth it. It gets harder each time, not easier, like you told me it would get, like it was for you. I knew I was going to call you this morning; knew it last night. As soon as I got up, I couldn't wait for Bob to leave. That's wrong, Chris."

"Isn't it good for you? Sure seems like it is."

"It's too good." Her eyes reddened. "I don't know what to do."

"All I know is that it's good for both of us, and I don't want it to stop. Why can't you just enjoy it and, every once in a while, allow yourself a few minutes of, I don't know, liberation?"

"Chris, your words, you, are like a siren's call, but it's a trap. I hate myself so much afterword...I just gotta stop." She ran into the bathroom and dressed. When she came out, he was sitting forward over the coffee table, his head just millimeters from the glass. As the last trace of white dust disappeared into his nose, he looked up slowly and poked a vial of the powder toward her.

Her hand started to lift but jerked to a stop. "No, never again. Chris, you're throwing your life away. I'm so scared it's already too late for me, but what you do from now on is your business. All I know is that it's going to catch up with you, and you obviously don't give a damn. And I'm not letting you take me down when you crash." She spun toward the door. As the lock opened, tears coursed along her cheeks. "Goodbye, Chris."

As the door closed, he looked up and hissed, "You called me, remember?"

Gauthé slept through much of the afternoon. He awoke at 5 P.M. so hung over, he stumbled and fell as he got up to go to the bathroom. His eyes passed over the cell phone on the coffee table next to the still-open vial of powder. His heart clutched as he saw there had been several calls, but when he checked, not one was from Krystal. He muttered, "Bitch," and was about to toss the phone back onto the couch but recognized several of the numbers as having come from the University Hospital's Emergency Department, from the surgical pre-op area, and finally, two from the surgical department chairman's personal cell. He shook his head trying to remember if he had done surgery that morning or, maybe, late last night. He was reasonably sure he had not. Then he wondered if he had been on call that day and slept through it, so he started on the bottom of the list and worked his way up the increasingly impatient messages. After the third threatening call, he emptied some of the powder onto the coffee table and relaxed for a few moments.

Things seemed, somehow, to clear in his head. He pieced together that a patient who had undergone his new procedure three days before had taken a bicycle ride, fainted, and fallen. She presented to the ER as white as a sheet, clearly bleeding internally. The surgeon on call refused to make any decisions beyond ordering a transfusion and trying to get Chris on his personal line. The messages became more and more menacing until the final call, from the Chairman of the Department of Surgery ordering Chris to appear at the hospital immediately. That last call was two hours old.

Gauthé ran through the shower, dressed in jeans, drove to the hospital, and charged up the stairs to the surgical recovery floor. His patient was still groggy from the major open procedure the on-call surgeon had heatedly done to stem the internal bleeding.

Gauthé called the chairman, protesting, "Alex, I didn't appreciate your tone. If you're not on call, you're not supposed to be on call. Are you available 24-7-365? It so happens I was flying in a friend's plane out in the mountains. No cell coverage. What did you want me to do?"

The man was silent for a moment. "Look, Chris, you're the one who took on this experiment—tip of the spear, sexy vanguard, and all that crap. It doesn't come for free, throwing this stuff in everybody's face. You wanna change the profession, have procedures named after you, it's gonna cost. We'll talk about it on Monday. The man hung up without another word.

Chris went to his car and sat for a few minutes, thought of calling Krystal, pulled out his phone, but grunted, "Fuck 'er," and instead called Khai. "Hey, Kiddo, how you doin'?"

Her gut clenched, and all she could hiccup was, "Hey."

"Just got done at the hospital. Awful day. Sitting in my car freezing. Bet you are too, in your place. How about dinner—Metro Grill? Been there?"

"Nope. Not in my budget."

"Well, it's in mine. How about it?"

The awful taste in her mouth from that morning lingered, but it was not as bitter as the loneliness. "Okay. Sounds great. Should I meet you at the restaurant?"

"Nah, let me pick you up. Dumb to take two cars."

She hesitated but inhaled slowly. "Okay. Half an hour?"

"Perfect."

Chris drank five glasses of wine. Khai stopped after one. Two hours later, Chris put his credit card in the leather folder and stood to go to the men's room. He wobbled about for a moment before walking off. When he came back, he stood behind Khai and put his hands on her shoulders. "Ready, Kiddo?"

She sat stiffly for a second. "You know, Chris, I don't think you should drive, nor should I. Let's take a cab, or two. My treat."

"Pretty lady, that's not a bad idea, but what if you drive? Take me home, and you sleep in the bed, in a locked room, and I suffer alone on the couch. Just like I promised last time. I'll drive you home in the morning. Have to go on rounds anyway at the U. It's perfect." She shook her head, but with a smile.

Gauthé mumbled. "I understand but sit in my car for a minute and talk some more. I just love to hear your voice."

He started the engine, turned on the heat, and adjusted the radio to a classical station. Nana Mouskouri was singing "Amazing Grace." They sat breathless for a few seconds until he reached over and touched her hand. She flinched, though he soon wrapped her hand with his. With his other hand, he stroked her face. She trembled but did not when pull away when he kissed her, nor when he gently stroked her breasts through her coat. She didn't stop him when he unbuttoned her coat and caressed her breasts with both hands. This went on for just a minute, until he brought his lips to her nipples. With that, she suddenly stiffened and pushed him away, though softly.

"Sorry, Chris. Give me a call when you're free. It never ends well. It can't."

She touched his face and left to call a taxi.

CHAPTER TWENTY-NINE

Social Security had denied Sabrina's request for disability benefits beyond a bare-bones, motorized wheelchair, a ramp into their home, and modifications to allow Sabrina to ride in the van Mike had bought thirdhand. They refused to grant her a monthly benefit for total disability. No explanation was offered, though Mike read on the internet it was almost a rule that the first time a person under fifty applied for Social Security benefits, they would be refused. The site recommended the family obtain all the hospital records before trying again but warned the copy fees could come to nearly a thousand dollars, and the wait for archives might be months when the patient's admission had lasted for so many weeks.

Mike left school for the hospital during his prep period the morning after he met with Scott Bialek. The clerk had him fill out several forms, took two pieces of ID, then found the account on the computer. She winced and turned her head in confusion as she mumbled, "I'm sorry, sir, but there seems to be a hold on these records. Would you mind waiting in the lobby while I get someone to check on this?"

"Okay, but I need to get back to school. I'm a teacher."

Fifteen minutes later, an older woman in a barrel dress marched up to him. She queried brusquely, "Mr. Maddingly?"

"I am."

"I'm Odette Camerata, Administrator of Records for the corporation. You see, we will be happy to release the documents to you. They do, however, have to be appraised before we can hand them over."

Mike bristled. "Why is that?"

The woman took a step backward and held out a palm. "I'm sure you can understand that the case was very complicated, and we have the legal right to determine if there are records that should be withheld."

"What are you talking about? I want every word written about my wife. Those are my records. I know my rights."

She took both palms and pushed them down in front of her, repeatedly as if calming a man with a gun. "I assure you, sir, we will go through the process with perfect attention to the legalities. I can also tell you that if it takes longer than thirty days, we will give you a written explanation as to why there has been a delay. You can appeal the decision at that time."

"How do I appeal it right now? I need those records for my wife's Social Security claim. She's already been turned down once. They said they want every word. This is not right. And why would there be any of the file withheld?"

"I'm sorry, HIPPA and all that. We can't discuss that with you. In fact, I'm afraid I must terminate this conversation. Good day, sir." She pivoted and disappeared behind the cloth partitions.

That night, Mike called Scott Bialek for the number of the lawyer who had helped him. Two days later, he sat in the man's aged office just blocks from the county courthouse in McKinley.

Harrison Jennings had begun practicing law in that very clapboard, timeworn house forty-five years earlier. Mike walked up creaky stairs onto the front porch and knocked on the plain wooden door. When there was no answer, he opened it cautiously, immediately confronted by a tiny, shrill Schnauzer cowering behind an older woman sitting to the right of the door. She laughed, "Oh, don't mind Cyclops. His bite is much worse than his bark." She giggled and extended her hand. "I'm Shirley. You must be Mr. Maddingly—sent by Scott. What a good man. Lousy break. Can I get you coffee?"

Before she could stand, though, Harrison Jennings hitched through a narrow passage past Xerox boxes in progressive stages of yellowing. There were mounds of them, piled four and five deep. Each was marked by a broad-tipped magic marker with initials and the years that case had been active. Mike's jaw dropped when he saw one marked 1967-1972.

Jennings shook Mike's hand warmly and turned to the rear of the tiny house. As they weaved through narrowing tunnels of ancient records, the final path was barely thirty inches wide, walls lined by shelves of dusty, faded, legal tomes. Mike trailed the diminutive attorney, smiling to himself reassuringly as he studied the man's shiny bald patch.

In the small office, Jennings pulled a chair from the corner and had Mike sit just inches from the desk. He laughed, "Gotta keep you close. Nearly deaf." Mike looked at the man's ears and saw the hearing aids. "Yeah," Jennings laughed, "VA specials. Not worth a damn. On the other hand, I will give the VA credit. They're the best money can buy. Free, and free batteries for life. What a deal!

"I understand you feel you have a problem with our friends over at Mitchie-Sterling. That right?"

"Yeah, on several levels."

"Okay, start at the top of the list. Worst first."

Mike spoke of the night he took his wife to the ER. Jennings shook his head. He stopped Mike every few sentences to ask questions, writing furiously on his yellow legal pad, turning pages so hurriedly, Mike worried he would run out of paper before the whole story had been revealed. Nearly an hour later, his voice hoarse, Mike told Harrison Jennings about the warning that all the records might not be forthcoming from the hospital.

Jennings thought for a moment and took out another pad, titled it, "To Do—Maddingly," and started scribbling a numbered list. "Well, Mr. Maddingly, that is quite the story. I've been around since before the flood, thought I'd seen it all, but the administration over there is setting world records for poor behavior. On the other hand, let me warn you, poor manners, by themselves, are not actionable. On the face of it, they clearly damaged your wife—gravely. But a court of law takes nothing 'on the face of it.' And they shouldn't. You, apparently, clearly understand that the obstacle facing us is the problem your wife was, unfortunately, born with. They will pull every stop to get experts to convince a jury that sooner or later a major neural tube defect, or some other problem associated with it, will cause drastic problems. And they may be right. On the other hand, they would have to survive cross-examination and convince a jury that the two problems are one and the same. From what you've told me, it seems there is medical evidence to the contrary.

"Now, as I am sure Scott told you, this whole thing is a process, and a very strict one at that. The t's have to be crossed and the i's dotted. The first step is for me to shift through all of this and see if there really is a problem—legally, that is—then define it, and think hard if it is worth your time and money, and mine, to go to the next step and get an expert to review the records. You will have to pay up front for the records and the expert. Figure six to seven thousand by the time just the initial step is all over."

Mike sighed. "Yes, sir, Scott told me that was where his case foundered. Poor guy. Just doesn't seem fair."

Jennings snickered unsmilingly. "I'm afraid you need to understand one thing from the outset. If you want fair, go to Puyallup." He waited for Mike to laugh, but all he did was turn his head in confusion. "You really are new to the area, aren't you?" Mike smiled. "Puyallup is where the Washington State Fair is held in August. Pigs and cows and chickens, funnel cakes, on and on. County and state fairs are a big deal out here. Bottom line, though, you better understand that there is nothing fair or just about American justice. First day of law school, they smirked and told us, 'If you're here to learn justice, please step through the doors at the rear of the lecture hall. If you're here to learn the law, you may keep your seat.' Problem is, it's worse everywhere else."

Mike thought for a moment. "Yes, but it's a travesty, what's happened in that hospital."

"Yes and no. From your standpoint, it is horrible. From Scott's, pardon me for saying it, it's even worse. While I'm an entrepreneur, I tend to stay away from cases based simply on bad outcomes in the emergency room. There's always another side to the story. Their mission, I mean in the ER, isn't like any other specialty. First, and foremost, they are there only to save the life of any comer, no matter how hopeless. If a battered soul gets pushed through the door with a heartbeat, it is expected they will resuscitate him. It's unreasonable, but it's just the way it is. They can't be looking years down the pike thinking about a patient's quality of life when someone bleeding to death gets plunked down in front of them.

"Their work is largely algorithm-driven. I mean, you see this medical sign, you do that. Blood pressure is x, you do y. Doesn't matter why the blood pressure is crashing, you fill up the tank with something as close to blood as you can get your hands on that minute. It isn't their job to decide if you've been without blood flow to the brain nine seconds or nine minutes. You do what you must to get the blood pressure back up. It's pretty much like that for all the emergencies they face. How could it be any different? They don't have the luxury to sit and ask questions and do an hour exam to find the source of the low blood pressure. That comes later, when the internists and surgeons are summoned to stand around and cogitate."

Mike shook his head. "But, Mr. Jennings, in this case, they should have taken Sabrina into the back the moment we walked into the ER waiting room. They knew we were coming. That guy, Cardozo, was angry at another doctor, so he ignored us. That's not what you're talking about, sir, or I don't think it is."

"No, it isn't. But it is so hard to say just when the actual problem began..."

Mike interrupted. "Excuse me, Mr. Jennings, but it seems to me Sabrina's blood pressure was okay the first hour we were in the waiting room. She was talking, even laughed at all the hubbub. There was this old man peeing in the corner 'cause the bathroom door was locked—some guy inside shooting up. She said, 'They'll probably send him down to me for a psych eval.' I said, 'Probably send 'em both.' I didn't want to make trouble, so I kept my mouth shut until this young gal, who's been pacing back and forth, comes up to me and says she has bugs in her ears, and they're drivin' her nuts. Her nurse comes out and pulls her into the back. Meanwhile, Sabrina and I are still sitting there."

"Why didn't you say anything to anybody?"

"I did. I went to the desk and told them we had been sent by the doctor in Evanston. She goes in the back, and someone else comes out and tells us to take a seat. The place was a zoo. I couldn't keep bugging her. Then they really would get mad and keep us out there forever, which in the end they did anyway."

"This is different, Mr. Jennings. I'm no doctor, but I've found out that it is very hard to start an IV on someone whose blood pressure is extremely low. Five minutes earlier, that Cardozo would have been able to start the central line, and I wouldn't be sitting here pleading with you, and Sabrina's life wouldn't have been destroyed. All over some inadequate, obstinate, emasculated asshole." He heaved a deep sigh as his shoulders dropped.

Jennings cupped his palm over his mouth as he stared past Mike. For a minute, no one spoke. The old man finally drew a deep breath. "Okay, Mr. Maddingly. I will look at this in a different light. I certainly don't have enough information to dismiss the case out of hand. That's the problem with malpractice cases. Takes so long to get all the facts together. Worse, the other side is deceptive and smart. Hospitals have evolved into virtuosi at covering up really egregious behavior.

"Now, let me caution you. Even if we go ahead, a small percentage of malpractice cases ever win. Something like two-thirds are dismissed, dropped, or withdrawn. Of the third that make it to trial, eighty percent are won by the doctor. That's eighty percent.

"And please forget about those huge settlements and jury awards you hear about. They're rare. The median award, last time I looked, was around $500,000. Then, start subtracting my fees, the fees for experts, court fees, filing fees, and you really wonder if the years you, I mean you and Sabrina, put into it are worth it. That time and effort would be better spent by you teaching driver's ed after school.

"But, on the other hand, more people in the U.S. die from hospital mistakes than AIDS, breast cancer, or car accidents, and that doesn't include deaths from medical errors made in doctors' offices and clinics. So, there is a market for the services I provide. It's just that I have to be thoroughly convinced before I commit. Make sense?"

Mike nodded. "Sure does. No more beseeching from me. What do you suggest I do to help you?"

"First, cancel the request for your wife's records. They already told you they will withhold some of the documents. And they will, but not after I file a subpoena for an ongoing lawsuit."

"Yeah, and why can they do that? I thought we were entitled to the records."

"Well, it turns out you may not legally be entitled to all of your information, but it's only in a few special cases. If one of the doctors decides something in your file might endanger you or someone else, the doctor may not have to give this information to you. For instance, during an admission for a standard appendectomy, a woman is found, incidentally, to have a sexually transmitted disease. Suddenly, the hubby gets suspicious and demands the records. The woman warns her doctor that he's a violent man and will certainly harm her, like he has in the past. In that case, the hospital may decide only to provide the records associated with the surgery. That's the game they're playing. Problem is, in this case, you don't know what you don't know. You wouldn't have a clue which records were being withheld.

"They can't do that, however, if we enter litigation. But filing a lawsuit remains to be seen." He stopped and looked at the papers on his desk. "Let me do some thinking and get back to you. There's plenty of time."

"Yeah, but I need the records for Sabrina's Social Security. Another battle."

"You trying to do that on your own?"

"Yes."

"Won't work. That, I can help you with. We'll have to find the right doctor to examine her. One who knows the Social Security ropes. Just another game, I'm afraid. Let Shirley out there have you sign the records release forms, and I'll get what they'll give us from the hospital. It'll be enough for Social Security. She'll also have you write a check for a thousand dollars to cover the copying costs. Anything we don't spend, I'll return, but we may ask for more."

CHAPTER THIRTY

Six weeks after the end of the ECT treatments, Sabrina scheduled a meeting with the department head and her old friend Pete Hegge, Dean of the School of Medicine. Mike drove Sabrina to the University of Washington, where she motored down the ramp in the back of their van onto the ramp leading to the mezzanine. She wore a crisp white blouse, navy slacks, and the sapphire earrings and matching necklace Mike had bought at Tiffany's for their fifth anniversary. Three days before the meeting, Mike had gotten a stylist to come to the house and cut Sabrina's hair. Both Dean Hegge and the department head rose to their feet as Sabrina rolled through the door. The dean gushed, "My God, Sabrina, you really are better, aren't you? So, so happy to see it."

Marion Nixon, the department head, let her jaw drop theatrically. "You look mavelous, dahlink!" She bent forward and hugged Sabrina, asking, "If I remember correctly, Dear, you like jasmine tea. Is that right?" Sabrina smiled and nodded. The woman poured a cup from a tea caddy on the sideboard, and Sabrina reached for the cup, though awkwardly, and a swish of hot tea spilled into her lap. She almost cried out but bit her lip and stared straight ahead. The dean jumped to his feet and brought a napkin from the sideboard. Sabrina pushed the cup forward slowly for him to hold as she used her right hand to pat the spill. After the hesitant transfer of the cup back to Sabrina and the napkin to the dean, Sabrina filled the uneasy silence pretending to sip the tea. Finally, Marion folded her hands in her lap and spoke with a tentative smile. "Well, Dr. Maddingly, we have missed you. Your patients have missed you. So, let's look at

168

the opportunities we have for you to rejoin the department. First, I have to ask about the mechanics. How would you travel from Evanston all the way down here? Would Mike have to drive you?"

Sabrina smiled. "Marion, I know this is a big deal. Last thing you need is to be babysitting an employee. Your plate is as full as it can get; yours, too, Peter. I'm sorry to add to that load. But here's our plan. As I mentioned to you, Marion, my dream is to return two days a week at first. Work six hours and increase to a third day in a couple of months; sooner, hopefully."

"Mike will drive for the trial period, but we are looking at Community Transit after that. They have wheelchair lifts, and they stop right outside the building here. There are enough ramps around to service an army of us. Seeing patients should not be a problem, and dictating notes is a simple matter. Mike is going to fit my chair with a dock for the recorder and switches on the steering bar to turn it on and off. The recorder is compatible with Dragon, which Dragon says is compatible with our electronic medical records—curse them, the EMRs, that is."

Marion and Peter spoke together, "Amen."

Sabrina smiled, genuinely this time, and Carla's shoulders relaxed a bit. Carla went on. "The only problem I can see is the transferring to use the bathroom. We have so-called wheelchair compatible bathrooms here, but I have been told they are not easy to use with only one arm."

"Well, I'm getting better and better at getting in and out of the chair. There is, though, a device, actually a pole that has a stirrup that moves up and down by a pneumatic something or another. You grip the handle for dear life, up you go out of the chair, onto the potty, then up you go again back into the chair. We have one at home. Mike and I will be glad to pay to have one installed here. It's very usable."

Marion interrupted. "We will pay for it. Not a problem." She hesitated for a moment. "Well, it seems you've done your homework. I do have to ask, and please don't take offense, but have you had occasion to sit in one place and concentrate for six hours? As we both know, post-stroke patients get tired easily."

"I am practicing every day, studying the basics again, and also reading journals and doing my Psychology Continuing Education credits. Quarter and half hours every morning, and then again in the evenings on the internet. I can do it."

"I'm sure you can." She drew in a deep breath. "Well, when do you want to start?"

Sabrina's eyes reddened. "How about first of the month? That'll give me more time at the books until six hours'll look like a kindergarten project. Also have my PCE requirement done for the next ten years!"

For six weeks, Mike and Sabrina left home at 5 A.M. to make the drive to the University. It took better than an hour, and after watching Sabrina motor into the hospital, he turned around and fought the traffic to school. The principal let Mike reduce his schedule to point-eight, and the vice-principal made changes allowing Mike to take his prep period from 7:30 to 8:30. It was, nevertheless, barely enough time to get back for his first class.

The medical school co-opted a resident on-call cubical for Sabrina if she needed to rest between patients. The modification with the lifting pole in the restroom worked perfectly, but there wasn't one in the residents' on-call section a building away. The department assigned a psychology intern to help Sabrina transfer to the toilet over there.

At 3 P.M., after six hours of seeing patients, she wheeled her way to the eighth floor on-call room to wait for Mike's call that he was twenty minutes out. They got home at seven, both so exhausted, they usually had just a slice of toast and were in bed by nine.

At the end of the six weeks, they began to take the bus. Mike rode with Sabrina to and from the U. twice a week. The wheelchair lift on the Community Transit coach took days to master. More than a couple of her fellow travelers puckered impatiently with the litany of Sabrina's false starts. Her eyes reddened, and Mike scowled as she wheeled into place and fumbled about, grasping for the levers to lock herself in place.

Three weeks later, though, she told Mike during the cocktail hour that she was ready to make the trip on her own. He drove her to the bus stop at the end of their block and waited until she was settled, waved goodbye, and steered away toward school. A block later, he did a U-turn and followed her to the University. Mike watched from a distance as she worked her way into the medical office building, then he ran across the skybridge, beating Sabrina to her office. She sobbed when he stretched his arms forward with a dozen roses.

Sabrina added a third day to her schedule, and for a month, she came home floating, euphoric. During the cocktail hour, she regaled Mike with stories of patients suffering from psychiatric syndromes that curled even her toes. Mike chuckled at how much easier he had it with the panoply of teen angst and inscrutable life decisions he faced from the first period to the end of school. Some nights, Sabrina laughed aloud.

Even the bus ride become a social event. Several of the commuters jumped to their feet as they approached Sabrina's stop to ease her aboard then dropped to their knees to lock the wheelchair into its station. She brought cookies but did not tell her new friends Mike had made them.

CHAPTER THIRTY-ONE

On a Thursday morning in late autumn, nearly a year after her Thanksgiving hospitalization, the wind and rain once again besieged the streets of Western Washington. Sabrina, though, ignored the weather and pushed on, her slacks sodden by the time she made it up the ramp into the hospital. As usual, her gloves were soaked as well, her hands trembling so, she was barely able to wrap her fingers around the brake lever. The ice had not been fully cleared, and by the time she closed her hand on the brake, the chair skidded into the glass doors. The thud was so loud, a patient ran outside and insisted on wheeling her up to Psychology. In the elevator, one of Sabrina's colleagues stood mortified and demanded she call him right before the bus arrived. He would come out with an umbrella and escort her into the hospital. She agreed but made him promise not to tell Marion.

It was hours and hours before she stopped shivering that day, and her clothes were still damp when her friend took her out to the bus under an umbrella. Mike was at the stop in Evanston. As he lifted her out of the chair into the car, he grumbled, "Jees, Sabrina, your hands are freezing."

At 1 A.M., she awoke with a sore throat. Mike brought her two Tylenols. By morning, it was so painful to swallow, she skipped her cup of tea. Her temperature was one hundred. With two more Tylenols, though, she felt well enough to motor to the bus with Mike holding an umbrella. She coughed a couple of times at the stop, and Mike asked her to come home and call in sick. She shook her head.

By noon, the cough had worsened to the point her third patient, a medical doctor, stopped the session and recommended she be seen at the ER. "It's just an elevator ride down and thirty feet through the tunnel to the hospital." She refused. When her colleague came at the end of the afternoon, she began shivering before they reached the bus stop. He, too, recommended she be seen at the ER, but she took his hand, thanked him, and rolled onto the bus lift.

At 9 P.M., her temperature spiked to 103.6, and her shuddering was causing the floor of the living room to vibrate. A pain deep in her chest worsened when she coughed. Though Sabrina asked him not to, Mike called Khai Weathersby. She was just leaving the clinic but insisted he bring her over.

The instant Khai laid eyes on Sabrina, she was struck with the pallor of the woman's face and quickly placed a clip on the tip of Sabrina's index finger. Khai mumbled to herself, "Ninety-one—borderline."

Mike's face tightened. "What does that mean? Is that her temperature?"

Khai held up an index finger. "Hang on a sec." She lifted the back of Sabrina's damp sweatshirt and listened with her stethoscope. Mike watched her eyes, searching for a glint of emotion, but Khai hid it well. He began to fidget as Khai closed her eyes, listening more and more intently to Sabrina's breathing.

Finally, she looked up. "Definitely some fluid on the right side." She pointed to the clasp on Sabrina's index finger. "You remember this little clip?"

Mike shook his head. "Not really."

"It measures how much oxygen is in the bloodstream. Actually, it tells you how full the red blood cells are with oxygen. We call it percent oxygen saturation. Should be around ninety-seven or ninety-eight percent if you're breathing regular old room air. But if there's an infection in the breathing sacs, that draws in water from the bloodstream and blocks some of the air that's supposed to diffuse into the blood. If that happens, the hemoglobin in the red cells passing around the outside of the breathing sacs picks up less oxygen than it should. All the sacs don't fill with fluid, but even a little causes a major blockage, and that tells us pretty much how compromised the lungs are, I mean how widespread the pneumonia is. Sabrina, your saturation is ninety-one percent. Sounds okay, like an A minus, but it's really a D plus—barely acceptable. So, I wasn't terribly surprised to hear a lot of congestion growling around in your lungs. Let's put you on oxygen. You remember those nasal prongs from the hospital? That should be enough to get the numbers back up near normal. And we'll also get an x-ray."

Khai had taught herself basic radiology, and she muddled through a chest film. As she expected, Sabrina's right middle lobe was opaque, a sign water had been drawn into that lung from the bloodstream, the body's attempt to dilute the infection. Now she had audio proof, the crackles she heard with her stethoscope, and visual proof, the chest x-ray, to make a solid diagnosis.

Khai shook her head. "Right middle lobe pneumonia. No surprise. That's the same area as last year's pneumonia. It seems one weak area in the body takes the brunt each time there's a stress. People sprain the same ankle, break the same bone and, here we are, suffer infections in the same places, over and over again. This is not unusual at all."

Sabrina had begun to shake again, early rigors, tremors so violent, people in the next rooms often felt the quaking. It was the final sure sign of a serious lower pulmonary infection. She took Sabrina's temperature again. It had, that quickly, risen to 104.7. Khai started an IV to rehydrate her and replace the fluid that was being drawn into the lungs, lost as sweat, and the extra she was breathing out with her serious fever. After a few minutes, with the help of the nasal prongs set at five liters per minute, her percent saturation rose to ninety-four.

"Mike, Sabrina needs to be admitted to the hospital tonight."

She watched his eyes closely but relaxed when he sighed, "Of course. It's just that, Dr. Weathersby, the thought of walking back into that ER, into that hospital, terrifies me. Is there anywhere else Sabrina can go?"

Khai thought for a moment. "At least, let's see who's working tonight." She dialed the emergency room and put her hand over the mouthpiece. Her eyes rolled, and she laughed mockingly, "Guess who?" She thanked the clerk and hung up. "I'm going to have Sabrina transferred to the U. That's going to make your life just that much more impossible, but I have a feeling Mitchie-Sterling might want to transfer her down there anyway, given her history.

In the ambulance to Seattle, Sabrina's breathing became more labored, her cough weaker, and her oxygen saturation dropped to eighty-nine despite the nasal oxygen. In the ER, she was started on intravenous antibiotics, and a proper x-ray was taken. It showed early infiltration of fluid into the right upper lung as well. There was no question that Sabrina was experiencing a multi-lobular pneumonia, and she was admitted to the intensive care unit. Sabrina's oxygen saturation level rose to ninety-four after she was settled, but she became increasingly weak as soaking sweats replaced the shivering. Mike slept next to her in an easy chair.

The next morning, she was feeling a bit better, fever down to 102.2, and the coughing controlled with medication that also dulled the burning pain in her chest. She ordered Mike to the cafeteria to eat something. As he stepped into the elevator, there were but two figures aboard, at opposite corners, both in scrubs. Mike sensed they stared away from each other determinedly. His eyes did not lift to the man's face, his attention drawn to the rigidly-still, stunning blond. He forced his gape away and began to turn toward the door, though stopped when the man asked questioningly, "Mike?"

He looked back. Weakly, he sputtered, "Oh, hello, Dr. Gauthé."

Gauthé's face tensed as he looked at Mike's disheveled hair and slumped figure. He spurted bluntly, "What's going on with Sabrina?"

Mike's voice faltered. "Looks like she's got the pneumonia back...Ambulance brought her here last night."

Gauthé's shoulders sagged ever so slightly, but he quickly caught himself. "Well, I'll certainly stop by. What room is she in? Oh, and I'm sorry. This is Krystal Kaywood, my wonderful scrub nurse." Gauthé turned to her. "This is Mike Maddingly. Good man. His wife's had a rough course. Wait, you remember, Kris." He took a step to his side and touched her bare forearm. When she stiffened, he forced a weak smile and went on. "Sabrina was the patient we came down to see in the ER last year. Started a central line."

Krystal grimaced. "Of course. I'm so sorry. She's still dealing with all that?" Her hand reached out, almost in reflex, and squeezed Mike's arm. "Yes, I'll definitely stop by and look in on your wife."

The three exited the elevator together and walked toward the cafeteria, but Gauthé took Krystal's elbow and guided her rigidly toward the ER at the end of the opposite hall. He whispered, "I want to talk to you—alone."

Krystal pulled her elbow away and faced him, the top of her head barely at the level of his jaw. "Look Chris, I told you what was going to be from now on. I screwed up, but I'm going to try and save my marriage and my life. And I've decided to look elsewhere for work."

He glared down at her and was about to speak when she hissed, "A little problem when things don't go your way, huh?" She heeled about and walked to the other end of the hall, disappearing into the Human Resources office.

For nearly thirty minutes, Gauthé waited inside the cafeteria, hiding by the doors, until he saw Krystal walk out of HR, a ream of paper clutched in her fist. He followed far behind as she took the elevator to Three East, Sabrina's floor, then he ran up the stairs and walked into Sabrina's room a foot behind Krystal. The bed was empty and, seeing no one in the room, he grasped her elbow again, this time more roughly.

She pulled away, took a step further into the room, and spun toward him. "Listen, Chris, I'm not going to tell you again..." But she stopped abruptly as Mike, half asleep, dragged himself to his feet.

"Ah, Sabrina's not here. They took her for an x-ray." At that moment, there was stirring in the anti-room, and they turned, expecting to see Sabrina being wheeled in, but it was Khai putting on a mask.

She took a step into the room, her eyes locking Gauthé's for a trice longer than they should have. It was not lost on Krystal, who tried to smile, but Khai saw her pupils narrow. Chris introduced them, and Khai stiffly extended her hand, though she had a hard time pulling her eyes away from the nurse's blond hair, especially the roots, which were nearly as fair.

Chris explained that Khai was Sabrina's primary care provider. Krystal feigned interest then turned and spoke over her shoulder. "I better get back to work. Dr. Gauthé, don't forget, you need to do the op note on the last patient."

He laughed distantly, "Yeah, yeah, never ends. Good to see you, Mike." He nodded to Khai. "Dr. Weathersby," and when he was sure Krystal was gone and Mike wasn't looking, he put his hand up to his ear and mouthed, "I'll call you." He was gone before Khai had interpreted the message.

Mike shook his head. "Looks like those two are playing doctor inside and outside the hospital, but it's none of my business, is it? Hey, that's so nice of you to come by. Sabrina should be back in a minute." And in seconds, an orderly wheeled her into the room. Khai stayed for a few moments, quite relieved to see Sabrina breathing on her own.

Halfway along the highway toward home, Khai took a call from Gauthé. Though she said she was busy, on her way to return a sweater at Nordstrom's, he talked her into meeting him outside the store in an hour.

At Nordy's, she asked where returns were made. A clerk pointed toward the escalator. Three-quarters across the floor, Khai heard a bang, then screams, and she braced as people ran past her in the opposite direction. Instantly, she stopped and accessed the flow of traffic, her attention moving along the spokes of dispersion backwards, toward the focal point—the escalator. She moved cautiously at first, eyes eventually fixing halfway up on a thrashing figure, arms grasping desperately for the handrail. Khai ran forward, hit the emergency stop button, then bounded up the stairs to an elderly woman, face bloodied, her left wrist already swollen and deformed. Khai spoke softly to the woman, "It's okay, ma'am. I'm a doctor. Nothing scary. You're going to be fine. I promise."

As the woman began to sob, a hand reached from the stair above her to wipe the tears away and stroke her cheek. Khai looked up into the stunning green eyes of a very dark-haired woman. For an instant, Khai thought it was Cher, but when the woman smiled at her, she sensed softness.

The woman asked Khai, "Are you a doc?"

Khai smiled, "Yeah. And you are, too, aren't you?"

"Yep. Good, let's see what we can do."

Khai turned to the crowd, pointed at a well-dressed man, and spoke calmly. "Sir, would you be so kind as to call 911? Tell them," she enunciated carefully, "there's an elderly woman with a fractured arm and multiple lacerations on the escalator between the first and second floors at Nordstrom's downtown."

At the same time, the other doctor began asking: "Ma'am, what's your name? Do you know where you are? Do you have a list of your medications in your purse?"

As they waited for the medics, Khai placed the sweater she was returning under the woman's head as the other doctor draped her own coat over her. Their new patient looked up and smiled. "Two such pretty doctors. Aren't I lucky?".

Khai winked. "Everything's under control; you're gonna be dancin' in no time."

The woman started to cry, and they could barely hear her falter, "I wish I still had my Donald to dance with."

The other doctor looked at Khai, whose eyes reddened. "You okay?"

"I guess." She paused and forced a smile. "No matter, I'm Khai Weathersby."

"Sonya Laureano. Good work. I'm impressed. You're cool. Military?"

"Wow. You're pretty perceptive, and apparently not burned out. A caring doctor. Breath of fresh air."

"That's high praise from a colleague."

After the medics transported the old woman on a backboard, Sonya turned to Khai. "Hey, time for a cup of coffee?" Khai glanced at her watch, and Sonya added, "No problem, maybe some other time."

"No, no. Don't have to be anywhere for a while."

They walked slowly to the Nordstrom restaurant. It was quiet. Sonya asked, "I don't know you. Been around thirty years, but there are so many new faces. Can't keep up. Do you practice here in Seattle?"

"No, I'm up in Evanston."

"That's my neck of the woods—McKinley—Mitchie-Sterling Hospital." Sonya's jaw dropped. "Hey, aren't you the doc at the walk-in clinic? Yes!" She hesitated for an instant. "Dr. Weathersby, right?"

"You really are on top of things. Wow. Yep, that's me." Khai paused. "Are you shocked I don't have horns?"

Sonya Laureano laughed. "Not at all. I heard you're involved with the patient who had those multiple strokes."

Khai's head pulled back in uncertainty. "Multiple? I just saw her a few minutes ago. Pneumonia, but no new strokes. Wow. Is that what's going around at the hospital?"

"Yeah. That's what the board of directors is being told, that she had a number of congenital defects, and these strokes were just the latest of the complications. I've read through her entire chart—took days. Latest is that you overtreated that security guard, the one on duty that first night?"

"Sonya, if I may, that's not the case at all." But she stopped abruptly, worrying that she was about to talk about a patient without permission, and also that she was openly consorting with the enemy. "I'm sorry, Sonya, I probably need to think about patient confidentiality."

"Yes, yes, you do, but in this case, we have all the notes on the guard. He's State Industrial, so his records are available to his employer, i.e., the Board of Directors, for perusal. And guess who's on the board?"

Khai paused but quickly looked up at Sonya. "Imagine you want to hear the truth."

Sonya patted Khai's arm. "Only if you are comfortable telling me." She, though, suddenly hesitated. "Nope, you know what, I'll read the chart, and this time, I'll demand your notes. They weren't included in the morass handed over to the Board. Clearly, this thing needs fixing. I'm going to drill down to the truth." She hesitated again. "Khai Weathersby, it was, is, a pleasure to meet the real you. This was a special morning. So happy to see who you are, that you can obviously handle the crap my colleagues puke out around the clock. Good for you."

"Thank you, Sonya. That's quite flattering given the circumstances. A gift to meet you." She stood. "And now, I'll take my blood-covered sweater and deposit it in the hazardous waste bin at work."

"You're new here, Khai. This is Nordy's. They'll take it back even if you bought it at, say, Macy's. They're amazing business people."

"I've heard that. But this one's too much. Not going to have them handling blood."

"How is it I'm not surprised? Hope we can get together again."

Khai walked back toward the parking lot and stood numbly outside the main doors. When Chris pulled up, he reached across and pushed the passenger door open. Just as Khai slid in, Sonya Laureano drove out of the parking garage. She could not have missed Khai disappearing into the Carrera, nor could she have failed to recognize it as Chris Gauthé's, or the red and white Mitchie-Sterling Hospital doctor's parking sticker.

CHAPTER THIRTY-TWO

By the beginning of the next week, Sabrina was breathing comfortably without extra oxygen. Her percent saturation on room air was ninety-five, and her fever had abated. As Mike wheeled her toward the hospital exit, they passed Chris Gauthé, though his stare was so remote, he did not recognize them. Seconds later, Krystal Kaywood walked by. Mike's eyes met hers, but they, too, looked straight through him.

In the car, Mike mentioned it to Sabrina. She thought for a moment. "You mean the guy we just passed in the hospital? I saw him, too. Didn't recognize him, but now that you say so, I guess it was him. I even commented to myself that that's the cost of years in the hospital—sucks the life out of you. Makes me scared sometimes. I don't want to end up that way."

Sabrina began home physical therapy once again. She pushed and pushed, but by the time Mike eased her into bed, her body hurt more than the night before. She lay awake hour after hour, restlessly shifting those limbs that still worked. With the lack of sleep, her mood darkened, and she stopped reading her psychology journals, instead, staring for most of the day at the same AOL screen. The cocktail hour once again degenerated into a contest with herself to see how fast she could muddle her brain with deeper and deeper swigs of wine. A few weeks later, she stopped eating for several hours before the cocktail hour, the alcohol to be drawn into her that much faster. Mike convinced her to start seeing the psychiatrist again.

Two mornings later, Dr. Darling thought for a moment and suggested

Sabrina be admitted straightaway to Mitchie-Sterling's psych unit. Mike tensed. "Dr. Darling, excuse me. Ah, we weren't supposed to say anything, but our attorneys filed a lawsuit against Cardozo and the hospital. Do you think it's wise to continue using the hospital, even across the street?"

She thought longer this time. "Well, you've got a point. I'd like to say, 'don't be silly', but I imagine everyone'll know, and some'll try too hard to stay in your good graces. Then there's the jerks. They'll act super rude to prove they're not afraid of you or your lawyer, and they'll do little things, mean things, behind your back, to get even. Meal comes an hour late, wake you up an extra time to get vitals. That's the hospital for ya—not very godly, I'm afraid.

"What we'll do is admit you to Warm Hills General. Small, but a good staff. We should plan on seven or eight days; give you any notes you need for the teacher, both of you.

CHAPTER THIRTY-THREE

K rystal Kaywood gave Mitchie-Sterling four weeks' notice. She had been offered a full-time administrative position at the U, two buildings away from the operating theatre Gauthé used for his gall bladder surgeries.

In McKinley, Gauthé interviewed half a dozen senior scrub nurses to replace Krystal but had made no decision with only three days left on her contract. During the first surgery of that morning, Gauthé bristled into the operating room late and gowned impatiently. He ignored the circulating nurse, who hummed, "Aw come on, Dr. G, it's good to be alive. Let's see those sparkling eyes,"

He spun on his heels and snapped at Krystal, "And I don't want any of your sunshine bullshit today. That clear?"

Her eyes clouded, and she turned to the door but halted, straightened, and snapped back, "Yes, sir," then began setting an array of instruments on her tray.

After that surgery, Krystal knocked on the nursing supervisor's door. "Abby, I will not work with him for one more procedure. I know I've still got three days to go, but enough is enough. I quit as of this minute. I'm going home. You can sue me." She turned and left the office without shutting the door.

Abby followed her out but couldn't keep up. Instead, she marched, unannounced, into CEO Harp's office. "Norman, I need to talk to you about the Dr. Gauthé thing. Krystal Kaywood just walked out. Refused to work with him one more minute. Not like her at all. Wouldn't say why, but it's obviously some sort of sexual harassment on his part."

"Abby, I've known you for, what, eight or nine years now? Every conversation we've ever had has been about sexual harassment of one my surgeons on one of your girls. I respect you and all that, but a joke or two in the heat of battle over a dying patient, or a little pinch on the butt as a thank you for a good job handing over instruments; well, I thought we were going to foster a live and let live ambience in the OR."

"That's fine, and I don't give a damn about the run-of-the-mill stuff. Half the time, it's the nurse baiting the surgeon with her own touchy little hands, usually just to get me going, stir the pot. It's a boring little department, you know, dealing with one near-cadaver after the next. You don't even know if the carcass on the table's male or female, just that it bleeds red through the little hole the surgeon spends two hours sticking his fingers in. Have to generate some excitement over there, especially now that the board has, in its infinite wisdom, decreed we can't play rock and roll in the OR.

"But this is different. Here we are with patients on Gauthé's schedule for the rest of the day and tomorrow and the next day, and no scrub nurse good enough to use a laser that is well known to cause irreparable harm in the wrong hands, in any hands for that matter. I don't trust that thing at all."

"I'm familiar with your Luddite sympathies, Abby, but the laser is here to stay."

"Lud-what? All I know is a tiny slip of a laser cost that hospital in California three million. And the one in Utah, what was it, two point five? Remember?"

He smirked. "You certainly know how to get right to a man's heart, but you also know the rules—come to me with a problem, better have the solution in your back pocket."

"Yeah, Norman, I have a suggestion. Tell Gauthé to choose a nurse today and work with her after hours; teach her to keep her paws off the laser and to step back from the table when he picks the damn thing up. And, best of all, you teach him to keep his paws off her. It's the best we can do, given the mess he's got us in."

Harp called Chris to the office. "Dr. Gauthé, thanks for coming up. I know you're in the middle of your surgery day." He waited for a nicety, but when Gauthé just stared, Harp's shoulders tightened, and he spoke flatly. "I understand it is hard to accept that you're going to have to train a new girl, but it happens to every one of us. Looks like we've run out of time. Is there anything I can do to help?"

"Norman, it isn't a problem at all. I'm just not taking one of the department's rejects. I mean, that's who they are—somebody else's dirty laundry."

"No one's asking you to accept garbage, Chris. Each of the girls you interviewed has three times the experience of Nurse Kaywood. And she's been giving night classes on how to use the laser, so they're ready to go, any one of them. I know they may not be so pretty, little saggy here and there, but once they're stuffed into a bra, and then a scrub suit, and add an OR gown, they're all pretty much the same." He laughed, waiting for Chris to chuckle, but when Gauthé looked away, he grumbled, "We need to make a choice right away. We helped underwrite your project, and I'll be damned if we're going to drop it. Make us look like fools, like we discovered some big hole in the procedure and bolted when our shill spotted a cop. That's not who we are."

Gauthé hissed, "Oh, and who we are is an ethical organization who fights to the death to dodge paying a penny when our doctors fuck up patients for the rest of their lives. That who?"

"You know, Dr. Gauthé, it really isn't necessary to use that language in my presence. I don't appreciate it, and I don't think the board of directors will either."

"Well, you can tell them at your emergency meeting du jour that they can go fuck themselves, and the horses they rode in on. You, too." He was out the door before Harp's jaw reached the bottom of its plunge.

Harp phoned the medical director. "Harvey, hey, I just had a less than cordial conversation with our Dr. Gauthé. Refuses to make a decision on the nursing thing. Got quite aggressive. Lot of profanity and threats. Can I ask you to reach out to him and see what's brewing? I'm not totally convinced he's fit for duty, but, of course, I'll leave that to you. My sense is that he's a legal liability at the moment."

Fifteen minutes later, Christopher Gauthé pushed red-eyed into OR-6. A nurse, already scrubbed and gowned, greeted him at the door. "Hey Dr. Gauthé. Guess who you're stuck with?" There was giggle from a new circulating nurse but no other sound in the room, other than Gauthé asking the anesthesiologist if the patient was sound asleep. With her nod, he snatched a scalpel off the scrub nurse's tray and opened the patient's belly with just a few swipes. He worked quietly, grumbling occasionally for an instrument, mostly just reaching over the scrub nurse and picking tools sullenly from the tray. After the final staple, he turned tersely and barged out of the room.

The same scenario played out through the week, a pall tainting the entire surgical suite. It worsened each day until late the next Monday afternoon, when he knocked a tray of surgical instruments to the floor because a scrub nurse handed him the wrong sutures. Five minutes after the end of the case, the trembling OR team was standing over the nursing supervisor's desk. She called Harp, who called Klat, who called Gauthé, whose phone went straight to voice mail.

CHAPTER THIRTY-FOUR

The Director of the County Medical Society had also received a call from Harp. He, too, tried to phone the errant surgeon. This time, Gauthé had actually gone beyond cell range and sat huddled against the cold in his Carrera, staring at Mt. Rainer. The harder he tried to discover his future in the lenticular clouds swirling above the snowcap, the darker and more violent the shadows churned. The eyes of his children and his wife were veiled by the images of so many women, he saw nothing more than a morass of meaningless faces.

He cursed himself for not having planned routes of escape, though he realized, at that moment, none of what he had dropped onto himself was the product of a strategy; it had all been spontaneous, one tryst after another, the bareness of his life erasing any notion of consequences. He thought back to his residency, where he had also been out of control, but in a different arena, one surgical case after another—all day, all night, every weekend, year after wretched year—packing as many victims under his belt as he could steal from his fellow trainees, and even his professors. This was the stuff of a surgery residency, cutthroat, never an admission that you were in over your head, that you were not sure what you were doing with the hapless patient on the stainless-steel slab in front of you. Never admit the slightest weakness, never a single question about who was right—you always were. The internists and family doctors and the dermatologists, the fragile, not one had undergone in three years of residency the trial by fire you'd endured every couple of weeks, and for five or seven years.

But there was a pot of gold at the end—a successful practice, a pot of gold to be raided for a boat, a mansion with pillars, a new Carrera every three years—just for the new safety features, mind you—and a private apartment twenty miles from your wife. Chris Gauthé was where he had fought like a dog to land. He was on top, looking up from the bottom.

He drew his eyes back into the car and pulled from a slit in the padded visor a tiny plastic bag of white powder. He stared at it for a minute, and then more intently, his mind focused only on the coming detachment. He did not hear the car pull up behind him, nor did he see the state trooper approaching. The man knocked on the fogged window, and Gauthé startled so, he dropped the bag of cocaine onto the floor.

"Just checking. Cold out here. You okay?"

Gauthé flushed so deeply, the cop's face tightened. "Oh, yes, officer. I'm fine. Just enjoying the view."

"Sir, do you have your driver's license with you."

"Of course, but am I doing something illegal?"

"Not at all, but to be honest, you just seem pretty darn nervous."

"No, sir. Just in the middle of a bad divorce. Was thinking about my kids when you knocked on the window."

"That's fine. Just let me take a look at it real quick." Gauthé's legs slowly came together, hiding the floor as he reached into the back pocket of his jeans. He handed over the license, and the trooper smiled. "Hang in there, I'll be right back."

He was on his computer for a while and came back with a scowl. "Looks like you got an unpaid citation."

"I do?"

"Yes, sir. Eight months ago. Single occupancy driving in the diamond lane on I-740. Speed, also."

Gauthé's voice was tremulous. "Excuse me, sir, but that is not correct. I explained to the officer that I was a trauma surgeon on my way to do an emergency procedure. He gave me a written warning."

"Did you read the citation?"

"I don't remember, officer, probably not, because it was a warning."

"Okay, this is what's going to happen. You've been polite to me. I believe that you misunderstood the other trooper. You have no other traffic violations over the past three years. And, if I ever need you in the middle of the night, I don't want you saying, 'I know this prick.' So, I'm going to write you a sort of warning. A real one this time. Doctor, just pay your ticket and be done with it. It's no big deal. Fair enough?"

Gauthé looked up to thank the man, though he had about-faced and was gone just that fast. As the patrol car pulled away, Gauthé tossed the warning into the back of the Carrera and drove deeper into the mountains. He pulled off a gravel road into a cleft in the forest, pushed his seat all the way back, picked the cocaine from the floor, and slowly opened the tiny plastic bag, forcing himself to wait just a bit longer. Once again, he did not hear the crunch of gravel approaching his window. When the figure cast a shadow, Gauthé's chest felt as though it would burst, his fear dulling his consciousness. Without thinking, he started the engine, ready to burst away, but he slowly rolled down the window, sighing almost in relief that it was finally over. As he turned submissively to the figure, he realized it was not a cop but an old man whose face barely showed through a tangled, grey beard. Gauthé's shoulders dropped, happy, and then maybe not so happy, with his reprieve.

"Hey, man, handsome car. Don't see many of those out here in the mountains." The man spied the bag of cocaine, nodded toward it, and laughed sadly, "But you see a lot of that out here."

Gauthé grit his teeth and hissed at the man, "What can I do for you, pal?"

"Nothing, nothing, my friend. Just admiring the car. Didn't mean to upset you. I don't very often get to speak to people who can afford a Carrera. You look like a doctor."

Gauthé flushed a deeper red. He dropped the bag into his center console. "Nah, just a businessman."

"Business of medicine, huh?" He eyed the Mitchie-Sterling Hospital and University of Washington Hospital parking decals in the windshield.

Gauthé face tightened in anger as he reached for his seatbelt. "Have a nice day."

The man shook his head and smiled. "No need for all that. Just looked like you had a lot on your mind. I didn't come over here to hurt you. Recognized the stickers. So happens, I was a doctor, too, once—upper-crust Bellevue. You can look me up on the internet when you get back in range. Like I said, miss talking with colleagues, but not enough," he laughed sarcastically, "to ever go back. Too late anyway. Too much has changed."

Gauthé relaxed a bit. "You live out here?"

"Yes, I do. Up the road, in a cabin at the base of the mountain." He stared into Gauthé's eyes. "Bet you'd like to see the place." When Gauthé's face relaxed, the man smiled, "And I'd like to show ya. My rigs not that far."

"Yeah, I'd like to see it. But I think I'll just follow you?"

"You may not get very far."

"Well, I can't just leave the car out here."

"Okay. I drive ahead. Flash your lights when you've had enough."

The man's rusting Bronco crept out of a thicket of trees, moving slowly over the worsening gravel road until it became more freezing mud than rock. They turned up a path that was barely a couple of worn tracks in the brambles and deadfall. The farther they went, the bottom of the Carrera scraped on branches and small rocks, but the man had slowed his 4X4 to a crawl, and Gauthé was able to negotiate the rest of the road.

Half a mile up the path, they came to a cabin resting in a narrow cut of forest. The cedar roof was nearly obscured in pads of moss and fern, the fronds so long, they reached into the hanging branches that sheltered the cottage from the sky, and the world. The rapids of a nearby river muted the hums and jangles of the woodland.

The man stood by the door of his pickup until Gauthé made his way through the mud to his side. The two looked at each other for a moment, and the stranger stuck out his hand. "Anton Milton."

Gauthé took it but paused before nodding, "Chris Gauthé, and thank you for your openness. This is really quite unusual...breathtaking."

"Yes, it is." Anton held the unlocked door open for Gauthé. The St. Vincent DePaul relics were dust free, the glass of the gas lanterns and the pellet stove, without soot. "Please have a seat." He gestured to a castaway recliner covered in a red, white, and blue quilt. "My mother made that during the War, waiting for my pop to return. Coffee?"

"Thank you."

Milton turned on the two-burner stove; the scent of burning propane filling the six-hundred square feet with a memory of his father's workshop. He pushed a button on the wall, and the hum of a generator wafted into the cabin. He toggled another switch, and the room filled with light. "Electricity...I'm just not sufficiently robust to give it up. When I built the place, I found a couple of generators and converted then to propane. Gas company's good enough to deliver out here, though the prices, Lord, might as well be burning eighteen-year-old scotch."

He gazed toward a wall behind Gauthé. "Like to read." It was covered with textbooks—medicine, physics, math—and rows of novels, some ancient, some by Jodi Picoult, Abraham Verghese, and Steven King.

Gauthé stood and asked, "May I take a look?"

Milton smiled. "Of course. Can even borrow a couple if you like."

"Dr. Milton, excuse me, but what the hell are you doing out here?"

Anton laughed. "No one's called me Doctor Milton in years. Maybe Doc, the polite ones; mostly they just nod and don't call you anything, but they also don't bother me. They do their meth and heroin, and I do my wine, occasionally, but I've never been so free. Like I said, too much has changed, and I don't mean electronic medical records and high-field 3Tesla MRI scanners. Too much has changed in me."

"How long have you been here?"

The pot began to whistle, and he pulled it from the stove. "Milk and sugar?"

"Sure."

He took a quart of milk from a tiny refrigerator under the kitchen cabinet. "Nine years."

"May I ask what happened?"

"Of course. I have no secrets anymore. Not like before. As if my skeletons are so earthshattering. Same as everybody's. Not what you think, Chris. No scandals at work. No ripping off Medicare or patients. Nothing like that. Just got tired and came out here to camp for a few days. Met a guy, a former Boeing engineer, if you can believe it. Invited me to some weird-ass ceremony—worship the mountains, cull the spirits, become whole again, whatever the hell that means. Not a lick of science behind it. Hey, stop me if I'm boring you, please."

"Are you kidding? I'm on the edge of my seat."

"Well, don't fall off and get hurt, I don't take Blue Cross." Gauthé smirked without a trace of humor. Milton stopped and looked at him sadly. "Pretty burned out, huh?"

"Not all that happy, to be honest. Is it that obvious?"

"Like seeing myself in the mirror before I came out here. You know, after thirty years of doctoring, you get pretty good at reading people. I'm sure you can just look at a patient and have a medical diagnosis in fifteen seconds, then a psych eval by the end of the first minute. Hard to hide despondency from a doctor.

"But, anyway, as I was saying about my dubiously mystical pal, I went with him at dusk in late May few years ago. Trudged partway up the mountain. Figured it'd just be the two of us lambs. There's a depression in the granite, a cave of sorts. As we got near, I could see a flickering light, then gritty sounds—woo-woo—sounded like an owl retirement home. Just about turned around and ran back down to my car, but curiosity got the best of me. There were a dozen of them sitting around a fire. Looked like they were stoned, but they weren't. Just letting the anger and sadness come out, or so I learned. Each one had a story, a tale of endless fighting to shed the emptiness. I stayed and learned from them, all professionals, all smart as whips. I'm the dullest, by far..."

Gauthé interrupted. "Yeah. I can see." He pointed to the books."

"Never read a one. On the shelf when I got here."

"Right. You said you built the place."

Milton laughed. "I guess the books were what finally convinced me to leave practice, especially the novels. None of what I did in that life was real. I was on the board at my clinic. Everyone of 'em hiding secrets, tossing and turning night after night that someone'd find out, and that would be the end. Was already divorced, kids grown, took up with a nurse. She was unmarried, but CEO had me in for a chat. 'Don't get your meat where you get your bread, and don't dip your pen in company ink.' The affair was consuming so much real estate in my head, I became angry all the time. Lose my livelihood because I fell in love with a woman? Lose my retirement? I had no one. So lonely.

"And the whole time, every one of 'em was doing it, and the CEO knew, but..." He paused and stared out the window. "Funny, I read an article on the internet..."

Gauthé interrupted again, "You get the internet out here?"

"No. I'm terrible. Once a week I go in for groceries. Stop off at the library and use their computers. They think I'm homeless. One of 'em stands behind me to make sure I don't look at porn—God forbid. Anyway, I found a list of professions that draw sociopaths, like honey draws bears."

Gauthé laughed. "Friend of mine told me about it. What was it, CEOs, lawyers, and surgeons?"

"Yep, especially the CEOs. Power, money, autonomy, command, and status. Heartless bastards, willing to fire dozens or hundreds at a time to preserve their kingdoms. Look what's happening at the hospitals, even the good ones. University of Washington got caught with their fingers in the Medicare cookie jar. They blamed the doctors, said the administration was blameless. Real virgins, I'm sure."

"So, did you join the Wiccans?"

"We're not Wiccans, and laugh if you choose, but oneness with the divine isn't such a clichéd concept. That's what the books over there taught me, especially the biology and nuclear physics. We great scientists know nothing of the real secrets of life. You got one side saying it's God's hand; the other, that it's nothing but chemical reactions and two billion years of DNA mutations, nothing but pure chance. And that's grounds to fight and kill each other over who's right. What a joke. Nobody knows a damn thing. I'm getting better on my own. Don't need 'em anymore. Happy to move onto the next level without their help. Glad I'm done dealing with moron zealots on both sides. You a surgeon?"

"How did you know?"

"Pristine hands, smooth movements, Carrera. I will say, you guys do some good, 'specially the trauma guys. Rest of 'em, me at the top of the list, pretty much beating our heads against a rock, sorry to say."

"Doctor, are you sick?"

"Yeah, I guess you'd call it sick. When I started going downhill, losing weight, loss of appetite, food tasted terrible, pain deep in the gut, I figured it was pancreatic cancer. Runs in the family. Went to my colleagues, my friends. They hung their heads and became very mechanical. Deep sigh and a hard face. They didn't know shit from shinola about what was going on. Tried to explain it to me like I was a ten-year-old. They talked in circles, made up stupid answers for my stupid questions. Finally had me follow-up with a PA. Let her deal with the difficult, know-it-all patient. Shoot, I was in practice before she was born—before her parents were born—and she's managing my care? Then more biopsies and tests. Took 'em a week to get back to me with the results. Dr. Gauthé, they could have had the results phoned to them that day. I checked; the films are read immediately, and the pathologist got the slides read before going home for the night. But they didn't care enough to understand that I was dying, waiting to see if I was being sent to Death Row or was just a hypochondriac. It was worse than the disease. And mention it to them? Talk about defensive posture—I thought they were going to call security.

"Put me on steroids for the anti-inflammatory effect. It was a shot in the dark. After a few weeks, I hemorrhaged, melanotic stool at first, then bright red blood per rectum. Wound up in my own ER. Eight units of packed cells. Surgeon cauterized a patch in my duodenum that looked to all the world like a fungating malignant mass. 'Cancer for sure, at least now we know,' the gastroenterologist said. Tell you the truth, I wasn't all that sad. Had had about enough. Imagine the mavens at the clinic had had about enough of me, too. A pushy, dissatisfied patient. My body? Yeah, I'm impatient.

"Turns out it was the meds that opened an erosion in the gut wall. No tumor, wasn't cancer. It had been bleeding for months, occult, off and on, and they never caught the bleeding just right with the stool tests. How they missed it on the imaging studies is beyond me.

"Took some time off and came back out to the mountain to clear my head. Thought about my friends, your Wiccans, but I was so sick, and indoctrinated, I started to laugh at them. Decided to give work another shot. I'd be a better doc, now, make sure I'd never use a dangerous medicine until I was a hundred percent sure I knew the diagnosis. Man, I began to feel like I was healing the ill. Lasted two whole months. Nothing had changed, except me. Administration still pigs at the trough. My productivity sucked; I will admit. And here I am."

The Board of Directors at Mitchie-Sterling granted Gauthé a ninety-day leave of absence. He took a few thousand dollars out of his checking account and bought a tiny cabin a mile further into the forest than his friend Anton Milton. Mostly he sat by himself, but once every couple of weeks, he drove out for supplies and to call his kids. He spoke to no one else for three months.

When he returned to McKinley, the medical directors and CEOs of both hospitals met with him and, cautiously satisfied the man had regrounded himself, allowed him back to work with the stipulation that his first several procedures be observed. Within four days, his surgery schedule was nearly full. For ten days, he spoke to no one outside patients and scrub nurses. But by early the third week back, he scrolled through his contacts on his cell phone and pushed the call button.

He and Khai met for coffee. Two nights later, they had dinner at Sergio's. By the weekend, Khai had spent the night at his place.

CHAPTER THIRTY-FIVE

On the sixteenth day of Sabrina's admission to the psych floor at Warm Hills General, she sat across from Mike and monotoned, "I'm ready to go home. I don't want anymore. This is sucking from me what life I have left."

Mike sat, head hung. "But you're getting better every day, Sweetheart, it's not time to give up, ple..."

He stopped abruptly as his eye caught movement at the door. Dr. Darling braced. "I'm sorry, would you guys like your privacy?"

Sabrina looked up. "No, Doctor, not at all. We're happy to see you."

"Well, I'm flattered. Thank you." She paused and thought for a moment. "I think I have some good news. Maybe lift your spirits a bit." When Sabrina and Mike locked her eyes, she smiled. "Just got off the phone with Dr. Weathersby. She presented your situation to a neurologist who works at a FES, Functional Electrical Stimulation, lab. They're part of a study with young stroke patients. Looks like you've been chosen to participate. FES, have you heard of it?"

Both shook their heads.

"Well, we know that you have been having increasing muscle fasciculations in your left arm during your treatments here. That's a good thing. Means there are motor nerve pathways open from the brain to the muscles in your arm. Those are the specialized nerves that tell the muscles to work. At least some are still connected to your brain. Problem is, not enough voltage is getting through to cause the muscles to contract on their own. Apparently, though, when you get a voltage boost from the outside, like from the ECT, more of them fire and you get movement. It's like getting a jump-start from the Triple A guy.

"Past few decades, electrophysiologists have been working on implanting a device that amplifies the tiny currents that are still getting through from the brain. Problem is, I mean, you can make a muscle jump by hooking it up to a battery for a second, but it's just a gross contraction—no value. Didn't you do that with a frog leg in science in 9th grade?"

Mike laughed. "I do that with our cat every night."

Sabrina reached out with her right arm to thump his leg. "Ignore him, Dr. Darling. We don't have a cat."

Mike laughed. "Little do you know. I stole two kittens from the neighbors three nights ago to play with in my lab."

Dr. Darling wagged a finger at him. He dropped his head, and she went on. "With the miniaturization of computer circuitry these days, they can actually choose a particular nerve fiber, boost the signal, and most important, set the progression of firing so that selected muscles down the line get the message in sequence. That produces coordinated movement. They can even get reverse flow from the skin back toward the brain. You know, like when you pull your hand away from a hot surface.

"From what I've learned, this group is using a series of electrodes implanted along the upper arm. Earlier forms were using stimulators on the skin, but they weren't able to elicit fine movement. There'll be wires under the skin, and naturally, a small computer somewhere. Sensors pick up the faint message from specific nerves coming into the arm, amplify them just enough, and, most important, coordinate them until, they say, she'll able to shift her hand freely. There might even be some movement of the forearms, though, I have to be honest, they warned me they haven't had a patient with a spinal cord problem on top of a stroke.

"I don't want to get too far ahead of myself, but they're implanting sensors in the legs. They claim to have had some patients relearn to drive."

PART THREE

CHAPTER THIRTY-SIX

Sabrina and Mike came to see Harrison Jennings on the Friday before the start of the trial. He stuck a pipe in his mouth but did not light it. Mike asked wryly, "Mr. Jennings, I didn't know you smoked."

"I don't. Haven't for the past thirty-some years, except the days before a trial. But I still don't light the thing." He took the pipe out of his mouth and pointed into the bowl. "That ash down there, untouched for the past three decades, no fire since Ronald Reagan was president. Just something to keep my hands busy while I'm thinking—if that's what you can call it.

"So, tell me, Sabrina, where are you right now, I mean in terms of what you can and can't do. That'll give me something to hang my hat on when I deliver my opening remarks."

She stared at him for a moment then turned her head in thought. "Mike, why don't you tell him?"

Mike's eyes opened with a mild start. "Oh, okay." He spoke with the first hint of dejection Jennings had ever heard in him. "I am sure you can see the atrophy in Sabrina's left arm. She really hasn't got any use back since the last time we saw you. We tried FES, functional electrical stimulation."

"It didn't work?"

"It did, but the insurance company said it was still experimental. At least the form we were using was. They implanted microelectrodes in Sabrina's forearm, and she got some use of her hand, but that part was paid for by the biotech company. Once they proved it had helped Sabrina, that was the end of the grant money for our participation. The plan was to get our insurance to cover the ongoing cost. Insurance company refused, sited data from studies that the results were too short-lived. Biotech company offered us a good deal, but what we could afford was far below their cost. Great guys, but they had dozens of people in our same situation. They would have gone out of business if they tried any harder to help us. My union guy raised hell with the insurance company, claimed they were withdrawing care that was working, but they said they weren't refusing care at all, just not paying for it."

Jennings agreed. "That's the loophole in the law. They never contracted to cover care they consider experimental, and they reserve the right to make that determination internally, and secretly. We can't even subpoena the documents from them—proprietary. All in the contract you signed. Nothing really to be done.

"Now, when we win our suit, you'll be able to pay for the treatment, and I bet the biotech company will still give you a deal. We'll make sure they do. That'll give you some time to raise hell with the insurance company."

"Mr. Jennings, not sure I have a lot of hell left in me to raise. We're trying stimulation with the electrodes on the skin. Nowhere as good as the implanted electrodes, a bit of movement, but insurance pays for it, and they say we need to give it time—a lot of time."

"Quite understand. Are you guys still doing the PT?"

Mike glanced sideways at Sabrina, but she turned her head away a few more degrees. Mike exhaled through pursed lips. "Well, I guess some of it got too painful. Sabrina would wake up on PT days crying. She hated it. We made the decision together. It wasn't working for her arm or her leg. Why should she suffer just so we can say we did every single thing we were told to do—like good little puppies. Why, because that horrible woman, Rhonda Uft, tried to take what's left of Sabrina's spirit during the deposition? I'll never forgive her for calling her the '...big victim in all this, aren't you?'"

"Again, I hear ya, but you aren't doing it for the trial. If it isn't working, then by all means, it's time to stop. No one's here to torture you."

Mike added, "Sometimes I wonder. I'll will say, however, part of the PT is working on coordination of the flickers. That doesn't hurt, so we're still doing that. It's something, at least."

"Look, we are going to beat them without taking any more out of you. You do what you think is right, not what you guys think others expect of you. I'll make the case with whatever we have. Let me handle them." He paused. "And about the depression—you see any change?"

Again, Sabrina looked away. "You know, Mr. Jennings, there was an improvement after the ECT, and it's lasted, but things have levelled off. No further improvement. I guess we're happy for what we got. Oh, and Dr. Darling suggested we add one of the atypical antidepressants, but Sabrina was really scared about the weight gain, especially with her sitting all the time. She couldn't try Wellbutrin because of the chance of seizures."

Jennings asked, "And about work?"

Sabrina turned to him. "I tried two days a week, like we discussed, seems like a long time ago. It felt great to get back to practice—better antidepressant than all the pills and lightning strikes combined. Taught me a lot. Made me feel I really do have something to offer. But after a week, I was so darned tired by afternoon, I had to take a nap. They put a couch in my office but getting in and out of the chair to lie down was such a pain, took fifteen minutes to get onto the couch, then fifteen to get back into the chair, and just that fast, lunch was over. Head of the department told me to call my helper. Just couldn't do it. I'm not some damn cripple." Both Jennings and Mike tensed. Sabrina felt it. "Yes, I am." She laughed flatly.

"So, they placed me on indefinite, unpaid leave. They continued my medical and dental insurance. They shouldn't have, I mean paid for medical and dental. A few good folks left in the hospital administration. I'm just lucky Mitchie-Sterling isn't part of the University's medical corporation. Just think, if they were, I'd be suing myself."

Jennings laughed and stretched. "Well, I called you here today to go over what to expect next week. That's if you want to hear it." They both nodded. "And I'm going to be detailed, so there are no surprises. Every trial is different, of course, but the flow chart remains the same. I have to be able to walk into any courtroom in Washington State and know the exact agenda and rules. No surprises.

"Okay, here we go. Trials are broken into six phases. First, we will choose a jury. I'm sure you know about the voir dire process. We can refuse a few people for no reason—don't like the cut of their slacks—and we can refuse a million if we can convince the judge that the potential juror is prejudiced. I mean, if there's an emergency room doctor in the pool, defense'll want him, but we won't, and the judge will go along with us. That one's a no-brainer. Gets touchier with, let's say a physical therapist who works in the community and gets referrals from the ER. What we want is people who have a history of long hospitalizations. That's ideal, because no matter how well you're treated, it's a nightmare. Nobody's fault, just the way it is. Next, we'll look for empathetic folks for other reasons. Parents of handicapped kids, elderly women taking care of their bedridden husbands."

Sabrina looked toward Mike and then Harrison Jennings. "And the opposite, like the guy sitting right here."

Jennings laughed. "He's a keeper, isn't he?"

Sabrina smiled, "Like you, Mr. Jennings."

"Let's see how you feel about me after the war—the trial. It can get pretty nasty in there. As you know from the depositions, I can't shield you from all the barbs. Anyway, what we don't want is people who see a disorderly world that needs strict rules to maintain order. They see life as a bedrock of chaos. To their way of thinking, there have to be iron-clad rules that everyone must follow. No room for feelings. If things go wrong, it was because the rules weren't followed."

Mike raised his hand. "Isn't that what we're arguing? That Cardozo didn't follow the rules?"

"That's the point, Mike. He did follow the rules. There is no rule for calling out the Army Rangers when all you get for orders is a voice on a phone claiming to be a company commander, and it's the middle of the night, and you've never heard the name before. I mean, there is an argument that Cardozo shouldn't have even taken the call from an unknown source, and let's be clear, at that moment, Dr. Weathersby was just a voice on a cold and stormy night. Think about it from a lawyer's perspective. Think how Cardozo opened himself up to litigation just discussing the case with a phantom. HIPPA, and all that.

"So, what we don't want is cops, ex-career military, coaches, and of course, no medical personnel. We want women who will sympathize with a woman who fought her way to success, and with a handicap, only to have it all taken away by a doctor who heard a female's voice, ignored her, and even used misogynistic epithets. Pretty damning."

Mike sighed, "You know, Mr. Jennings, sometimes I think maybe the hospital is getting the short end of the stick because of Cardozo. Besides that CEO, the rest of them worked pretty hard to help us—most of them. Makes you wonder why we're suing them along with that jerk."

"Mike, listen. He's a very bad man. Shouldn't be a doctor. Loose cannon. And please, don't feel sorry for any of the players. There are standards in how civilized people treat each other, and several of the administrators forgot those rules along the way. The hospital knows exactly what happened that night. They don't care. They will dodge their responsibility by every means under the sun. Just wait until the case starts. You saw how Rhonda Uft treated you in the deposition—how she degraded you two simply because her client can pay her more than you guys can. Remember how she picked at you until even I wasn't sure if Dr. Weathersby was the real culprit or not? She's very good at her work—to twist the truth until no one knows what one plus one equals. She's aware of exactly what happened that night, and what the hospital administration did to cover their tracks. Everyone knows, but she will spin it at your expense. Doesn't care who she hurts. She'll tell you it's not personal, just business, that every defendant deserves the best defense they can get, I mean pay for, and maybe she's right. But the bottom line is, business or not, she represents uncaring, greedy bastards on the hospital's board of directors who cherish nothing but their income."

Mike nodded. "She's good—you're better. A lot better."

"Thanks, Mike. And, I plan to be next week. Okay, back to the trial. After the jury is selected, it'll take a day at least, there will be fourteen of our peers perched in the jury box, twelve regulars and two alternates. But you know all that. By the way, in some states it's only six souls.

"Anyway, Judge'll start the proceedings by telling the jury what to expect. It's Arthur Galanter. He's a straight shooter; not intimidated by the, shall we say, 'vigorous' attorneys from the big city. Nice thing for him, and for Rhonda Uft, is that they probably won't be in front of each other again any time soon. But that also means the gloves are off. She's got nothing to be scared of. No need to lick his shoes. Here in town, we locals face the same judges day in and day out, year after year, for decades. Got to mind our p's and q's. She, on the other hand, will likely never see him again except at a party. And he doesn't need her contributions when it comes time to get reelected.

"Anyway, he'll greet the jurors politely and instruct that they must not discuss or make any decisions on the case until they sit down at the end of the trial and look at the facts. He'll probably say that several times, and then get real huffy about how, if there's conflict between the lawyers, he'll decide who has the law on his or her side. He'll apologize that sometimes he'll have to excuse the jury to allow arguments. And, he'll be pretty clear that if he tells the jurors to disregard a statement here and there, he means it.

"Phase Two: Each lawyer makes an opening statement. It's a road map for what he plans to prove with his or her witnesses. I go first, then Rhonda Uft'll tell the jurors how full of it I am. Usually, the judge doesn't allow the other attorney to interrupt during opening remarks, but if things get out of hand, he'll speak up. Guarantee our Ms. Uft will find a way to get him involved.

"Next, when she's done with her opening statement, that starts the third phase of the trial, actual testimony. I start bringing witnesses to the stand to make our case. Some will be on our side, some not. If I call a witness, I am the first to question that witness. It's called direct examination. When I'm done with that witness, she gets to do her cross-examination. That's when things start to get nasty. She has to show the jury that the witness is a moron and has no idea of what really happened that night. She'll suggest they're liars and in it for some personal gain. When she's done, I may or may not do a re-direct. But if I do, I can only refute what she said on cross. Can't bring in anything new, like if I forgot to say on direct that the witness saw the defendant operate on the wrong leg three times, I can't bring that up. Then she gets a shot again, called re-cross, but she can only challenge what I asked in re-direct."

Mike laughed. "When does it end?"

"Good question. Pretty soon, the jury gets tired of the games. They're not stupid. Re-cross is usually the last hack at the witness, and like redirect, usually relatively short.

"When I'm done calling witnesses, we'll say to the judge, 'The Plaintiff rests.' Then Rhonda Uft stands up and starts calling her own witnesses to refute everything my witnesses said. Same program, but she does the direct, and I the cross, ad nauseum.

"Finally, the defense'll tell the judge they rest, and the judge will call for the next phase of the trial, closing arguments. Some people call it summation. We go first. This time, the lawyers are allowed to speak directly to the jury and claim we proved what we promised we would in our opening statements. Then the defense. Then, if we want to, we can take a final bite of the apple. It's called rebuttal. Again, I can only comment about what she brought up in her summation. But she can't talk after that.

"Next phase—jury instructions. Judge tells the jury what the legal issues are, the real issues, and how the law applies to the issues, not what the lawyers want you to think, or what you think, they are. He sends them off with a piece of paper that has a place for them to write the verdict, and also, if the plaintiff wins, how much they award for loss of income, future medical bills, pain and suffering. They add it all up and divide it based on what they think each guilty party must pay, how much for Cardozo, how much for the hospital, if they find the hospital guilty."

Mike's lips twisted. "They can find Cardozo guilty and not the hospital?"

"Or the other way 'round, or any combination thereof. A jury is inscrutable. Lock twelve people from every walk of life in a small room and tell them they ain't gettin' out until they agree on a complicated, emotion-ridden question, and see what you get. Gave up trying to predict jury outcomes my second year in practice.

"On the other hand, what you put into a project often predicts what you get out. And we've put in a lot. Still weighing allowing you to testify, Mike."

Mike rolled his eyes. "What's your inclination?"

"Thought about trying to figure out a way to ring the bell on what you saw through the window that night. Still working on it. I filed another motion for the judge to allow you to set the scene, at least describe in layman's terms, but Judge Galanter ruled against us again. Rhonda Uft has him flummoxed. Convinced him that there are no circumstances that you could understand, medically, what you were seeing in the ER that night through the window. He won't allow you to say 'boo' about squirting blood and needles flying around and cursing and screaming, on and on. You are not a trained medical person, and she's argued that even a doctor, let's say a psychiatrist or a pathologist, would have no idea if what he saw was proper procedure or a Keystone Cops production. And, you know what, she has a point. If we have you testify to what happened, in your eyes, she will eat you alive on cross. Make you look like a fool. Make all your testimony suspect, every word of it."

"But they can't argue that I didn't see Dr. Gauthé say 'Keystone Cops.'"

"Mike, be serious. Think about this. She'll have you on the stand, put a doctor in front of you, and have him mouth Ketosis, or ketones, or Keebler Cookies, something along those lines. She holds up a sign to the jury of what he mouthed, and then she'll ask you what he said. How are you going to answer? You're not a lip-reader. She'll humiliate you. You don't want that. We don't want that.

"If you testify, we will stick to you telling the court what happened in Dr. Weathersby's office, how Sabrina was looking and feeling when you got to the

Mitchie-Sterling Hospital parking lot, during the pregnancy test, on the walk upstairs to the ultrasound lab, and then back down to the ER. I'm going to ask if you guys were talking while you sat in the ER. Was Sabrina alert, making good sense..."

Sabrina raised her right hand and pointed at Mike. "Don't you dare, Michael."

Mike grinned, "Who, me?" then turned back to Harrison Jennings.

Jennings smiled and rubbed his hands together, but quickly became quite serious. "Like I said, I haven't made up my mind if you are going to testify at all. How are you going to respond to her on cross when she demands an answer to the question, and I'm sorry to bring this up, 'Now, Mr. Maddingly, what were you thinking when you signed the AMA release?' Then she'll turn to the jury, 'Against Medical Advice.' And let's be honest, you did, Mike. 'And you didn't drive immediately to the emergency room? How sick did your wife have to be before you considered her more important, sir, than tomorrow's lunch for your fellow teachers?'"

"Mike, you can't answer that in any way that is going to help our case. You're an impressive man, Mike, but no matter what we come up with, her next question will just deepen the wound. Suddenly, she's the innocent party—you're your own executioner. Look, she makes a living out of crafting situations in which people hang themselves."

He gazed at the ceiling for a moment then turned back to them. "You know, I'm sitting here talking myself out of calling you to the stand. Anyway, let me finish telling you what happens at the very end of the trial. Before the judge sends the jurors off to deliberate, he will admonish them not to vote on what feels good, but what the law says, that is, what he says the law says. They will retire to the jury room and negotiate and take votes until they come up with ten people out of the twelve who vote for us, or not. If they can't come up with ten, we lose."

Mike asked, "Mr. Jennings, I thought a jury had to be unanimous."

"Not in a civil matter. In Washington State, the number needed to find for the plaintiff is ten. Different in different states. Yes, in a criminal trial it's all the members, and that grows out of our need to make sure we don't take a person's freedom, that is, put a person in jail unless we are absolutely sure of guilt. For civil trials, almost one-third of states only require a majority for a verdict. Some states require a majority if the money at issue in the trial is below a certain amount, and a unanimous verdict all other times. Here in Washington State, we're in the middle; we need to convince ten jurors.

"If we get ten, they have to come up with a total amount of damages. We measure that in money. In some countries it's land; some, camels; in some it's indentured slavery—whatever's the prevailing way to pay a debt in that society.

"First, the jury writes down medical expenses—that's in a document prepared ahead of time by the hospital, doctors, physical therapists, on and on. Then, lost wages. That's easy. The lawyers get a statement from the employer giving salary and lost days. What's harder is calculating pain and suffering. There's a cap on that in Washington State."

Mike asked, "Mr. Jennings, I thought the jury decided on pain and suffering by how angry they are at the defendants."

"No, Mike. Not at all. It's all very mechanical. Couldn't be any other way. When the judge sends the jury off, he gives them a standard form with a place to put down their decision about who is responsible for the harm, and, if they find for us, there is a strict formula how they calculate damages. If we win, they continue down the form and put numbers in a column to the far right for medical expenses, those already accrued, and future medical costs, all that stuff given to them by the bean counters. Then they put down the lost wages."

Sabrina lifted a finger. "Does that include Mike's? He's lost a lot of time."

"Not really. He's on a salary, and has sick leave, had donated sick leave, and you were granted coverage by the Family Leave Medical Act. No double-dipping."

Sabrina shook her head. "But Mike had to give up his coaching job. That should be covered."

"That's a good point. We can still add that to our demand for damages. Or we may not. I'll tell you why in a minute. Anyway, if they find for us, we will definitely ask for an award for pain and suffering. But this is a bit of a gray area. And, now, there's a cap on P and S. Plaintiff's lawyers hate it, but it really was getting out of control, especially in medical malpractice cases."

Mike interrupted. "They should hate it. How can a defense lawyer know what people are going through when there's been a tragedy?"

"They don't, but we're always trying to improve the delivery of justice, and things were getting out of hand in the Eighties. You've heard of 'runaway juries' and 'The Great Tort Lottery'?"

Mike laughed. "Actually, no, but I'm sure we'll walk out of here knowing."

"That you will. Let me give you an example. Forty-year-old woman in Virginia gets her tubes tied. You know where this is going. She gives birth to a healthy baby. She admits she loves the kid but sues her OB-GYN for damages. She was told before the surgery that there is a known, and legally-accepted, two percent natural failure rate for tubal ligations. Tubes can re-connect by themselves. Hard to stop procreation. Given that, the birth was not conclusive proof of negligence. But the mother had an expert witness who testified that the OB-GYN used the wrong clamp. He convinced the court, and the jury, that it really was a case of negligence. Jury found the doctor liable and found economic damages of $39,000 for medical expenses, the cost of the birthing, and $9,000 in Mom's lost wages. But, in Virginia, the cost of raising the child to adulthood is not recoverable, so the jury sidestepped that and came in with a total award of $1,800,000. That means $1,752,000 was awarded for pain and suffering—for a child that was loved and perfectly healthy, and a happy 6-year-old at the time of the jury verdict.

"Second case. Woman with multiple allergies complained to her physician about shortness of breath. She provided a list of her known drug allergies, was diagnosed with asthma, and was administered an inhaled steroid by the physician's staff. Unbeknownst to the patient, one of the primary ingredients in the medication was precisely a steroid to which she had a known allergy. Negligence, in other words, was abundantly clear. Patient suffered an allergic reaction. Had to go to the ER. It was bad. They had to intubate her because the swelling closed down her throat. Ten days in the hospital. When she went home, she could not swallow solid foods and could not recline. Her voice was hoarse, her hair fell out, and she had two surgeries to correct laryngeal scarring and tracheal narrowing. She was out of work for six months. She had economic damages of $43,000 in lost wages and $97,000 in medical and hospital fees, for a total of $140,000. She agreed to a settlement of $627,868, including, therefore, roughly $387,000 for pain and suffering. Clearly the plaintiff's competent counsel feared they'd recover less if they rolled the dice and went before a jury. If you're not sure, better settle. Let's remember that.

"So, what's the moral of this story? Pain and suffering for experiencing the joy of a totally loved and healthy child after a procedure that might or might not have been negligent: $1,752,000. But disfigurement, two surgeries, inability to eat normally, and permanent disability after pretty blatant negligence: a mere $387,000. Looks like pretty clear evidence that somethin' ain't right. Is that equal justice?" They shook their heads. "So, there had to be a cap.

"Here's the way it's done now. The jury figures out how many years of work-life the plaintiff has left. In your case, we'll argue you could have easily worked until near seventy-three. So, that's, say, forty years. Then they take your salary, in your case, one-fifteen a year, and any bonuses you are getting. You'll have to tell me that. And here's where the jury has all the leeway. Somehow, the legislature divined a magic number of point-four-three. That's forty-three percent. They multiply that by the yearly salary and bonuses. In your case, that comes to roughly fifty thousand dollars. Then they multiply that by the number of years left to work. Forty times fifty thousand, and that's, for argument's sake, around two million." He stopped for a moment and looked up. "Forty years to go. God that seems like a long time! Better you than me, Sabrina."

She raised her right hand and pointed at him. "Trade ya."

"Truth is, Sabrina, I wish I could. Make it probably the best thing I've done in my career. You two are special people. I've had a great life, all in all. Believe it or not, you two are just starting out. My race is run. It hurts me to see you guys taking a hit so early." He stopped and stared back at the ceiling. "But we're gonna do something about it. As we used to say in my college fraternity, 'Watch me now.'"

There was another pause, and Mike drew a deep breath. "Mr. Jennings, as far as Sabrina and I are concerned, you haven't left the starting blocks. You're a prince in our book. And win or lose, we'll never forget you. We'll be just fine."

"I know you will. And thank you." He pulled at his pipe for a few seconds. "Okay, so let's finish off here. I've calculated what we're asking for. Going strictly by the book. No inflation. Some jurors hate that. Don't blame 'em.

"Now, remember, the jury doesn't have to use the full point-four-three. That's their prerogative. They can say your Agent Orange issue was part of the problem and that you had pain and suffering before the present case. But if we keep it real and don't look like we're there for a mammoth payday, most juries would see your situation as pretty clear evidence of very close to the full award— that's if we win. That's why we probably won't be nitpicking for all the extras, like Mike's lost coaching stipend.

"And, think about it this way. If you put your share of the award in bonds and safe stocks, that's about six percent per year. If you leave it alone, at that percent it will double every twelve years—rule of seventy-two. Divide the percent return into seventy-two, and that's how many years it takes to double your money. So, after expenses, you'll have two-some million in twelve years, four and a half in twenty-four years, and over ten million when you decide to retire.

"But as I said a while ago, no matter what case we put on, you can never tell what a jury is going to do. Look at O.J., and that little girl who was murdered by her mother. What was it? Yeah, Casey Anthony. Another outrage, but it's just the way things are when you put together a jury. Then again, this system has been being honed for many hundreds of years. Cumbersome, maybe, but no one's come up with a better set of game rules. In fact, whether you win or not, it works pretty well—in the greater scheme of things, juries usually get the right answer. Problem is, you can't tell on an individual basis.

"One more thing to go over. Part of that piece of paper the judge gives the jury has a place to put down who's responsible for what percentage of the damages. Say the jury finds Cardozo eighty-five percent responsible. That means he owes around three-point-five million. But he only has a million in insurance coverage. We get the million and can demand he sells his skis and his mountain bike, but we won't get a damn thing, really. It'll cost more to go after him personally than it's worth. So, we need to depend on the hospital being held culpable to some degree, maybe one or two percent. I have to make sure my presentation is good enough to convince the jury of that." Mike started to raise his hand. Jennings laughed. "And you're not thrilled about the one or two percent, right?"

"Right."

"Wrong! There's such a thing as joint and several liability. That's where even though, in our case, say Cardozo is eighty-five percent liable, since he can't cover the full amount, any other party involved in the suit, anyone who has acted in concert with him, has to make up the difference. Again, in most states this is the law, but some don't have it. We're lucky that Washington does."

Sabrina shook her head. "Hardly seems fair."

Jennings thought for a moment. "Maybe, but the spirit of the law is that it is better for a culpable defendant to overpay than for the injured plaintiff to be undercompensated. And there's another legal point. Maybe the hospital shouldn't have been acting in concert with a known jerk. Pick your friends more wisely.

"Anyway, what happens then is that the insurance company for Cardozo and the one for the hospital fight it out. Good, let 'em kill each other. Couldn't happen to nicer folks.

"The theatrical problem, for me, is that Cardozo's such an embarrassment, so unsympathetic, the jury is going to hate him and will want him to pay the whole kit and kaboodle. You saw him act like a horse's patoot at the deposition. Betcha that'll pale compared to what he's going to do at trial. I have to make sure there's a smidgen of guilt on the hospital's hands.

"So, that's about it. Now, you two have been to law school. Any questions?"

Mike raised his hand. "What if we win, but they appeal, just like on letting us see the ultrasound files for that night. They didn't win, but it took forever, and we finally gave in."

"We won't give in, Mike. If the jury gives us the damages we're asking for, Rhonda Uft will meet with us and offer a settlement of much, much less. If we accept, we get the money right away. End of hassle—very tempting. If we refuse, they'll threaten to appeal. They will cite a bunch of questionable calls by Judge Galanter, and they're certainly there, always are, but he's a pretty wily old coot. He'll be careful, make his rulings on the sticky questions pretty bulletproof, but may look like he's erred on the simple ones. Puffs up the lawyers, makes them think they have him by the neck, that an appeal is a sure bet; and then when they spend all that money, it'll be clear that the mistakes would not have changed the outcome, and the appeal will be denied. It's all a game, I'm afraid.

"Problem is, appeals process takes a couple of years, if not more, and it'll cost a lot in legal fees because we'll need to get a proper appeals attorney for that. Too much money involved for a general practice lawyer to do it." Both Sabrina and Mike frowned. "I know, I know, but that's just the way it is.

"On the other hand, if we win at Superior Court level, and they appeal, Galanter'll be cool. He'll accept the challenge like a gentleman and pretend to be very matter of fact about it. But you can be sure he'll be madder than a wet hen, and when the review gets turned down at the appellate level, they'll return it to the trial judge to rule on paying our legal fees for the hassle. I'm sure he'll award enough to cover every penny of that.

"Then, there's also interest on the original amount the jury awards us. Courts don't like to go above twelve percent per year, but I'll bet he'll be miffed enough to give us ten percent, maybe better. Not bad, given the recent interest rates. Interest'll come to more than half-a-million, better if it takes more than two years. I figure, more than three-quarters of a million if it gets dragged out for three.

"Question becomes, can you wait that long?"

Sabrina lifted her head. "Mr. Jennings, we'll be just fine. I will be back at work, and Mike's very secure at school. Do you think the appeals court will be mad at them for wasting their time again; I mean, will that be the reason they deny it?"

"Not supposed to happen that way, ideally, everything according to the law; but they're human, human with especially oversized egos, and they are an impatient lot. No one questions a judge at any level. They simply can't admit a mistake, a weakness. Missing that gene. And since they can get away with it for a full career, they just get more obstinate. So, yes, that's why they'll deny the appeal."

He was quiet for a moment. "Anyway, let me tell you about the final thing that can happen in a trial. The judge can reverse the jury's verdict. That can happen when the judge believes there were insufficient facts on which to base the jury's verdict, or that the verdict did not correctly apply the law—you know, when the jury decides the law is just plain wrong. Jury can't do that, at least in theory. Problem is, how do you read the minds of twelve jurors on what they considered in their decision?

"And a judge can even order the jury to come to a specific decision. That's called a directed verdict. All sorts of possibilities. He can even stop the trial and, usually at the behest of the defense, as soon as the plaintiff has presented its case, just rule that there is simply not evidence to find the defendant guilty under any circumstances. Usually, the cases are weeded out long before that, but, believe me, I've seen it all. Anything is possible in court. It's unbelievable. But none of that's going to happen here. Our jury is going to listen to two well-presented cases and see that Mitchie-Sterling Hospital screwed up."

He stopped and thought for a minute. "You know, Mike, my decision is made. Like I said, you're imposing and well-spoken, but we need to base our argument on hard medical facts, not on our belief that they are skunks, which they are. I recommend you do not testify. You two can override me, but that's my professional recommendation."

Sabrina laughed. "No, I won't override a single decision, and, Mike, don't even think about it."

Mike nodded. "Okay, but I sure wanted to tell them about that crappy CEO refusing to see me, and they wouldn't give Sabrina some pain killers. She was hurting so bad."

"Mike, again, Rhonda Uft'll tell the jury, and convince them with witnesses, that you were a rogue family member running through the hospital like a madman, demanding the staff practice medicine the way you think it should be. If we don't bring it up, there's no point in her dragging people to the stand to show that you love your wife, but you broke all the hospital rules; rules, I might add, they'll show are in place in every hospital in the free world. Let's leave it alone."

Mike started to interrupt, but Jennings put up his hand. "Hear me out, again, please. There are times when a nurse can't give any more opioid pain medication. If there's already a certain level in the blood, a small additional amount may cause the patient to stop breathing. That's all a heroin overdose is. You know when you try to hold your breath for too long, you must take a breath. No human can avoid it—not possible. But with just a little too much opioid in your system, you lose that essential drive. If you've passed out from the drug, there's nothing telling you to breathe, and you suffocate in minutes. Can you imagine if they did that, threw your wife into respiratory failure? Had to rescue her again, save her life again, resuscitation teams and resuscitation carts? Mike, they have good medical practice on their side. Whether Sabrina was anywhere near that opioid precipice is not something you can say you knew. You had no idea. You can't win that skirmish, my friend, but we will win the battle."

CHAPTER THIRTY-SEVEN

That Sunday, the morning before opening arguments, Norman Harp summoned his board of principals. "As you know, testimony begins tomorrow. I've been advised that only I may attend as an observer. If we fill the peanut gallery with our friendly Mitchie-Sterling doctors, there'll be an outcry from the other side. Some of our providers will be recognized by members of the jury, just fodder for an appeal. Any questions on that tidbit?"

When no one responded, Harp turned to Weegun. "Doctor, our Ms. Uft says it's too late to call the security guy to the stand. He was going to be important—show just how unreliable that woman and her husband really were—loose cannons, caused the delays that led to her problems. What do you know about that?"

Weegun shook his head. "Norman, the guy missed his deposition. Was in jail, or don't you remember?"

"I remember he was in some dutch locally, but what was the outcome?"

"Well, first, he finally made his way up to Evanston, to see our favorite lady doctor. Apparently, she treats a lot of industrial injuries. Anyway, she gave him another month off work and put him on pain meds, OxyContin, I believe. Sure enough, he got hooked..."

Harp snorted, "Not surprised. Not surprised at either one of them."

Sonya Laureano raised her hand, though spoke before being recognized. "Norman, that's not quite how it happened. And Worth, you know darn well that's not the story. Did you bother to read the guy's chart notes?" He took a breath to defend himself, but she continued, her voice hardening. "Just be

212

quiet and listen for a change. All of you.

"The security guy went out to see Dr. Weathersby, yes, and she gave him a week off to go to physical therapy. He didn't show up once, excuse after excuse, so she signed papers to send him back to light duty—sit in the office and do the dispatching. He said it hurt too much to sit, so she told him to stand and sit alternately. He claimed he could only do that if she gave him more prescriptions of Vicodin. He got abusive and stormed out. Gave the receptionist the finger on the way, which is typical, no, absolute proof of drug seeking. They all do the same thing. As if they read a book. She gave him all of six Vicodins on the first visit. Six, Norman, that's it. Never gave him one OxyContin. And you don't get addicted on six hydrocodones—period.

"Before he marched out of the clinic, he pocketed one of Dr. Weathersby's prescription pads. He had taken a Xerox of the only script she had given him, so he'd have a copy of her signature. Started selling the blank scripts, so the buyer could enter their drug of choice.

"Didn't get very far. Pharmacy in town called her and asked if she had written that many scripts in a day. And our pal wrote one for sixty oxycodone. Dr. Weathersby had never given more than ten pills per script in the time she'd been practicing there. Pharmacist called the cops. Took the jerk away in cuffs.

"Got probation, said his back was hurting so much, he couldn't do any time. Judge bought it. So, the genius goes home and starts writing scripts for a safe twenty-five. Moron couldn't figure out twenty-five's an odd number. You take them two at a time, so it's almost always an even number.

"This time the judge throws the book at him—three days in the county lockup and a one hundred dollar fine. The deposition is for a week after he gets out, but he misses it and tells Rhonda Uft it's because he was in the midst of a serious legal matter. Just thank your lucky stars he's not on the docket. Defense attorney would have him for lunch. You have anything to add, Worth?"

Harp shook his head. "Let's calm down, Sonya. You sound like you're head cheerleader for that quack lady over in Evanston."

She rose from her chair. "Norman, she's not a quack. I'd take my grandkids to her long before I would to a lot of my colleagues in this place. And don't call her 'lady' again. She's a doctor, not a lady or a girl." She did not take her eyes off of him. "I hope we don't have to visit that again. And that goes for the rest of you, too." She pivoted away from the table and walked toward the door but stopped short. "No, I'm staying in your august company. I want to hear every word of bullcrap that pukes out of your collective mouths."

Harp stared at her. "Sonya, that type of behavior is unacceptable in a professional meeting..."

"That's Doctor Laureano to you. When you spend thirteen years after high school, then go through getting into medical school, paying tuition, and working a hundred hours a week for most of those years, then you can call me Sonya. Got it?"

Harp rose. "Gentlemen, I will continue this discussion privately in my office." He bristled out. Several of the doctors stayed behind with Laureano.

Sonya Laureano drove home. She searched her purse until coming to Khai's cell number. The small talk did not last long. "Khai, in medical school and residency, what did they teach us was the kiss of death in a malpractice case, for either side?"

"Altering records?"

"Bingo. I can't discuss the coming malpractice case, but I can say one word."

"And that word is?"

"Ultrasound. Now, I gotta get goin'. Wish I could be there when you testify, but I can't. We were ordered not to attend. On the other hand, you can be sure I'll be there in spirit, hovering about sixteen inches behind you. God bless." She hung up without another word.

CHAPTER THIRTY-EIGHT

The trial commenced that Monday morning at exactly 9 A.M. An elderly man emerged from chambers and limped to his bench. The bailiff spurted, "All rise for the Honorable Judge Arthur Galanter." Within a minute, the jury was seated, and after very few words of greeting, and warning, Harrison Jennings was summoned to make his opening statements.

"Ladies and gentlemen, thank you for being here. Your presence is crucial to our way of life." He paused before twisting toward the Plaintiff's table. "Let me introduce Dr. Sabrina Maddingly." When her eyes dropped, he shook his head almost imperceptibly and turned back to the jury. "On the evening of November 25, two years ago, Dr. Maddingly suffered a devastating stroke at Mitchie-Sterling Hospital, a disorder of the brain that took away all use of her left arm and most of the use of her left leg. That stroke put her in the wheelchair to which she is confined most hours of every day, and likely will be for the rest of her life. Worst of all, though, that stroke robbed her of the spirit that had made her a truly remarkable woman." He took a step toward Sabrina but stopped and turned back to the jury, his body as taut as a bowstring. "Your critical mission over the next days is one of the most important in our society. You will listen to the facts, think hard, and make a decision regarding who is responsible for this tragedy." He swept his arm toward Sabrina. She reflexively dropped her head further and tugged nervously at the dark blue blanket that covered her legs. "That, ladies and gentlemen, is who you and I and this court are here to serve, to ensure justice for, Dr. Sabrina Maddingly.

"Let me tell you what happened to Dr. Maddingly two years ago, on

Thanksgiving Eve, the disaster that has sadly brought us here. And let me assure you, we are here despite our best efforts to settle this amicably with the Defendants, Dr. Cardozo and the corporation that runs Mitchie-Sterling Hospital. We are here despite the fact that Dr. Maddingly's case would never have gotten to this final step in our justice system if a court-required panel of experts hadn't first reviewed the case meticulously and found it had merit. And despite the obvious tragedy sitting before you, Mitchie-Sterling Hospital has pushed us to this final step simply to protect the corporate coffers, i.e., their money. Does that surprise you, perhaps make you uneasy, to think of a hospital, not as a gathering of selfless healers, but as a run-of-the-mill, for-profit corporation that exists in the end for one purpose—to make money? They're just better at hiding it than Bank of America.

"I want you to know that it is a big deal to get a medical malpractice case this far in the justice system. The bulk of these cases, when presented to malpractice lawyers, are refused as meritless. A percentage of the cases that pass that first step, to find a willing lawyer, are dismissed by that court-mandated panel of experts I mentioned a moment ago. Of the very few that pass the review by experts, some are dismissed by a judge as without merit when the case reaches superior court. Most of the rare cases that survive the winnowing process are settled without the need to empanel fourteen citizens. Like I said, it is a big deal to get this far. But Dr. Sabrina Maddingly's chronicle cleared all those major hurdles. Her case is for real, and so horrifying, Steven King could hardly come up with a tale so nightmarish."

Harrison Jennings glanced surreptitiously at the defense table. Rhonda Uft's head was turned directly toward the jury, eyes rolled so far up, Jennings chuckled to himself that she should audition for the *Night of the Living Dead.* He looked back at the jury and went on. "So, let's go back to Thanksgiving Eve two years ago. Dr. Maddingly, a 30-year-old, previously healthy woman with a Doctor of Psychology degree from Harvard, got an early start on the Thanksgiving meal she was preparing for twenty-some of her husband's fellow high school teachers. Putting the turkey in the oven at around 8:30, she bent over and felt an excruciating pain in her back. Her husband, Mike, a local high school teacher and head football coach," he stopped and gestured toward him, "took her to a local walk-in clinic. The doctor, who you will have the privilege, and I mean privilege, of hearing from during this trial, examined Dr. Maddingly methodically. She quite astutely sent Dr. Maddingly and her husband to the

Defendant Hospital to see if the pain was a result of an ectopic pregnancy, more commonly referred to as a tubal pregnancy. If you don't know much about tubal pregnancies, like most of us, don't worry; we will be learning a lot about them from the witnesses we are going to ask help us ferret out the truth. You will be impressed by how the walk-in clinic doctor made her diagnosis, alone, late at night, without all the fancy tests available to the doctors at the Defendant Hospital.

"But what is critical to note at this point is that Dr. Maddingly walked on her own, without help, without a cane, without a wheelchair, into that small clinic on Thanksgiving Eve two years ago. Then she walked out on her own to their car and was driven to the Defendant Hospital by her husband Mike, where she walked, unaided, downstairs into the hospital lab for a pregnancy test, then walked, unaided, across the hospital into the radiology department for an ultrasound. Then she walked back across the hospital, several hundred feet, into the waiting room of the emergency department, where sat down and waited for medical care. It was the last time she ever took a step, the last time she ever would."

When Jennings paused, the jury's gaze shot again to Sabrina, though her head was turned toward the wall. The lawyer's voice hardened, and all eyes snapped back to him. "She took that seat in the emergency room and waited. And she waited. Sometime between when she sat down on her own for the last time in her life, and the hour and a half later when she was finally brought back to the treatment area, the tubal pregnancy ruptured, burst—the worst-case scenario that the original clinic doctor feared might happen. You will hear how unlikely there was any internal bleeding when she reached the hospital; how unlikely there was any internal bleeding when she had her blood drawn at the lab; how unlikely it was that there was any internal bleeding when she had her ultrasound; and how unlikely it was there was any internal bleeding when she walked, on her own steam, into the emergency room, when there was still time to save her, lots of time.

"Unbelievably, a random hospital employee, a receptionist going off duty, was walking to the restroom a final time, when she passed Dr. Maddingly and her husband. The young woman was shocked to see how pale Dr. Maddingly had suddenly become. She had walked by the Maddinglys several times during her shift, impressed by the gentility with which they held each other. She, not the people trained, paid, and trusted to be medical specialists, realized the sudden change. She was the one who raised the alarm and urged that Dr. Maddingly be brought into the treatment area of the ER. It was, though, too late."

He stopped and gazed away from the jury for a moment. When he restarted, his voice softened. "A little bit about Dr. Sabrina Maddingly. She used to drive to work from Evanston every morning, fighting the traffic like the rest of us—on her own, in a normal car—then parked in the staff lot at the University of Washington. She did not have a handicap sticker, or even a close-in parking pass. Why would she? Just like the rest of the employees, she walked, carrying a briefcase and a purse, a quarter of a mile to the hospital complex. When she got there, she chose to ignore the elevator and, daily climbed three flights of stairs, without the use of a walker or cane, to her office at the University of Washington Hospital, where she was an Assistant Professor of Psychology." He looked directly at her. "She had been able to walk completely normally for all of her life.

"In fact, ladies and gentlemen of the jury, she is now on indefinite, unpaid, leave from the University of Washington, not only because she can't get to work, but because the stroke she suffered at Defendant Hospital caused a major personality change, just like what happens to most people who suffer severe strokes. She tires so easily, she has to sleep fourteen hours a day. She can barely use the bathroom and cannot bathe on her own. Their medical insurance company has stopped covering visiting nurse and home physical therapy services. The insurance executives shake their heads and tell the Maddinglys to apply for Social Security. That, ladies and gentlemen, is an insult. Social Security would barely cover Dr. Maddingly's medications, medications she never took before the nightmare at Mitchie-Sterling Hospital. Would Social Security help them save their home, that is now up for sale, to meet their unending medical bills?

"But, Ladies and Gentlemen, that is not the point of this lawsuit. Let's back up and talk about that night again. I want you to know who you are going to be seeing on the witness stand. I want you to know that, despite the fact that we are suing a number of doctors, there are some superb physicians in practice right here in our community. You will meet Dr. Khai Weathersby, the first doctor the Maddinglys saw that night. She had just finished a twelve-hour day when the Maddinglys came to her for help. She did not turn them away, despite the fact that her clinic was already long closed. No, she saw them and sent them to the hospital where Dr. Maddingly's life could potentially be saved. A lesser doctor would not have opened the clinic door after hours; a lesser doctor would have ignored them, snuck out the back door, and driven home. But, no, she didn't. She waited in her clinic until Thanksgiving morning, by the telephone, to make sure Dr. Maddingly had all of the necessary tests done on an emergency basis. In other words, she sat there prodding the hospital to do what was necessary to save her patient.

"When Mr. Maddingly called Dr. Weathersby from the hospital and told her that his wife had a strongly positive pregnancy test, Dr. Weathersby sent them for an ultrasound to see just where that pregnancy was located. She spoke personally with the radiologist, who told her he did not see a fetus in the uterus. With a strongly positive pregnancy test, that meant a baby was growing, but not where it was supposed to. Dr. Weathersby knew well it was almost certainly in the fallopian tube. That, ladies and gentlemen, is a tubal pregnancy. Again, don't worry, you will be experts on all of this before we are done.

"So, Dr. Weathersby told both of them to walk to the emergency room and sit there until she, Dr. Weathersby, could call the Defendant emergency room doctor and tell him a seriously ill patient was sitting in his waiting room.

"And now we are at the point where this malpractice case against Defendant Mitchie-Sterling Hospital and its employees begins. I bring to your attention the name of one of the specific defendants in this case, Peter Cardozo, M.D., who is employed by, and on the staff of Defendant Mitchie-Sterling Hospital. He was the lone doctor working in the emergency room that night. Dr. Weathersby and Defendant Cardozo had never met and never spoken or had professional or personal contact before the early morning call of that Thanksgiving Day.

"Though they were both medical doctors, both from American medical schools, both from residency programs in the United States, it will be pretty clear to see that not all doctors who take the Hippocratic Oath, and swear to treat all sick people, take that pledge equally sincerely."

Harrison Jennings looked quickly at Rhonda Uft, who twitched as if she was about to raise her hand but settled back in her chair, her expression souring.

Jennings went on. "Well, Dr. Weathersby called the emergency room, and after two dropped calls, and despite having made the clerk understand she was a medical doctor referring a desperately ill patient, was denied access to Dr. Cardozo—twice. On the third try, Dr. Weathersby's fourth call to the ER,

Defendant Cardozo was so angry, he grabbed the phone from the clerk and began a diatribe against Dr. Khai Weathersby, who he knew to be a fellow physician.

"You will hear from that clerk that Defendant Cardozo's language was, to be frank, ladies and gentlemen of the jury, unprofessional. And that's being generous. It was profanity-laced, and I mean real profanity, the kind you might hear during a drunken brawl down in Pioneer Square. Don't believe me? Wait until we present some of the witnesses to Defendant Cardozo's side of the call.

"Now, you will likely be presented with all manner of excuses by Defendant Mitchie-Sterling Hospital's attorneys that Defendant Cardozo was very busy that night—patients with heart attacks flying around all over the place. Is that sufficient cause for Defendant Cardozo to refer to Dr. Weathersby using the 'C' word, out loud and directly to Dr. Weathersby?

"Again, this is despite having never heard of each other, and despite the fact both were medical doctors, and were talking about the same, very ill patient, who, by the way, was still sitting—ignored, unattended, dying—thirty feet away in Defendant Cardozo's waiting room. This is also despite the fact that only a single emergency room doctor is on duty at Defendant Hospital on the great majority of nights, especially major holidays, when ER traffic is expected to be very low. There was no one else to field that call. He was the man.

"We will show you, by presenting witnesses, that this behavior is endemic to Defendant Mitchie-Sterling Hospital's corporate culture. You will hear from employees who refuse to," he raised his fingers to make quote marks, "'take it anymore.' Why, Ladies and Gentlemen, has Defense Counsel not objected to this claim? It's simple: because these are the statements employees made under oath during their depositions for this court case. You will hear their claims that they were urged by the Defendant Hospital to consider very carefully what they were going to say before this court. You will be able to make up your own minds about why these potential witnesses were counseled to do that by their employer, the Defendant Mitchie-Sterling Hospital, before their depositions.

"You will hear, I'm afraid in graphic detail, what transpired the night Dr. Maddingly was finally treated in the emergency room by Defendant Cardozo. You will hear from an eyewitness that the bag of blood for a transfusion intended to raise Dr. Maddingly's crashing blood pressure wound up sprayed all over the walls and the floor of the operating room. Not a single drop of it got into Dr.

Maddingly. In fact, under Defendant Cardozo's deficient care that night, not a single drop of blood or any other life-saving IV fluid got into his dying patient. You will hear evidence from others that Defendant Cardozo was simply unable to start an IV in the arms, or even a central line IV. An emergency room doctor who can't start central line IV!"

Rhonda Uft jumped from her seat so aggressively, her chair slid backwards and tipped onto the floor. She hissed, "Objection, Your Honor. First, Counsel is referring to Mr. Maddingly, who is not a medical professional. This has been ruled on in pretrial motions. By your order, Plaintiff's husband will only be allowed to testify about the circumstances that brought the Plaintiff to the hospital, and only that he witnessed the ER staff moving rapidly to save his wife's life. Counsel is suggesting that the jury will be allowed to draw conclusions about the medical specifics of what he thinks he saw. He has no idea what that wonderful staff was trying to do when they saved his wife's life. He's a schoolteacher, not a doctor. I want this nipped in the bud.

"And number two: 'Blood all over the walls,' is clearly hyperbole. A treatment bay in an emergency room was never intended to be neat as a pin. Everyone knows and understands that speed is the primary assignment in the ER—neatness falls far down the list of priorities. They were trying to save her life, which they did.

"And, third, Dr. Cardozo started several IVs in the Plaintiff that night. I object to Counsel's characterization."

Before Judge Galanter could rule on the objection, Harrison Jennings interjected. "Beg your pardon, Your Honor. I never mentioned Mr. Maddingly testifying. Now that Defense Counsel has introduced the matter, I move to allow Mr. Maddingly to testify in full."

"Mr. Jennings, overruled. This is opening arguments. I will allow both of you latitude. And you will have ample opportunity to request the court reconsider the limits of Mr. Maddingly's testimony. And, Ms. Uft, your second objection is overruled. Perhaps other witnesses will comment on what the treatment area looked like. And number three is overruled. You will have ample opportunity to demonstrate the Defendant's skills and to peruse the medical record for evidence of successful procedures as the trial proceeds."

Her assistant leaned back to right the chair, but Mrs. Uft began to sit before it was in place. She stopped her fall by grasping the table, but that sent several books and folders winging from the table. Sabrina and Mike barely hid smiles.

Harrison Jennings waited, hands behind his back, swaying ever so slightly until all the items were rearranged, with deliberation, on Rhonda Uft's desk. "Thank you, Your Honor." He turned to the jury. "Since the night Dr. Maddingly suffered her stroke, she has been hospitalized for meningitis, several episodes of pneumonia, and admission after admission for severe depression."

Jennings paused again, straightened his jacket, and turned to the jury, his toughened expression marshalling their attention. "Ladies and Gentlemen of the jury, let's change directions for a moment. Let me present the most important question in this case. That Dr. Maddingly suffered a stroke at the Defendant Hospital, and that her present condition is a direct result of that stroke, is not in question. What the Defendant Hospital will use to try and convince you of their innocence is that Dr. Maddingly was so sick when she earned her PhD at Harvard, was so sick when she took a job at the University of Washington, was so sick the night she was preparing Thanksgiving dinner for twenty-some friends, was so sick when she walked into the hospital and then into the ER on her own, that anything that happened in the hospital was her fault.

"Let's get the cards on the table so you don't get blindsided by what you're going to be exposed to by the Defendant Hospital's lawyers; or should I say pummeled, if you will, by Defense Counsel with distortions..."

Rhonda Uft was on her feet again. "Objection, your Honor. Again, I respect that this is opening arguments, but characterizing me or my clients as professionals who would twist facts is prejudicial and inflammatory. I do not intend to distort a single detail to the jury. They will be presented strictly with the truth. And I will not allow my clients and their witnesses to distort anything. Let's get that straight up front."

The judge peered down at Harrison Jennings. "Sustained. As I said, I will allow latitude, sir, but statements denigrating the truthfulness of Defense Counsel, without basis, are not going to be tolerated. The jury is to disregard Mr. Jennings' characterization of defense Counsel's or her clients' integrity."

Jennings nodded sharply. "Yes, Your Honor. Well, ladies and gentlemen, as I said, I want you to hear the story from me first. Let's get the truth out now so that you can make a just decision.

"Dr. Maddingly had a weak left arm before her treatment at Mitchie-Sterling Hospital on the night of 25th November. Notice I say weak, not paralyzed. Dr. Maddingly was able, for all her life until that night when she entered the Defendant Hospital, to use her left hand to steady herself, to cook meals for her family, to drive! Why, just hours before this tragedy, she was holding a twenty-pound turkey in a heavy Pyrex dish, standing straight up on her own before bending forward to place it into the oven. She can do not one of those things now.

"But that is just the beginning. Dr. Maddingly wasn't confined to a wheelchair before Thanksgiving Eve two years ago. Oh, no. In fact, she had never been in a wheelchair in her life, not ever held a cane or touched a walker in her life. Why? Simple: she had normal legs, no limp, no weakness, none of it until the night she was admitted to the Mitchie-Sterling Hospital. She could run, ride a bicycle, ice skate, dance, climb stairs, even go bowling. I hope you will remember that above anything else you might hear during this trial.

"Let me tell you what the defense is going to argue. You will hear Ms. Uft tell you that all of Dr. Maddingly's problems stem from a defect in her spinal column. Yes, she was born with a small hole in her spinal column. And who cares? It was a stable problem, one that had not changed a single iota for the three decades since her birth. And that spinal problem had nothing on earth to do with Defendant Cardozo's ability to start a life-saving, stroke-preventing IV. And, I say again, we will prove, with Dr. Maddingly's hospital records, that Defendant Cardozo did not start a single IV in Dr. Maddingly that night. Period. Her spinal problem had nothing to do with letting her bleed until she was just a just a fraction of an inch from death. There is not a single thing wrong with Dr. Maddingly's veins. Nothing!

"Look, we all have internal problems—every one of us. Is that grounds to ignore a patient and leave them in your waiting room until they nearly bleed to death, all because you don't like the doctor who sent the patient to you?"

The jurors' faces perked.

"That's right. Just wait until you hear." He paused. "And, Ladies and Gentlemen, finally, you will learn how hard the Maddinglys sought to settle this matter without the need for a trial and to impanel jurors for a matter that could have been resolved amicably and fairly. But, of course, the hospital did not want to pay for its mistakes, and they may get away with it, for they have all the money in the world for lawyers and appeals...and here we are. I hope you won't allow a second injustice to befall the Maddinglys."

CHAPTER THIRTY-NINE

G alanter looked down. "Ms. Uft, your opening remarks please."
Rhonda Uft marched center stage, halfway between the judge and the jury. Though her hair had been frosted, the very back was marked with uneven patches of dusty gray. She wore a cylindrical black top over a cylindrical black skirt that extended to her ankles—it made her appear more a can of Raid than one of Seattle's highest paid jurists. She nearly genuflected to the judge then turned to the jury and smiled plastically. "Ladies and gentlemen, you have heard from Mr. Jennings that the Plaintiff in this case suffered medical problems that began out of the clear blue on the unfortunate night of November 25th, two years ago. He alluded to the Defendant as a perfectly healthy woman descended upon by an uncaring, incompetent team of callous health workers who conspired to destroy her life." She stopped and rolled her eyes. "May we take a step back, please? You already know that isn't true. We will provide you with more than sufficient evidence to prove that the Plaintiff was, unfortunately, born with many congenital deformities; some of which had already manifested themselves, and some that only became evident as a result of her tubal pregnancy. This is the cause of her unfortunate state, not the exceptional efforts made by Mitchie-Sterling Hospital to save her life.

"All her present problems grew out of the treatment she was provided that night? Quite the contrary. Plaintiff's Counsel has already stood before you and admitted to a major, major preexisting problem. Yes, he tried to sneak that by as a trivial little annoyance; but a hanging arm since birth, one the Plaintiff could not use to lift to brush her teeth, use a knife to cut her food, brush her hair, or even lift a piece of paper? Please, that is hardly trivial. Her birth defect was devastating quarter of a century before Mitchie-Sterling Hospital saved her life. I promise each and every one of you folks that we will provide expert testimony to make your job as triers of fact quite straightforward. Mitchie-Sterling Hospital provided Dr. Maddingly with, if anything, superior care."

She stopped and straightened her shoulders. "But her underlying birth defects were only part of what has forced us together. I am about to present you with the most important factor in this trial. And it is painful to say this, but the Plaintiff's own husband willingly delayed bringing his wife to the hospital. You'll see."

She turned and looked at Mike Maddingly. "You know, guilt is a funny thing. It can be so painful, it often makes the shamed person harden their position that it was the other guy's fault; harden it to the point that they will force the local government you're paying for with your taxes into an incredibly expensive trial, with the inconveniencing of fourteen fellow citizens, just to escape responsibility, and maybe make some money for themselves as a bonus. Then, as Plaintiff's Counsel told you, if their side loses, they can blame it on the fact that the Defendant had more money for attorneys. That exonerates the lawyer, but most importantly, the guilty husband walks away again blaming someone else, maybe the judge and jury, for his awful mistake.

"That deliberate delay on the part of the husband, combined with the Plaintiff's unfortunate birth defects, Ladies and Gentlemen of the jury, is why the Plaintiff is confined to a wheelchair and we are here today. Period.

"Well, you might say, we are talking about modern medicine, with all of its miracles. We will show that medicine remains an inexact science, and we are not yet to the point that physicians and hospitals can correct every defect caused by a patient, her husband, or her parents' lifestyle.

"That is why we have in this country what we call the standard of care. I'm sure all of you know very well that means the level at which the average, prudent doctor in a given community would be expected to practice. It is how similarly qualified practitioners would have managed the patient's care under the same or similar circumstances. In our case, here in this court, the Plaintiff must establish that standard of care. The burden falls on them to do so. And then they have to prove to you, the jury, that the standard of care was not reached. Again, you are the triers of fact. You must listen to each witness's account and decide if it is fact, a guess, a simple mistake, or perhaps even a false statement.

"Though we don't have to, we will evaluate the care provided to this Plaintiff with the care expected, not just locally, but that expected at the most famous hospitals in the nation. I daresay, the care for a tubal pregnancy provided the Plaintiff here in McKinley, Washington, was the same as it would have been for the First Lady in Washington DC. The Plaintiff received that level of care, if not higher.

"Again, every reasonable adult knows that doctors do not cure every illness. Doctors do not have the ability to take back thirty years of aging and questionable life choices made by patients and their parents. We will share with you some of those choices. And, more importantly, doctors do not have the ability to erase congenital, that is, birth defects such as those we will prove to you were unfortunately suffered by the Plaintiff. No doctor or hospital will produce a brand-new person upon discharge, and, sometimes, the best a doctor can do for a patient, given the circumstances Mitchie-Sterling Hospital faced, is save her life. Why, she's has even spoken of returning to her important work as a health provider at the University of Washington. In fact, this is the best outcome anyone could've hoped for.

"And that's all I am going to say. I will not talk to hear myself speak. I've spelled out the truth.

"Thank you."

CHAPTER FORTY

Judge Galanter peered down at Harrison Jennings and muttered, "You may call your first witness."

Khai Weathersby took the oath from the bailiff. Jennings began softly, gently, and with a warm smile. "Dr. Weathersby, please state and spell your full name for the court." Jennings continued, "Please give the jury a list of your educational degrees. Why don't you start with your undergraduate degree?"

"I graduated from the United States Military Academy at West Point and spent eight years on active duty as a United States Army aviation officer. I then attended and graduated from Yale Medical School and completed a three-year residency in internal medicine at Massachusetts General Hospital in Boston."

"Was that a Harvard residency program?"

She answered softly, "Yes."

Jennings smiled toward the jury. "That's very impressive, Dr. Weathersby. I have to ask, while in the Army, did you spend any time in combat in the Middle East?"

"Yes, sir, I did."

"Where was that?"

"I did one tour each in Iraq and Afghanistan."

"Did you receive any medals for your service?"

"Yes, sir."

"And the medals you earned, Doctor?"

"The Distinguished Flying Cross."

"Is that considered fairly high in the ranking of medals? I mean, is that for bravery in the face of enemy action?"

Rhonda Uft looked up without standing. "Objection. I believe we're here to discuss Dr. Weathersby's medical findings on the night in question, not to be bewildered with a military cavalcade."

"Overridden. I believe this goes to the credibility of the witness as well as her quality as person. I want to hear it. Go on, Dr. Weathersby."

"I can only say that it is not awarded frequently. It is granted to a member of an aircrew who distinguished him or herself during combat operations. As far as I'm concerned, it was my crew who deserved the DFC."

"Thank you, Dr. Weathersby, and thank you for your service. I do have one more nonmedical question, and I hope the court will bear with me. Your first name is Khai. That is an unusual name, and I wonder if you would mind telling the court where it comes from."

"My father, who is a medical doctor now, was a combat officer in Vietnam. But he spent the second half of his tour living in a primitive village as a civil affairs officer. One night, during an awful battle, he and the village chief, with whom he had become great friends, were under bombardment by the Vietnamese communist forces. He promised the village chief that if they survived the night, he would name his first child after him. The man's name was Vu Van Khai."

"Thank you again, Doctor. Now, is it correct that you were the sole physician on duty at the Evanston Medical Center on Thanksgiving Eve two years ago?

"Yes, sir."

"In the carrying out of your normal duties, did you see Dr. Sabrina Maddingly that night?"

"Yes, sir."

"What was your first impression of Dr. Maddingly that evening?"

"Dr. Maddingly appeared to be in moderate distress."

"What does that mean?"

"Well, she was hunched somewhat forward with her hands on her abdomen."

"Let me stop you there. Were both of her arms on her abdomen?"

"Yes."

"Did you place her arms there?"

228

"No."

"Did her husband place them there or, perhaps, your nurse?"

"No."

"Thank you. Go on, please."

"Dr. Maddingly's face was clearly tense, though she made no verbal complaints of pain. She was able to walk without difficulty. She remained fairly quiet when I questioned her about her pain but was completely alert, cooperative, and was an excellent historian."

"What do you mean by 'historian'?"

"That means she remembered her medical history in great detail, easily providing all the information I needed to continue treating her."

"What did she tell you about her medical history?"

"That she was born with a deformity in her spinal cord that had caused her to have a weak left arm and hand."

"Let me stop you there. Did she report any weakness in her legs at any time in her life?"

"No."

"Did she report any difficulty speaking at any time in her life?"

"No."

"Did she report any history of clinical depression?"

"No."

"Did she inform you that she had had a recent physical exam?"

"Yes."

"Tell us about that."

"That night, she told me about the only two medical problems she had. First about the arm, and second that she was told she could not conceive, but she had never had single medical test to determine if that was true. After seeing Dr. Maddingly that night, I gathered her prior medical history and went over it very carefully. There were essentially no records, aside from the usual GYN records all young women have."

"Were any abnormalities noted?"

"Again, the patient reported that she was told by a nurse at Mass General Hospital in Boston that she could not conceive. I did not find that in the sparse records from that hospital. I did see in those records that she was judged to have two-plus out of five weakness in her left upper extremity—that is, her left arm and hand. No weakness was noted, as I said before, elsewhere."

"What does two-plus out of five mean?"

"We rate weakness on a scale of zero to five. Five is totally normal strength. Zero is no muscle contraction at all. Two is active movement, but you can't resist gravity. So, you can wiggle your fingers or even move your wrist a bit if the arm is hanging at your side. Three is active movement against gravity, so you could move your hand, but couldn't, for example, lift something as heavy as a coffee cup. You might be able to raise the arm a foot or two to wave. Dr. Maddingly was between two and three according to the hospital in Boston. We call that two-plus."

"Meaning that she could lift paper?"

"Easily."

Jennings glanced sideways at Rhonda Uft. "Glad we have that off the table. Now, did you review any other medical chart notes regarding Dr. Maddingly's prior medical history?"

"Yes. Three months before the night in question, Dr. Maddingly had a physical at the University of Washington in anticipation of her new position as a staff psychologist. Aside from the weakness in her left arm, which, by the way, was rated as three by the doctor at the University, the exam was totally normal."

"Let me ask, Doctor, why would they rate her strength higher than they did at Mass General?"

"Most likely, it was just a different doctor doing the evaluation. Like in most of medicine, judgment is a factor you can't predict. Really makes no difference, two-plus or three. There's even a three minus some compulsive doctors have invented. Basically, she was between two and three, and closer to three."

"Have you examined her recently?"

"Yes."

"When was the most recent evaluation?"

"Two weeks ago."

"What would you rate her strength at this point?"

"One, at best."

"Which means, again?"

"Perhaps the slightest flicker of movement."

"Did you examine her on the night you first saw her?"

"No, not specifically."

"What do you mean?"

"I was far too busy dealing with her ectopic pregnancy to do a neurological exam."

"Do you, though, have any sense of the strength in her left arm and hand that night?"

"I can say that she was able to help herself onto the exam table without assistance. And then I saw her use her left arm to steady herself on the table as she lay back for the exam."

"What about her ability to walk?"

"She was fully mobile in the office."

"Did she limp?"

"No."

"Was her speech slurred?"

"Not at all."

"And did she have a history of depression or any mental disease?"

"On the contrary, she had been touted by the professors in her residency at Harvard, and her mentor at the National Institutes of Health, where she did her fellowship, that she was the best resident and..."

"Objection, stating facts not in evidence."

Galanter spoke unemotionally, though there was the slightest upward roll of his eyes. "Sustained."

Jennings pulled the various letters from his binder, the ones speaking of Sabrina's superior work ethic, her exceptional intelligence, and her bedside manner. After another thirty minutes vaporized with the documents being admitted into evidence, Jennings had Khai read them to the jury. Then he asked her to read the psychiatric notes by the hospital staff and those from Dr. Darling. That frittered away another forty-five minutes.

When done, Jennings shook his head subtly and spoke with a finality, as if he was sure that chapter was finally put to rest. He knew, though, it was far from over. "Okay, let's talk more about her level of pain that night." He paused, waiting for Rhonda Uft to object and go back to the psychiatric history, but the woman was silent, smug, having fooled the old man into breaking his own momentum. "Well, Doctor, let's get back to the meat of the trial. You noted in your deposition that Dr. Maddingly described her abdominal pain as coming and going but never leaving completely. Is that correct, and what does that mean?"

"Yes, sir. By the time she left, though, she was actually feeling much better."

"Is that typical of someone who is already bleeding?"

"I am not an obstetrician, but in general terms, pain that comes and goes is not typical of a bleed that is progressing. And at the time, we weren't thinking about bleeding, especially when the pain faded to next to nothing in a few minutes. Every one of us has had belly pain that causes us to double over for a couple of seconds and then just fades away."

"Well, let's get back to the level of pain she was experiencing at the time you first saw her. What did you find when you examined her?"

"She was very tender over the left adnexa, the left portion of her pelvis where the ovary and fallopian are found." She pointed to her own abdomen.

"Did that mean she had strained her back?"

"No. I felt that Dr. Maddingly was suffering from a problem in the abdomen or pelvis. Could have been gas in the intestine, most likely; perhaps a twisted ovary, less likely; or even a tubal pregnancy on the left, which would have been down the list of possibilities, but had to be considered."

"So, you didn't feel that Dr. Maddingly was in imminent danger of rupturing a blood vessel and dying?"

Rhonda Uft growled, "Objection. Leading."

"Sustained."

"Then let me ask, what were you fearing at this point?"

"Well, I had to imagine the worst-case scenario—that's what doctors do. So, I worried about the unlikely chance that this was a tubal pregnancy."

"Doctor, were you afraid that Dr. Maddingly would die if she didn't receive immediate care?"

"No, because she was quite stable when she left my clinic."

"Then why did you ask her to go to the hospital?"

"First, I needed to find out if it actually was a tubal pregnancy. They can only do that at the hospital. And, second, to be sure that Dr. Maddingly would be in capable hands if a rupture and bleeding was imminent."

"Maybe this would be a good time for you to tell us about tubal pregnancies: what they are, how they occur, and the danger associated with them."

"Yes, sir." She stood and walked to an easel Jennings' secretary had unfolded, half facing the judge, half toward the jury. Rhonda Uft waited until Khai began speaking before coming to her feet and objecting that she could not see the exhibit.

Judge Galanter sighed, "Bailiff, please position the exhibit to allow Defense Counsel a better view."

There were several adjustments before Rhonda Uft grumped, "I suppose that will have to do." The easel was, by the end of the exercise, canted mostly away from the jurors. It forced them to crane their necks. Khai's gentle expression, though, did not change. She turned the easel back toward the jury and drew the female reproductive organs. First, she sketched the ovaries—the size and shape of big almonds—then the thin, winding fallopian tubes that led down from the ovaries to the plum-sized uterus. She traced the normal course of a ripened egg erupting from the ovary, floating into the fimbriae—nature's funnel—its filamentous fingers arising from the top of the fallopian tubes, rippling constantly to gather the egg. Slowly, she traced the ovum's path as it started down the first third of the fallopian tube, where it would meet the sperm if a pregnancy was to be consummated. She explained that in the normal course of events, the fertilized egg would, days later, leave that spot to course down the rest of fallopian tube into the uterus, where the fetus would be nurtured for nine months.

When Khai finished speaking, she turned the easel toward Rhonda Uft, pointed at the path of the egg, and waited for the woman to take a cursory glance at the exhibit. When the attorney looked down at her papers, Khai shifted the diagram back toward the judge and jury.

With that, Rhonda Uft coughed, though Khai ignored her, as did the judge. Khai sketched again with her Magic Marker, explaining, "As it turns out, for Dr. Maddingly, hers was a tubal pregnancy, which means the fetus became locked in the fallopian tube." She drew a small pocket of dividing cells, high up in the tube, and added, "In this case, the tiny, early fetus never made it down to the uterus. By the way, this process had been going on for several weeks. And let me assure you, there was no way for her to know. The first hint that she was pregnant was when the fetus grew so large, it began to erode through the tube. That may or may not have hurt at first, but as it grew even more, it caused the tube to stretch to its limits. That brought about the tearing of blood vessels, just a few tiny ones at the beginning, not enough to cause a life-threatening loss of blood, but maybe enough to cause some pain, and yet maybe not. A little bit of internal bleeding often goes unnoticed by a patient. And even when the bleeding increases, the pain may come and go, no different than bowel gas. The pain from bleeding or bowel gas or stomach flu is the same, no matter the cause. It's the body's way of telling us there's a problem and to look into it. The point is, she was not bleeding seriously when she came to my clinic."

Jennings put up his hand. "Doctor, how can you be sure?"

"First of all, her blood pressure, pulse, and coloring were fine. Next, her thinking was crystal clear, and she was able to move quite normally."

"Let me stop you there. What was her blood pressure?"

"First time I took, it a little bit before 9 P.M, it was 132 over 88, and her pulse was 88."

"What did that tell you?"

"Normal blood pressure and pulse, especially for someone in pain. Certainly no evidence that she was bleeding internally."

Jennings posed, "What was your medical impression at that moment?"

"Well, even if it was the worst-case scenario, a tubal, in the literature you find that there is generally time after the onset of pain before the major rupture, that is, before the tube bursts open and the serious bleeding starts. Problem, is, you never know how much time.

"But let's take a step back for a moment and examine why there is such a danger of mortal bleeding in the first place. Don't forget, nature provides a lot of blood vessels, a lot of blood vessels, to a growing fetus. They're there to feed it because it grows so incredibly fast. Nature doesn't wait until there is a pregnancy to add new blood vessels, or even until the fetus is too large for its present blood supply. It's always ahead of the game; nature sort of keeps the pantry overstocked, far more blood vessels, that is food, available for the baby than it needs at that moment. Another part of the miracle.

"As I said, at the time I first saw Dr. Maddingly, I thought about all the possibilities that could have caused that sudden onset of pain. After asking questions, that is taking a history and examining her, I felt the most likely worst-case scenario was a tubal pregnancy. Of course, I wasn't a hundred percent sure, so I sent her to the hospital for tests."

Jennings put up his hand. "Doctor, please tell us what you would have done if you believed the bleeding had started or that it would be a matter of minutes before it did?"

"Small clinics don't have blood for transfusion. But if blood is leaking at a fair rate, you need to put *something* back into the bloodstream, at least temporarily; so I would have started an IV, added saline as fast as needed—

always careful not to overload the heart—put her on oxygen, called for an ambulance, and ridden with Dr. Maddingly to the hospital."

"Thank you. Dr. Weathersby, let me ask if you were certain that the fallopian tube had not ruptured and was not bleeding appreciably when you last saw Dr. Maddingly that evening?"

"No, sir, I cannot be absolutely certain. No one can. However, a very accurate test, short of surgery to look inside and see, is to watch the blood pressure and pulse. Dr. Maddingly had a normal blood pressure and pulse half an hour apart, which led me to believe, if it was a tubal pregnancy, that there was still time before the situation became critical. But, again, I did not know how much time, so I sent her to the hospital."

Jennings asked, "Let's go over what you had the Maddinglys do when they reached the hospital."

"As the Maddinglys left my clinic, I made several phone calls to Mitchie-Sterling Hospital in McKinley. The first was to the blood test laboratory. I asked for an emergency serum pregnancy test and for an immediate call back on the result."

"Then what did you do?"

"I called Radiology at Mitchie-Sterling Hospital in McKinley and asked them to be on alert with a radiologist present to do a stat, that means immediate, ultrasound if the pregnancy test was positive. If it was positive, it meant there was a fetus growing somewhere. An ultrasound of the pelvis would determine if the fetus was in the uterus or somewhere else. They were to call me back immediately with the result. While Mrs. Maddingly was walking toward the radiology department, I received a telephone call from Mitchie-Sterling Hospital laboratory indicating that the serum pregnancy test was strongly positive."

"What did that mean."

"Only that she was pregnant. It did not tell us anything about where that pregnancy was growing. I had to find out."

"What did you do next?"

"We went ahead and asked for the stat ultrasound."

"When you say 'we,' who do you mean? Was it up to the lab tech?"

"Sorry. No, it was me."

"What did the ultrasound show?"

"The radiologist called half an hour later. He told me he saw no products of conception, that is, no evidence of a developing baby inside the uterus. Unfortunately, the ultrasound was not sensitive enough to see a tiny embryo in the fallopian tube. He did tell me, actually warn me, though, that he thought there might have been a thickening in the left fallopian tube, just where I thought I felt a mass when I did my exam hours before. He simply was not sure."

"Let's stop there. Was there anything else the radiologist told you?"

"Yes. He said he could see no blood in the pelvis. He allowed that there might be a scant amount hiding behind some organ, but if it was there, it was meaningless. Certainly nothing was seen to indicate a ruptured tubal pregnancy."

"Did that surprise you?"

"No, not at all. As I said, her blood pressure was normal, she was walking around normally, so there had not yet been a full rupture and catastrophic bleeding."

"Wait, Doctor. How do we know that her blood pressure remained normal when she first got to the hospital and during the ultrasound?"

"Well, I was surprised to hear Dr. Maddingly's blood pressure was not taken at the lab or in radiology, but, in both places, she was walking, talking, and looked quite normal. I felt it was safe to tell the Maddinglys to remain calm and simply walk to the emergency room. There seemed no need to declare an emergency and have a stat team descend on Dr. Maddingly, dump her on a gurney, and pull out the cardioversion paddles. I've seen it many, many a time..."

Rhonda Uft roared, "There is no evidence whatsoever that the professional staff at Mitchie-Sterling would have," she rolled her eyes and raised her fingers in quotes, "'dumped' any patient anywhere."

Khai Weathersby, no longer unsettled by Rhonda Uft's theatrics, observed the woman's fingers trembling when she raised them above her head. There was also the slightest hesitation before she brought them down. Khai waited for a rest tremor, but Rhonda Uft had seen Khai's eyes on her and quickly tightened her hands into fists against her belly. That served to extinguish all quivering.

Khai asked herself what she would do if she became convinced Uft had early Parkinson's. Would she call the woman, perhaps write a note to urge she seek treatment, or just let it be? Her reverie, though, was extinguished by Galanter's grumble. "Doctor, please tell us only what you saw and heard that night. Thankyou."

She startled but quickly answered, "Yes, sir."

Harrison Jennings turned to the bench. "Excuse me, Your Honor, Dr. Weathersby is trying to explain why she made the very important decisions she did that night. If the possibility of madness in a hospital setting is in her medical experience..."

Rhonda Uft howled, "I object most strenuously to Counsel's characterization of the hospital deteriorating into," and with the fingers shooting this time toward the ceiling and immediately back down into fists, "madness."

Harrison Jennings saw out of the corner of his eye several jurors tighten in their seats, glaring at Rhonda Uft as she began to stomp toward the bench. He stood perfectly still in silence. Judge Galanter let his jaw drop in faux shock. "Madame, excuse me, but where are you going. I did not ask you to approach. Please retreat to the defense table. And, Mr. Jennings, a little less hyperbole, if you don't mind. Now, Dr. Weathersby, I might request the same restraint on your part."

"I understand, sir." She turned back to Jennings. "I was hoping Dr. Maddingly would simply walk to the ER on her own, quietly, not having her blood pressure shoot up in fear when a team of well-intentioned, ancillary employees arrived to," she paused, "help. There was clearly still time for me to call the emergency room doctor, explain the situation, and hand off the patient for calm and deliberate treatment."

Jennings spoke quietly. "Excuse me, Doctor, we'll get to your conversation with the emergency room in a minute. Let me ask you, what were you thinking at this moment?"

"Well, Dr. Maddingly was clearly pregnant, but there was no evidence that there was a pregnancy inside the uterus, and given that she had so much discomfort, particularly in the region of the left ovary and fallopian tube, it seemed pretty clear that this was a tubal pregnancy."

"Okay, but let me backtrack for a moment. Dr. Weathersby, did you say the radiologist told you there was no blood in the pelvis?"

"That is correct."

"Is there any possibility you heard the radiologist wrong?"

"None whatsoever. We talked about it for some time."

"Well, is there any possibility that the radiologist was mistaken in his verbal report to you?"

Rhonda Uft was on her feet. "Your Honor, this whole line of

questioning is a waste of the court's time. There is no way for us to prove or disprove what this witness heard from the radiologist. She can say anything she wants, given that the radiologist died within hours of the ultrasound."

As several of the jurors gasped, Khai Weathersby flushed and began to rise out of her chair, but Harrison Jennings winked at her, and she settled stiffly back into her seat. Judge Galanter growled, "Ms. Uft, overridden. Continue, Mr. Jennings."

Jennings spoke firmly. "Your Honor, given defense Counsel's innuendo regarding the witness, I would like to take another step back and reassure the jury of Dr. Weathersby's honesty. Her exceptional military serv..."

Before Galanter could look up, Rhonda Uft was on her feet. "Your Honor, just more waste of the court's time. There is no way to confirm the witness's conversation with the deceased. Period."

Galanter sighed, "Using that logic, Ms. Uft, why is there a need to swear any witness? Sometimes we need to use our sense of a person to decide the veracity of their testimony." He turned to Harrison Jennings. "Sir, there is no need to further establish the witness's credibility. The jury has sufficient maturity, intelligence, and common sense to decide on that matter for themselves. She swore to tell the truth. Let's move on."

Harrison Jennings resumed. "Well, Dr. Weathersby, the radiologist told you there was no blood. Is that corr..."

Rhonda Uft snorted, "Asked and answered."

"Sustained."

"Doctor, had there been free blood, do you think the radiologist would have put that in his report?"

"One hopes so."

Rhonda Uft stood. "Objection. Non-responsive."

"Sustained. The witness will answer the question."

Jennings nodded. "Thank you, Your Honor. Doctor, in your experience as a medical professional, do radiologists include findings of collections of blood where it's not supposed to be?"

"In my experience, they always do."

"In your experience, would a reasonable radiologist who graduated from Stanford University School of Medicine, did a full residency in radiology at the University of Washington, and was board certified with a certificate in ultrasound, have alerted you if there was free blood visible on the ultrasound examination of the abdomen?"

Rhonda Uft grumbled, "Asked and answered, leading, and assumes facts not in evidence."

"Sustained."

Jennings blurted, "Doctor, can you imagine a situation in which a finding of such importance would have been ignored by a board-certified radiologist?"

Khai answered as quickly as she could. "No."

Rhonda Uft took a deep breath to object but saw Jennings' subtle smile and remained seated.

Jennings marched to the Plaintiff's table. "Now, Doctor, I would like you to open your 3-ring binder to Exhibit H. Dr. Weathersby, have you ever seen this document before?"

"Yes, it was first given to me during my deposition.'

"What is it?"

"It is a radiology report of the ultrasound done on Dr. Sabrina Maddingly on the night of 25th November two years ago."

"You said you first saw this document, not on the night of 25th November, but at your deposition, a year and several months later?

"Yes."

"So, you are testifying that you never saw this report prior to it being handed to you by the Defendants' attorney on cross-examination during your deposition?"

"Objection, asked and answered."

"Sustained."

"Okay, Doctor, please read the findings. Ah, just the conclusions, if you please."

"Number One, there appears to be an abnormal fluid level in the pelvis. There is no apparent source of this fluid."

"Let's stop there. What does that mean?"

"Probably that there was blood in the pelvis at the time of the ultrasound."

"Why do you say 'probably'?

"I imagine it could have been ascites, that's fluid leaking out of the liver..."

"Let me stop you there. Why would Dr. Maddingly have fluid leaking from her liver?"

"She wouldn't unless she had end-stage liver disease, which she didn't and does not have, and if she had had a liver that sick to fill the belly with fluid, an abnormal liver would have shown up easily on the ultrasound."

"Where else could the fluid come from?"

"I don't know. Cancer, kidney disease, maybe congestive heart failure, all of which she did not and does not have."

"Does that mean that the only reasonable fluid in her pelvis was blood?"

"Yes."

"Which would mean, and I am asking you, does that mean the fetus had burst through the fallopian tube?"

"Very likely so."

"Okay, please go on reading."

"Number Two, no products of conception visualized in the uterus or the fallopian structures.

"Number Three, possible thickening in the left fallopian tube.

"Number Four, Bicornuate uterus."

"What is that, Doctor?"

"It simply means there are two what we call horns on top of the uterus. Means very little."

"How often is it seen?"

"They say one in two hundred women, but it's probably more common, as many women never find out they have a bicornuate uterus. They have normal pregnancies and deliveries."

"Okay, and the final note on the radiology report."

"Number Five says, 'Note: the attending physician was advised at 1:17 A.M. of these findings, and especially of the presence of a large amount of free fluid in the patient's pelvis.'"

"Doctor, did you take that call at 1:17?"

"No, I was on my way home."

"What time did you take that call?"

"I have cell phone records to confirm that call came at 2320, 11:20 hours on the evening of the 25 November. I was still at my clinic."

Jennings quickly added, "I want the jury to remember the time, 1:17 AM, when we examine Dr. Weathersby's cell phone records."

He pulled a document from a binder, had it introduced into evidence, and projected it on the courtroom screen. "Is this a certified copy of your cell phone records for that night?" He pointed to a notary seal.

"Yes."

"Dr. Weathersby, do you see your cell phone number, well, the area code for Boston, 617, and the last four digits of your number on this document."

"Yes, that is my number."

He pointed again. "Do you see this number from which your cell phone was called that night?"

"Yes."

"At what time?"

"Eleven-twenty."

Another slide went up, side by side, with Khai's telephone records. "Is this image a phone directory for Mitchie-Sterling Hospital?"

"Yes."

"Is 360-978-6260 the number listed for the Department of Radiology at Mitchie-Sterling Hospital?"

"Yes."

"So, did you receive a call from the Department of Radiology at Mitchie-Sterling Hospital at 11:20 PM?"

"Yes."

"How long did that call last?"

"Three minutes and thirty-nine seconds."

"Who were you talking to?"

"The radiologist."

"The entire time?"

"Yes."

"Were there any other calls from the hospital to you that night?"

"Yes. One, at 11:00 from the lab, to tell me the blood draw was done and that the pregnancy test was positive."

"Now, what is the number listed on the directory for the Emergency Room?"

"360-978-6266"

"How many times did you call that number?"

"Four times."

"In how long a period of time?"

"Three minutes.

"The final call lasted how long?"

"One minute and fifty-five seconds."

"With whom did you speak?"f

"A clerk who put me on hold and, finally, Dr. Cardozo."

"Had you ever before, or ever after that call, ever speak to Dr. Cardozo?"

"No."

"Oh, and by the way, where does the telephone company list the tower off which your phone pinged?"

"Evanston."

"At 1:17, where does your cell phone ping off of?"

"Between Evanston and Seattle."

"Let's go back to the radiology report. Do you see any indication that the radiologist said he, himself, informed the emergency room doctor of the results?"

"No."

"Okay, Dr. Weathersby, let me ask how you interpret that this board-certified radiologist made a statement on an official medical record that you were advised of blood in the pelvis, and you did not immediately inform the emergency room physician of that grave finding?"

"Mr. Jennings, I was never advised that there was anything abnormal on that ultrasound, other than the possible thickening of the left fallopian tube and a meaningless bifid uterus." She turned to the jury and hissed, "I hope that is very clear."

"Objection. Argumentative."

"Sustained. Please just answer the questions, Doctor."

Khai stared straight ahead inexpressively as Jennings asked with a persistent tone, "Okay, Dr. Weathersby, let me ask how you interpret that this board-certified radiologist made a statement on an official medical record that he informed you, a doctor miles away from the hospital, of blood in the pelvis, but did not immediately inform the emergency room physician of that grave finding on a patient within the confines of the hospital, when no other doctor was on duty?"

"I can't come up with an answer for that, sir."

"Well, Dr. Weathersby, is it true that physicians are extremely fearful of medical malpractice suits?"

"Yes."

"Dr. Weathersby, are you aware of a doctor or a hospital so frightened of being hauled into court for medical malpractice, that he or she or the hospital altered a medical document to make it appear as if he or she or the hospital was not guilty of having made a terrible mistake?"

The howl might have been heard as far away as Portland. "Objection! More prejudicial than probative."

Galanter summoned the lawyers. Uft barked, "Your Honor, Counsel is planting a seed that my client altered an official medical record. That assumes facts not in evidence, and," she went on, her face as tight as a heavyweight Olympic weightlifter's, "and that is not the case here!"

Galanter's demeanor hardened as he pointed a finger at Jennings. "Mr. Jennings, do you have sufficient facts to present to this court that the ultrasound report was falsified?"

"Isn't there enough already?"

Galanter shook his head. "Hardly. An error in citing the time in the middle of the night, by a doctor who had been on duty forever, doesn't cut the mustard."

Jennings nodded. "I understand your position, sir. But we will get there, and beyond a reasonable doubt, before the trial is over. You can be sure, sir."

Rhonda Uft stormed, "That's a damn lie. You've already had your own document expert declare the report was the standard form for that radiologist and for that radiology department."

"Yeah, but she couldn't determine a thing about the verity of the statements contained in the document, nor when or by whom it was dictated, or where it was printed, could she? And we can't call the radiologist as a witness, can we? Very convenient, huh?"

Galanter locked Jennings' eyes. "Well, until you present evidence to the contrary, you will cease and desist making insinuations about the hospital. Watch yourself, sir." He sputtered, "Step back," then turned to the panel. "Ladies and gentlemen of the jury, you are to understand that there is no question as to the authenticity of the radiology report. The conclusions on the document read by the witness are to be regarded as fact until proven otherwise. In other words, the jury is to disregard the suggestion that the radiology report has been altered. Continue, Mr. Jennings."

Jennings asked poker-faced, "Doctor, in your training, were you told about changing medical records to cover up your mistakes and avoid a malpractice lawsuit?"

"Yes."

"What were you taught?"

"We were warned that if a document is altered after it was originally signed, that was good enough to convict a doctor of malpractice, even if the doctor had done nothing wrong."

"Objection. Foundation. The witness is just making up the law."

"Sustained."

Harrison Jennings turned to panel and nodded, though his exceedingly subtle smile was not lost on the jurors. He began again. "Dr. Weathersby, are you absolutely sure you were not informed of the presence of fluid in Dr. Maddingly's pelvis?"

"Objection. Asked and answered."

"Sustained."

"Well, let me ask this, is it usual practice for a test to be ordered by a physician, and the results of that test not forwarded in hard copy to the requesting physician?"

"It is very unusual."

"Could one reason be that the radiology department at Mitchie-Sterling Hospital simply did not know your address?"

"By the end of the next week, the week after Thanksgiving, I am pretty sure everyone in Mitchie-Sterling Hospital knew my name, address, and probably dress size."

"Objection, Your Honor. Non-responsive, and there has been no evidence that anyone from the radiology section of Mitchie-Sterling Hospital knew the witness, or her whereabouts."

"Sustained." He sighed. "We've been at this for some time now. We will take a break and reconvene in fifteen minutes. I remind the jury that you are not to discuss this case between yourselves at any time other than when you receive the matter for deliberation. Fifteen minutes." He looked at his watch and at the bailiff, who had the court rise as the jury was sent to their room.

Khai left the stand, shoulders sagging, for the ladies' room. Jennings followed and pretended to be coming out of the men's room when she reentered the hall. He whispered to her to meet him in a corner far down the corridor. He laughed, "She's a handful, huh?"

"Guess she's just doing her job."

"Yeah, sort of like the Nazis pled at the Nuremburg Trials. 'I vas yust doink mine job, followink orderz.' Actually, all of her objections serve a purpose. First, she's throwing her weight around, trying to take command of the floor. Works sometimes. You know, trying to show the jury the other lawyer's a journeyman, doesn't know how to present a case. Keeps making mistakes. 'I have to keep correcting him.' Depends on the level of sophistication of the jury. Smart ones see through it. Average jury, who knows?

"Also, she realizes we have a good case, so she's setting the stage for an appeal. We'd win that, too, but it's just so much more time and money. Most people who are behind on their mortgage, like the Maddinglys, would agree to settle for pennies on the dollar without an appeal. And she's doing a masterful job of making the process of being in court so painful, especially with Sabrina locked in the chair all day, you'll do anything to get it over with. In the end, they save a lot of cash, maybe millions. Judge knows it, too, and he's going along with the act. He's no plaintiff's advocate, I'll tell ya—spent a career as a corporate lawyer. Got a wagonload of contributions from the auto insurance companies before the county elections. He's not going to be handing us any breaks, but so what, we've got the horses—great witnesses, like you."

"Thanks."

"Look, when she objects, let her blow her horn. In the end, it really doesn't amount to a hill of beans. But when cross-examination begins, don't let her make you mad. Just remain poker-faced, 'yes' or 'no' answers, and when you have to respond with a sentence, make it so short, she'll have to ask two or three times. That'll frustrate her. She's a charging bull, and all you have to do is step out of her way a few times, and she'll get tired. You stay cool, as if I had to tell you. You were great in your deposition. Made her mad, and she started making mistakes. She doesn't dare do that here, but she'll bare her teeth and try to scare you. I imagine you've been faced with overblown commanders in the past. In the end, they can't do a damn thing to you. We'll get her. After all is said and done, it'll be clear; she's all puff."

Mike pushed Sabrina down the hall and stopped to talk to Jennings. Sabrina looked up from her wheelchair at Khai. There was still a bit of slur to her voice. "You are one tough cookie. We're so lucky we have you..." she paused to catch her breath, and Khai reached forward to take Sabrina's hand, but Jennings shook his head subtly, though sharply. "Jury's not supposed to be able to roam the halls, but around here, don't forget this is County Superior Court—anything's possible. Lotta spies for the hospital. Dr. Weathersby, just turn around and head back into the courtroom. Mike, Sabrina, you two go in the other direction. Don't talk to anyone, not even in the bathroom, especially in the bathroom."

As Khai walked toward the courtroom, one of Rhonda Uft's associates shuffled into the doorway, head down, blocking her entry. He was pretending to be reading notes on a legal pad, and was so beefy, Khai could not see past him. He finally looked up and grunted, "Oh, excuse me, Doctor," and moved to the side. Khai saw Rhonda Uft's other associate walking away from the witness stand. When Khai took her seat, she noticed her binder was not opened to the last page from which she had read. In fact, she was looking at personal notes Harrison Jennings had made on her copy of the ultrasound report, and she recalled how frustrated he'd become trying to gather evidence that the report had been written long after the night in question.

Khai thought back to her deposition, when she was handed a mangled copy of a mangled copy of the missing radiology report. At the time Jennings subpoenaed the original report, the hospital maintained it could not be found, and the best Jennings could do was hire a document specialist to review the Xerox. The expert was able to confirm only that the document appeared to be a radiology report, but the quality was so poor, she was unable to authenticate neither where it had been typed, nor if had even been done in the transcription department at the hospital. The date of document creation was impossible to determine; even the printer on which it had been done could not be identified as one from the hospital's typing pool.

Jennings demanded the copy from the patient's electronic medical record. Two weeks later, it was delivered in the mail. The print was as distorted as the copy that had been handed to Khai during the deposition.

Jennings wanted to subpoena the young woman from transcription who had typed the record from the radiologist's dictation device, but the initials on the bottom were smudged and unintelligible. His document specialist was at a loss to provide anything other than the first letter was likely a K or an R. Of the twenty-three transcriptionists, two were named Renee, one Robin, two Kristin, and one Karen. Jennings wanted to depose all six, but in pre-trial motions, the judge refused and ordered Harrison Jennings to choose one. Instead, he deposed the head transcriptionist, demanding she bring with her the daily employee lists for the period between the ultrasound and the day the report was faxed to him. The woman complied, but it came out during questioning that several of the women had been caught trading shifts but using the initials of other transcriptionists to hide the goings on. And, finally, she allowed, two of the Ks had been let go, one for stealing a doctor's prescription pad and the other for conducting a personal transcription business on company time.

Jennings' final comment for the lead transcriptionist at the deposition was, "Tight ship you're running there."

Rhonda Uft immediately burped, "Objection. Inflammatory."

Jennings then subpoenaed for deposition the ultrasound tech. Because the radiologist was deceased, the judge allowed her to be called, but he also ruled she would be the last of the peripheral hospital personnel the Plaintiff could depose.

During her deposition, the radiology tech reported she was not sure if there had been blood in Dr. Maddingly's pelvis that night. After all, she had done hundreds and hundreds of ultrasound studies since that night. As she testified, Rhonda Uft objected every time Jennings asked about what fluid would look like on an ultrasound of the pelvis. Her argument was that techs were just that, trained where to place the ultrasound head, not to be able to read the actual study. "That's why it takes thirteen years of training after high school to become a radiologist and read the vital information."

Next, he requested the internal computer records that listed the dates on which each document in Sabrina's chart was entered into the record. It arrived a month later. The ultrasound report appeared to have been placed in her chart four days after her admission. It had, though, not been included in the massive packet of records he had been provided by the hospital when he filed the malpractice suit a year after the admission. Finally, he subpoenaed the IT department head, to query whether the date on the radiology report could have been manipulated. Rhonda Uft filed a motion that the Plaintiff was ignoring the judge's order to stop harassing the peripheral staff at the hospital. Galanter agreed. Jennings decided not to call the tech as a witness during the actual trial.

Khai had made several suggestions along the way as to how the ultrasound report could be authenticated, and some were still on the table. Those were the notes to which her binder was opened.

Trial resumed half an hour later. Jennings began his questioning by reminding the jury, "We were just asking Dr. Weathersby if she regularly received notes from other doctors regarding her patients. And my question was why she hadn't received the report of Dr. Maddingly's ultrasound..."

"Objection. Calls for speculation."

"Sustained."

"Okay, Doctor, let me ask, did you receive documents on a regular basis from the medical staff at the Defendant Hospital regarding the medical status of Dr. Maddingly after the evening of November 25th?"

"I have received some documents from various Mitchie-Sterling Hospital staff regarding Dr. Maddingly's medical condition."

"Some, Doctor?"

"I've called several offices and asked repeatedly for progress notes, but they have not been sent."

"Have you asked the medical director why?"

"Yes."

"What was the answer?"

"There was no reply—twice."

"Okay, moving on. Did you receive the radiology report?"

"Objection. Asked and answered."

"Sustained."

"Okay, no problem. Let me ask you, Doctor, is there one document that summarizes Dr. Maddingly's medical situation when she was discharged from the Defendant Hospital on November 25th?

"Yes."

"By whom was this written, and to whom was it sent?"

"It was written and signed by Harvey R. Klat, M.D., Medical Director of Mitchie-Sterling Hospital. A copy of this document appears to have been sent to various physicians on the staff at Mitchie-Sterling Hospital, to the CEO, Mr. Harp, and to the County Medical Society."

"Was it sent to you by the medical director?"

"He did not include my name on the mailing list."

"Where did you get it, then?"

"From the records you subpoenaed from the hospital."

"Doctor, do you know how many admissions there are to the Defendant Hospital every year?"

"It is over 25,000."

"Does each one of those admissions have a discharge summary?"

"Yes."

"Is it usual for the CEO to receive the discharge summary of a patient?"

"In my experience, it is not sent to personnel other than the directly involved health providers, unless, of course, there is a major problem with the care provided."

The objection was so strident, one of the jurors nearly fell from her chair. Ms. Uft bellowed, "There is no evidence on the record that there was a problem with Plaintiff's care. The CEO is not a doctor, but he or she is responsible for everything that goes on within the hospital. When there is the threat of litigation, as in this case with the Plaintiffs screaming malpractice within ten minutes of arriving at the hospital..."

The whack of Judge Galanter's gavel silenced the courtroom. "That's enough, Ms. Uft. Your objection is sustained, but I will remind you that you are not to launch into a dialogue of your theory of the case while expressing your objection. Please limit yourself to accepted legal jargon. Thank you. The jury is to ignore the witness's characterization of the care the Plaintiff received, and to Ms. Uft's sermon. Go on Mr. Jennings."

Rhonda Uft jolted into seated attention, drew a breath, but remained mute. Harrison Jennings looked at her and waited until her color started to fade before nodding at Khai. He smiled, "Now, Dr. Weathersby, is it unusual for the Medical Director to write the discharge summary of a patient's treatment at a hospital?"

"In my experience it is, unless he or she was involved in the case."

"Well, was Dr. Klat involved in Dr. Maddingly's care?"

"Objection. There is no way that the witness could possibly know if Dr. Klat was involved in the Plaintiff's care."

"Sustained."

Jennings asked, "Well, Dr. Weathersby, then why did you say you did not think Dr. Klat was involved in Dr. Maddingly's care."

"All I can say is that his name is not mentioned in the summary as a provider for Dr. Maddingly. I did not see any orders or progress notes signed by Dr. Klat. In fact, there was no gastroenterology consult requested, and Dr. Klat is a gastroenterologist."

"Who normally does write the discharge summary?"

"The attending physician writes the discharge summary in all the hospitals I've ever worked at."

"And have we agreed that Dr. Klat was not the attending physician?"

"From the records, he clearly was not the attending physician."

"Thank you. Now, please read the section of the document that mentions the ultrasound examination done on Dr. Maddingly on the evening of 25th November."

"There is no mention of the ultrasound."

"Is there mention of the pregnancy test done that night?"

"Yes."

"Are there any other laboratory or radiologic test reports from the first night of Dr. Maddingly's admission to Mitchie-Sterling Hospital mentioned in the report?"

"Yes. There are several standard lab tests noted, as well as an operative note."

"In your experience, is it unusual for the person who wrote the discharge summary to omit a study as crucial as the first ultrasound?"

Rhonda Uft blurted, "Your Honor, I object. Counsel is testifying. There were thousands of pages of records in this case. Dr. Klat could not possibly have noted every test."

"Overruled. You will have ample opportunity on cross-examination to establish which tests were crucial to the patient's care." He nodded to Jennings.

"Rather than entering a detailed examination of the discharge summary, one that is filled with medical jargon, please, for my sake and the jury's, read to us just list the diagnoses Dr. Maddingly left the hospital with."

"Number One: status post right hemispheric CVA..."

"Stop there for a moment, please. Dr. Weathersby, what does hemispheric mean."

"If you consider the brain a sphere, like the Earth, a hemisphere is half a sphere, or, in this case, it means the right half of the brain, the part of the brain that controls the left side of the body."

"Right controls the left? I don't understand. Could you explain that?"

"Sure. No one knows why in evolution this happened, but in all vertebrates, that is animals with spines, all of them have pupils and lenses in their eyes. Because of the presence of a lens, the image you see is really upside down, but the brain turns it right side up. Also, the images coming from your right side fall onto the left side of the retina of both eyes." She moved her index fingers to amplify her answer. "That's backwards when you think about it. One theory is that if you see a threat coming from your right, your right hand and arm should be able to react to your right side. It would be inefficient to have to reach from your left side to react to a hazard coming from the right. So, somewhere along the line, nature switched the path of the nerves going from the brain to the opposite side of the body. Or so we were taught in medical school. Bottom line is, whatever the reason, it worked well. And in nature, what works well gives that organism a small survival advantage. Slowly, but surely, over the millennia, that small advantage takes over, and the creatures that don't have it die out. By the way, the nerves from the eyes cross over in the part of the brain right behind the eyes, but the nerve bundles controlling the muscles of the body cross at the bottom of the brain before they get into the spinal cord. Must be a reason, but like I said, no one is sure. Yet again, the miracle."

"Okay, we know about hemisphere and nerves crossing, but what does CVA mean?"

"Cerebral vascular accident. In English, that means a stroke."

"Do you know why we call it a stroke?"

"Supposedly, historically, it was seen as a stroke of God's hand, it was so devastating."

"And what does that mean inside the brain?"

"The brain is just a bunch of wires. For the moment, think of it as the fuse box in your house. Wires go from the fuse box to the various lights, appliances, radios, and the like. If you burn out a fuse, everything on that line stops because the electricity can't get through to radios, lights, etc. It is exactly the same in the brain. Since the brain sends electrical messages to everything in the body, if a fuse blows, messages from that part of the brain can't get through; messages like, move your arms or legs, or move your mouth so you can speak. That's what a stroke is—a burned out fuse. A stroke in the left brain, the left hemisphere, causes the muscles on the right not to get the signal to move. What caused the stroke in this case..."

Harrison Jennings looked from the corner of his eye at the jury. Most were rapt with Khai's testimony. He held up his hand and smiled. "Excuse me, Doctor. We'll get to that very important testimony shortly. For now, could you please continue reading the discharge summary? Let's get that out of the way first."

"Okay, Number One, Status post right hemispheric CVA. Etiology unclear."

Jennings raised his hand. "Let me stop you again. Please explain the meaning of the word etiology."

"It simply means the cause."

"So, the summary is saying the cause of the stroke is unknown. Is that correct?"

"Yes."

"Do you agree with that?"

"No."

"Why, in your professional opinion, is that incorrect?"

"Well, there are several reasons. First, the night of the incident, actually very early the next morning, I went to the hospital to check on Dr. Maddingly. I spoke with the surgeon who operated on Dr. Maddingly for the ruptured ectopic pregnancy. He told me..."

"Objection. Hearsay."

"Sustained."

"Let me rephrase. Did you have any part in Dr. Maddingly's care in the hospital that night?"

"Not directly, but the surgeon who had saved her life and I discussed the case in depth after surgery. He asked me, as an internist, what tests I suggested to determine if Dr. Maddingly had suffered a stroke. I suggested a CT scan."

"Was that test done?"

"Yes."

"What did it show?"

"A large stroke, embolic, in the right hemisphere."

"Thank you, and, please, the meaning of embolic?"

"First, let me explain why the so-called fuse blows. The fuse, so to speak, is just a clump of brain cells that are fed by a small blood vessel. If that blood vessel gets clogged, or one finally bursts from years of high blood pressure, the brain cells in that cluster don't get their blood, and that means no oxygen. The cells suffocate and die, and very quickly—six to ten minutes. Any nerves, which are, again, really just electrical wires leading away from the dead cells in the brain to the muscles they control, no longer get the command to fire. The muscles are okay, but they get no message to move. As I mentioned, there are two basic types of strokes. Here, we are talking about a blood clot forming and blocking the artery to the bundle of cells in the brain that control the muscles. A clot is called an embolism. When the amount of blood in the body drops dramatically from, say, bleeding, the blood itself becomes stagnant, and that causes a clot to form, just like if blood spills on the ground. Blood has to be moving to remain liquid. If Dr. Maddingly had very low blood pressure from loss of so much blood in the emergency room..."

Rhonda Uft was back on her feet, steaming. "Objection! Introducing facts not in evidence. There is no evidence that the Plaintiff's bleeding began in the emergency room."

Jennings came to his feet. "Your Honor, we know Dr. Maddingly's blood pressure became dangerously low in the emergency room. That is not in question."

Galanter thought for a moment. "Well, I agree with Ms. Uft, that the answer your witness gave made it sound as though the bleeding *began* in the ER. You haven't proved that. Sustained."

"Thank you, Your Honor. We'll move on. Dr. Weathersby, would you read the next diagnosis, please?"

"Number Two: Ectopic pregnancy, left, ruptured with massive loss of blood."

"If I could just stop you there, Dr. Weathersby. Is the Defendant Hospital acknowledging there had been a massive loss of blood?"

"Yes."

"Is there any information as to when this blood loss occurred?"

"None is listed in the summary."

"Well, as a board-certified physician, can you give us an idea of when the blood loss took place by looking into the medical records written that night?"

"Yes."

"I ask you to turn to Tab 24 in your binder. What is this document?"

"This is the operative note from Dr. Gauthé."

"Who is Dr. Gauthé?"

"He is the general surgeon who was called on to operate on Dr. Maddingly that night."

"Excuse me. You said general surgeon. Isn't an ectopic pregnancy supposed to be operated on by an obstetrical or gynecological surgeon?"

"Yes, if there is an OB/GYN available."

"Do you have any firsthand knowledge why Dr. Gauthé did this surgery instead of an OB/GYN?"

"Yes."

"Please tell us why."

"To start with, I called around to the OB/GYN surgeons in the area that night right after I sent Dr. Maddingly and her husband to the hospital. I had a feeling there was going to be the need for surgery, or at least for a specialist to assume her care."

"What happened when you called around?"

"I was able to get ahold of only one OB/GYN who would talk to me. Should I use her name?"

"No, it isn't necessary. She's not on trial."

"Well, she was quite brusque, asking if the patient had insurance, but she finally agreed to go to the hospital. She ended the conversation with the statement, 'You better be right about the ectopic,' and hung up. When the hospital eventually called her that night, to get her in immediately, she did not answer her phone."

Rhonda Uft jumped to her feet, but before she could speak, Khai snapped, "It's all in the hospital records. Do you want me to read them aloud?"

The judge banged his gavel, and Rhonda Uft retook her seat. "The witness will answer only questions posed by Counsel. The jury is to ignore the witness's outburst. Go on Mr. Jennings."

"Okay, back to the discharge report. By signing that document, did Dr. Klat acknowledge that Dr. Maddingly suffered a stroke in the right side of her brain on the evening of 25th November."

"Yes."

"Is that a common complication of surgery?"

"If blood pressure decreases thirty-percent below that patient's normal blood pressure, it means there might not be enough pressure in the blood vessels to keep the blood moving fast enough to prevent clots."

"Explain again the clotting problem you just mentioned, please."

"As I said, slow moving blood sludges. That means gets thick and stops flowing."

"I'm sorry. This is critical information. That's why I've asked you to explain this again. Please tell us why sludging blood clots."

"Let's say you get a small cut. After a few minutes, as we all know, the blood becomes thick. Actually, that's a chemical reaction, not just a drying of the blood. Clotting is one of the most important events in the body. We would bleed to death, probably before birth, if we couldn't form a clot very quickly. On the other hand, if we clot for the wrong reasons, we would be having heart attacks and strokes before we were born. The process is amazing, but very complicated, as you might imagine.

"Let me explain. Blood is composed of far more than red and white cells. In the liquid part of the blood, the plasma, there are over 4,000 chemicals, some of which are involved in the clotting process. It takes a series of chemical reactions, basically thirteen, before a clot is allowed to form. When blood is exposed to certain triggers, the first chemical reaction takes place. This produces a very specialized protein. The sudden appearance of this protein stimulates the next chemical reaction in the chain, on and on—we call it the clotting cascade— until a clot forms. It is incredibly complex, and it is designed to only allow a clot under the absolute right conditions—basically, to stop bleeding when all else has failed.

"Sometimes, though, the cascade can start for the wrong reason. One of those cases is if blood stops moving, or is moving so slowly, those proteins think the blood has stopped. We all know that if you sit on an airplane for eleven hours without standing up, the blood pools in your legs and gets stagnant. If that inadvertently starts the clotting cascade inside a big leg vein, that's called a deep vein thrombosis, and a piece of that clot can break off and travel from the leg to the lungs. Can't go any farther, because it's trapped there. That's a PE, a pulmonary embolism, and it is deadly. Now, if the blood pools in the arteries as opposed to the veins...let me stop and clarify. Veins bring used blood back to the lungs to pick up a new supply of oxygen. Arteries, on the other hand, pick up that oxygenated blood from the lungs and send it to the heart, which pumps it all over the body. If a clot forms *after* the lungs, it is in the arteries and can go to the brain before it gets stuck. That is a stroke, and it's what happened here.

"To answer your question, Mr. Jennings, a blood clot is not common in surgery, but it happens often enough to make it the dread of all surgeons. They take precautions to prevent clots, though they are very limited in what they can do. If we give a patient about to undergo surgery something to thin the blood, even as simple as aspirin or ibuprofen, the surgical site will continue to bleed. We don't want that. We want the blood to clot at the incision but not in the legs. So, the best way to prevent clots during surgery is to keep the blood moving at normal speeds."

"How do you do that.?"

"Keep the blood pressure up."

"And how do you do that?"

"There are many causes of dropping blood pressure, but here, for Dr. Maddingly, the obvious cause was blood loss."

"But the patient wasn't bleeding. There were no wounds."

"Not on the outside. But she was clearly bleeding inside, internally, losing blood out of her blood vessels where the ectopic pregnancy had burst through the tube. The blood was no longer in the bloodstream where it was useful; now it was pooling in her pelvis, where it's worthless."

"How do you know that if you couldn't see it?"

"Easy, her blood pressure was dangerously low."

"Was this during surgery?"

"I would say it began in the emergency room because the blood pressures they recorded were so dangerously low. It likely continued into surgery."

Rhonda Uft crowed, "Objection. Speculation. How many times do we have to revisit this?"

"Sustained."

Jennings nodded. "Well, Dr. Weathersby, let me ask again, was a blood pressure below seventy sufficiently low to cause a clot to form?"

"Objection. We don't know a thing about the Plaintiff's blood pressure being below seventy.?"

"Sustained."

Harrison Jennings shook his bowed head subtly. "Dr. Weathersby, can we tell the exact moment the patient, Dr. Maddingly, suffered her stroke?"

"No."

"Could it have happened when she was having her pregnancy test or when she was having her ultrasound at the hospital that night?"

"Categorically no."

"Objection. Speculation."

"Sustained."

"Dr. Weathersby, what is your expert medical opinion regarding Dr. Maddingly's blood pressure when she entered the hospital?"

"Simple. It's common sense. She walked into the hospital, walked downstairs to the lab..."

Rhonda Uft rose. "Objection. The witness just told us you can get a clot while being very much awake and normal on an airplane. How do we know the Plaintiff didn't get a clot in her leg sitting at work that day, then sitting in the car..."

Judge Galanter raised his palm. "You are testifying, Ms. Uft. But your objection is sustained. Rephrase your question, Mr. Jennings."

"Yes, Your Honor. Dr. Weathersby, let me ask, why do you believe the clot began after Dr. Maddingly arrived at the hospital."

"Very simply because the clot I was talking about before, the one in the leg, is in the veins, the blood vessels that bring blood back to the heart. Venous clots do not and cannot possibly cause strokes. They only cause clots that go to the lung, and no farther. They get trapped there. You can die from them very easily because they clog the lungs. Dr. Maddingly's clot was in the brain. It could not have gotten there from a vein, only from low flow in an artery. Completely different problem.

"If Dr. Maddingly had had low enough blood pressure from a bleed, that is, low enough to form a clot in an artery, one that got into the brain and caused a stroke, she would not have been able to walk into the blood draw lab, sit down, then get up again to walk all the way to radiology, lay down on the table, then get up without assistance, and walk on her own steam to the emergency room."

"Let me stop you there again. How do we know she did all this without assistance?"

"There is nothing in the notes to indicate the patient was incapacitated. There was no call for a wheelchair by the blood draw staff or the radiology department, not even a reference in the notes by these two departments that Dr. Maddingly looked ill."

Jennings shrugged. "You can't expect them to write everything down, can you?"

"This is a hospital, sir. Human lives are at stake. Anything out of the ordinary must be recorded, dated, and signed by a responsible staff member. If a patient is incapable of moving her arms and legs..."

"Objection. The Plaintiff is not claiming she can't move her arms or legs."

"Sustained."

Jennings raised his voice. "How do we know that Dr. Maddingly could move her legs before the last step of going into the emergency department?"

"As I said, this is a hospital. If a patient can't walk on her own, even a volunteer on his first day would get a wheelchair to move a patient to her next appointment. It is hardly reasonable for Dr. Maddingly's husband to carry her around a hospital on his shoulder. And, again, there was nothing in the notes about this patient being in extremis, that is, at the point of death. This is a hospital. A patient undergoing an acute stroke, well, you would think some sort of note would have been made by the professional staff attending her."

"Objection. This is simply the witness's opinion."

Jennings snapped, "And we have established this witness is a board-certified physician who knows very well the rules in a hospital. She lived in several around the clock for many years."

Galanter muttered, "Overruled. Go on Mr. Jennings."

Rhonda Uft snapped back, "The court can be assured we will present witness after witness who will testify that the Plaintiff's blood pressure is a red herring. We will show that Plaintiff's underlying abnormal..."

Harrison Jennings growled, "Objection! Counsel is testifying."

Galanter sighed, "Sustained. Move on, Mr. Jennings."

Harrison nodded at the jury. "Dr. Weathersby, let's go back to the problem of a low blood pressure. Where would the decreased blood pressure most likely show itself?"

"The most important parts of the body, I mean, in any emergency, are the brain and the heart. So, if the amount of blood going to the brain and heart is falling, the body starts shutting down flow to unnecessary organs. In the usual case, this would be the arms and legs. Muscles can live a long time without blood flow. Brain can't."

"I have to ask again, how often does this happen during surgery?"

"I cannot give you a specific number. There is no way to know, as clots often happen, but they frequently dissolve by themselves without ever causing significant problems. They can also form tiny strokes that patients don't seem to recognize. Maybe they think the mild weakness is just part of recovering from surgery. Then, maybe those tiny strokes heal themselves, or they don't, and the family says, 'You know, Mary's never been the same since that hysterectomy.' On the other hand, even if it is a not a common complication of surgery, when it happens, as in this case, it can be catastrophic."

Rhonda Uft was on her feet. "Objection. That is pure hyperbole."

The judge turned to Plaintiff's Counsel. "Mr. Jennings?"

"Your Honor," Jennings began, his shoulders drooping in disbelief, "catastrophic is a commonly used medical term. When a patient has suffered the level of damage at the hands of the Defendant Hospital that Dr. Maddingly has, everyone calls that catas..."

Rhonda Uft brayed, "And objection again. First, that is just more hyperbole; and two, we have no testimony on the record to demonstrate the Plaintiff's present medical status. She is sitting in a wheelchair, but the jury, and I, still don't know why, or, to be frank, if the wheelchair is really necessary or just a theatrical prop."

"I am going to sustain that objection on the grounds that we do not know what those words mean when used by a medical professional. And I'm sure Mr. Jennings will be very forthcoming as to Dr. Maddingly's present medical status. So, we can move on."

Jennings dropped his head and hid an obvious smile. "Thank you, Your Honor. Now, Doctor, please tell us what the word catastrophic means to a physician."

"It means the patient has damage that may kill them, or at least essentially end their life as they know it." He purposely turned to Rhonda Uft, pretending to wait for the explosion, but she was silent, and he went on. "Okay, back to the question: did Dr. Maddingly's blood pressure drop to the point that it was likely a clot would form?"

"Objection. The witness is not a surgeon."

The judge growled, "Mr. Jennings?"

"Your Honor, Dr. Weathersby knows more about clotting as a board-certified internist with special training in hematology than any surgeon on the Defendant's staff."

"Objection. Foundation and stating facts not in evidence."

The judge thought for a moment. "We have testimony that Dr. Weathersby has advanced training in hematology, but we don't know what that means. So, Mr. Jennings, would you rephrase your question to address the term hematology?"

"Yes, Your Honor. Dr. Weathersby, with your advanced training in hematology...first, please define hematology for us."

"Hematology is the study and specialty of blood, particularly red blood cell and clotting diseases."

"Thank you. When blood pressure drops to 70, can clots form?"

"Yes."

"Is it likely?"

"Yes, if it goes on for more than a few minutes."

"Thank you. If this likely clot forms, what happens next?"

"Eventually, if it forms in the heart or the arteries of the neck, a piece of the clot—or maybe, in the worst cases, the whole clot—flows through the large arteries leading from the heart to smaller branches of the artery, which get smaller and smaller as they enter the brain, until the clot is bigger than the next artery down the road. That's where it gets stuck, and..."

"Let me stop you there. Could you please draw a diagram on the easel for us?"

Khai walked back to the tripod. She turned it as she had before and ignored Rhonda Uft's grunt. She drew a blood vessel that forked over and over until the last tiny arteriole. A purple magic marker drew an uneven blob, which she marked as "Clot." "You can see that, as the clot travels, it's eventually going to get to a blood vessel that's too small to let it through. The clot is actually quite soft, very much like a like a lump of grape jelly."

She took a brown marker and drew a human brain, then drew blood vessels penetrating it. "When the clot gets here, as far as it can go, all the brain tissue on the other side of the blockage is immediately starved of blood, and that means no nutrients and no oxygen. In a few minutes, that part of the brain dies, and the muscles, or speech, or balance that part of the brain used to control, will likely never function again, certainly not normally. That is a stroke."

There was a gasp and a moan from the jury box. All eyes fixed on Juror Number 4. An elderly woman stood from her chair and called out weakly to the judge, "I can't do this anymore." She placed her pad and pencil on her chair and started to walk out of the jury box. The bailiff puffed his chest and placed himself in front of her, blocking her exit.

The judge stood and called out, "Bailiff, let her leave!"

When the woman limped through the rear doors of the courtroom, the judge took his seat and banged his gavel until the chatter died out. He muttered, "That does happen sometimes during graphic testimony. We got started a bit late today, so we shall adjourn, with Dr. Weathersby retaking the witness stand tomorrow morning at 10 o'clock. The jury is admonished..." As they filed out, Galanter rose, making for chambers before the last juror was out of the courtroom.

Rhonda Uft watched intently and made a note on her legal pad.

CHAPTER FORTY-ONE

K hai felt eyes on her as she dragged down the steps of the courthouse. She looked up to see Chris Gauthé charging up toward her, his Carrera parked illegally just feet away, the engine running, both front doors open. He grabbed Khai's arm and pulled her down the steps, nearly stuffing her into the passenger seat.

As they pulled away from the curb quickly, Khai turned and mumbled, "Sergio's? God Only Knows?"

"Yes, and yes."

She was silent for a moment then laughed wryly, "And, so, Christopher Gauthé, M.D., not seen you since, since, let's see..." She put an index finger on her chin.

"How was court?"

"SOS. Same old shit. Done it a bunch of times already."

"Were they really nasty to you?"

"Nah, we didn't get very far before one of the jurors ran out yelling, 'It's too much for me.' Must've been when I began talking about how much blood was in Sabrina's belly. Not that I blame her."

"Not sure I do, either. You know, you get kind of blinded to what you see every day—calloused, really. Souls on the table in front of you, probably one of the worst moments of their lives, and you're chewing gum and thinking about a glass of good wine with a special friend when you get done. Kinda rote after a few years and a few thousand bellies full of blood. I imagine war is like that. Just get used to it."

"No, no you don't. Just want to get away from it fast as you can." Khai looked at him and screwed up her face. "Okay, let's have it, what are you doing here? And how did you know where to find me?"

"Ve haf our vays."

"No, really, how come you're here?"

"The truth, I really wanted to see you. Are you angry at me?"

"Well, I guess you didn't really want to see me for the last six or seven weeks, huh?" He didn't answer, and she went on. "Had to hear it through the grapevine that you were banished to the gulag. They must've confiscated your cell phone, huh?"

"Khai, look, it happened so fast. I was gone before I realized that if I didn't take a break, I might do something stupid."

"Rumor is your pal Harp forced the matter. Is that not true?"

"Not really. I mean, we had some prickly conversations—to say the least. But this was my decision. Things were closing in on me. The doctor wannabes in the front office tried to intimidate me, have me obey, but I reminded them it's the folks in the trenches, the ones working around the clock, who're making them rich. They don't like to hear that. Always a millimeter under the surface that they didn't have the right stuff to get into medical school. Never met one who didn't turn red in the face when I reminded 'em about it. I told them I was taking a 'sabbatical.' Fresh start. Isn't that why you said you landed here?"

She sighed, "Yeah, fresh start, but coming to the Great Northwest doesn't seem to be the best decision I ever made. Not what I imagined."

"What did you imagine?"

"You know, in the summer before medical school, I went down to Nicaragua, out in the mountains, medical mission, with a church group from Boston. I watched the doctors and the nurses very carefully, to try and be like them. Man, were they a difficult amalgamation of misfits. Of course, I kept my nose out of the conflicts, and it wasn't that hard to remain aloof. I figured, with what I had witnessed of life, I could do the same thing in the real world. Wasn't any different in medical school—arrogance and nastiness. And residency at Mass General, worse than Yale. Hate to say it, but the surgical residents and the surgeons, what a condescending, obnoxious lot. Came close to saying the hell with it. Thought of going back into the service, finishing my residency there, and becoming a lifer. I used to think back to when I was stationed at Fort Lewis, far more respectful than the East Coast, slower, gentler. But then there was a twist in my life. Always is, isn't there? So, here I am, three thousand miles away, and who pops up? Just the same cast of characters. I wonder why I left Boston. At least that was the devil I knew. So, Chris, I'm not all that far away from the way you're feeling. I'm sorry. I didn't mean to get on your case. It's your beeswax. Sorry."

Gauthé nodded. "I guess what we see in some of our colleagues is pretty disheartening." He laughed and gave her a gentle tap on the shoulder. "Yeah, but hey, you gotta work. You gotta do something for a living, and I may be guessing, but I would imagine anything you did was going to be around people who were especially bright and educated. Same in all the professions—at least the real ones. Nah, it's same in any job. Human nature."

"Yeah, maybe you're right," Khai shook her head, "but a doctor, that's supposed mean something special. And there you are. In the end, it sure ain't." She turned away from Gauthé and stared out the window. When she spoke again, her voice quavered. "I just never dreamed you or I'd become such targets. In medical school, they beat into your head: the patient comes first, always first. It's such bullshit. It's all just a big lie."

He laughed. "Well, you gotta admit that you've never been shy about sticking your head up above the crowd, have you?"

"Not sure what you mean."

"Well, let's say you were a man who went to West Point, became a pilot, served as a combat officer two different times, went to Yale medical school, and then probably the best internal medicine residency in the country. Then you comport yourself head-up, shoulders squared, yada, yada, yada. You think that would be enough to say you were sticking your head up above the crowd?"

"I don't know; it's just what I did, do. Never planned to set the world on fire. You want me to walk around with my head around my knees?"

"And you are a woman, on top of all that!"

"I guess, but it sure seems like an awful lot of hard work to be low creature on the totem pole, and at the mercy of some folks who aren't all that squared away, doctors and suits."

"Sounds like we're diving into a very viscous pity party."

She glared for a moment, but her eyes softened. "Okay, you're right. But I just don't know why I feel like this. Enough time's gone by to not feel so isolated."

"Do you really mean lonely?"

She did not answer. Chris slowed the car to five miles an hour and reached his hand over and took hers. Her fingers jerked for an instant, but she slowly closed them around his. They did not speak again until they had been seated at Sergio's.

Chris ordered a bottle of God Only Knows. Khai started to mumble the usual about having to drive, but Chris put his fingers to her lips. He whispered, "I'm doing all the driving tonight. I have some news."

"And, what's that?"

"The Big D."

"Chris, are you saying you're divorced?"

"We are basically done."

"What does that mean, Doctor?"

Gauthé declared, though coolly. "I'm free. Made the decision during my 'interlude.'"

Khai turned toward the window and stared at the planes in their descent toward SeaTac. She finally whispered, "What happened?"

"I had a spiritual experience. You're going to have to trust me."

Two hours later, he offered to drive Khai to her car, but as she was considering it, he smiled, "Let's stay in Soundview tonight. I'll drop you off at the courthouse tomorrow morning, and same deal; you get the bed, I suffer on the couch, and the bedroom door stays closed, locked, throw away the key if you like." She shook her head with a smile but then nodded.

At the apartment, they shared another bottle of wine. Chris gave her scrubs, and Khai started a wash. Fifteen minutes after she was settled in the bed, she got up, turned the light as low as it would go, opened the door, and crawled back under the covers.

CHAPTER FORTY-TWO

When Chris dropped Khai at the courthouse the next morning, he pulled deep into the parking garage and whispered, "I hate to let you go. Can I call you?"

Khai touched his arm. "You better."

She popped from the car and ran toward the elevator then stopped and raised her hand to wave, but he was already flying through the exit. Out of the corner of her eye, Khai caught Rhonda Uft getting out of her Cadillac. Khai turned quickly back toward the elevator, but when she heard Rhonda Uft's car door close and the beep, Khai darted to the stairwell.

Court did not adjourn until 11:30, ninety minutes late, most of the time vaporized by Rhonda Uft's perseverant demand that the case be dismissed, as the trial had been tainted by juror histrionics. She was finally overruled with the admonishment, "Ms. Uft, I do not find it unnatural for a reasonable citizen without medical training to be highly uncomfortable with the notion of massive strokes being brought about by the image of grape jam, the condiment she probably had on the peanut butter and jelly sandwich she ate for dinner the night before, because that was all she was able to force down, as anxious as she was about having to come back and listen to more of this unpleasant wrangling. Not every juror, madame, relishes how some in our profession seek to rip the throat out of every soul they encounter. Some normal citizens don't want to hear or see that. Can't say I blame them."

Rhonda Uft huffed, "So noted, Your Honor."

"Good. Glad it is." He paused, and Rhonda Uft turned her generous backside toward the bench to write notes at a furious pace, but Galanter snapped, "And furthermore, that juror was sitting here looking at a disabled, young plaintiff who had suffered that very stroke. That was not histrionics. That was an understandable human reaction, and the trial will proceed with the first alternate juror in her place."

Ms. Uft pasted a haughty smile on her face. "Your Honor, excuse me, sir, but I do not believe it is apparent from the testimony we've heard so far that the plaintiff is as disabled as she would have us believe, that the so-called stroke wasn't just part of the plaintiff's underlying abnormality, or, more likely, the natural progression of that process."

Mike, who had been sitting in the front row behind Sabrina, inhaled loudly. Harrison Jennings swiveled about instantly, saw the flush in his face, and raised his index finger into Mike's eyes. Mike sat back and glared at Rhonda Uft, who grunted and rolled her eyes.

The judge waited until the color in Mike's face cooled then spoke. "You are correct, Ms. Uft, that there has been no clear proof that the plaintiff is worse now than prior to her visit to Mitchie-Sterling Hospital, but it is very clear, from Dr. Weathersby's testimony, that the patient was able to walk and use her left arm, the latter to some degree, prior to the hospital stay, and could not when she left the hospital. That much is clear from the hospital records. What we must do is have all the facts placed before us, and the jury will be the trier of those facts, not me. That is their function in our system of justice. But be sure, Plaintiff will have to prove to the jury that any underlying issues are separate from the final outcome, and you will have the opportunity to prove them wrong. Overruled."

Rhonda Uft smirked. "Well, Your Honor, I intend to do just that."

The judge smiled, "I'm sure that will be something to watch."

Jennings stood. "Your Honor, apropos to this dialogue, I make a motion that summary judgment be granted on the basis of the doctrine of res ipsa loquitur."

Rhonda Uft drew so profound a breath, her face and shoulders inflated like a puffer fish squaring off against a squid. "Your Honor, that is outrageous. I won't even dignify it with a counterargument."

The judge sighed, "Mr. Jennings, don't push me too hard."

Jennings, however, took a step toward the bench. "Your Honor, excuse me. Res ipsa loquitur, 'The thing speaks for itself.' Dr. Maddingly was mildly impaired when she entered the hospital on her own steam, but within twenty-four hours of her admission, maybe thirty minutes of her admission, she became relegated to a wheelchair for the rest of her life. The law allows a presumption of negligence if the following three foundational facts are established. First, the plaintiff sustained any injury. And as you just said, sir, it is obvious from pretrial arguments, from the defendant's own records, and from testimony in open court, that the plaintiff has been injured.

"Secondly, said injury was proximately caused by an instrumentality solely within the control of the defendant or defendants—in this case a botched attempt to start an IV—and thirdly, such injury does not ordinarily occur under the circumstances, absent negligence on the part of the defendant.

"In other words, she walked into the hospital, but she had to be wheeled out. And as we discussed in pretrial motions, the chance of a so-called seasoned emergency room physician not being able to start a large bore IV is ridiculously low.

"I am not pushing too hard, Your Honor. I'm just reciting the law."

Judge Galanter's lips tightened. "Mr. Jennings, you do not need to teach me the law. Thank you. In fact, res ipsa loquitur can be used only under very limited factual circumstances. I hope you know that. Even if I granted res ipsa loquitur, all that accomplishes is to create a presumption of negligence and shift the burden to the defendant health care provider to prove there was no negligence. Given that there was some underlying physical compromise, which you have readily admitted, we are miles and miles away from the conclusion that such injury does not ordinarily occur under the circumstances, absent negligence on the part of the defendant. Overruled.

"Now, if there are no more motions, I see yet another morning has withered entertaining dubious matters of jurisprudential import. In other words, we've essentially frittered away half the day. We will break for lunch and resume at half past one. I fully intend to have the jury seated at that moment."

At 1:30, the jury was, indeed, in place, and it appeared, from Judge Galanter's demeanor, his mid-day meal had not been any more soothing than his breakfast. He grumbled, "Ladies and Gentlemen of the jury, I apologize for this morning." He glared at the two lawyers. "There were important matters to be hashed out, arguments that might have introduced bias into the trial. I will do my best to ensure it won't happen again. Dr. Weathersby, please take the stand and remember you are still under oath."

Harrison Jennings took a step toward the bench. "Thank you, Your Honor. However, considering the objections voiced by Ms. Uft regarding Dr. Maddingly's present status, I would like to excuse Dr. Weathersby and call two other witnesses to substantiate our claim that Dr. Maddingly is substantially worse than when she walked into the Defendant Hospital on the night of 25th November. I assure the court I will recall Dr. Weathersby and give Ms. Uft ample opportunity to cross-examine her."

Rhonda Uft's faced glowed cherry red. "Objection! I will cross-examine her now."

The judge called them to a sidebar. "Mr. Jennings, what are you doing?"

"Your Honor, look, I had believed Dr. Weathersby's testimony would be sufficient to establish Dr. Maddingly's physical and psychiatric deficits. Apparently, Defense Counsel does not agree. She is obstructing my presentation at every turn, somehow believing that if she repeats enough times the lie that my client has not been damaged, the jury will believe it."

"Excuse me, but that's crap, Your Honor. This whole case turns on, not whether the Plaintiff is worse, but if that problem could have been avoided by any reasonable doctor, given the Plaintiff's underlying flaws."

Jennings sighed. "A few minutes ago, she was bellowing that we hadn't established the presence of the deficit suffered by my client."

Rhonda Uft rasped, "I've rethought the problem. Proving that she has deficits now is a minor point. Parading three, or a dozen, physical therapists before the jury proves nothing about the underlying problems this woman suffers. I hate to say it, but being completely objective, the plaintiff is a deeply flawed organism, and that pathological process began long before she set foot in Mitchie-Sterling Hospital."

Jennings snapped, "Your Honor, I don't have to listen to this unprofessional rudeness."

"Ms. Uft, Mr. Jennings has a point. Let's keep it civil. But Defense Counsel has a right to cross-examine your witness at this juncture, if you are done with your direct examination. A lot of bells have been rung, and she's going to get a chance to mute them." He glared at both of them. "Questions?"

Both answered, "No, Your Honor."

Rhonda Uft waddled toward Khai Weathersby, not stopping until she was but inches from the witness and blurted, "Doctor, let's talk about your medical experience. Are you board certified?"

"Yes."

"In what?"

"Internal medicine."

"Is that all?"

"I believe the great bulk of doctors are boarded in only one specialty."

"Let me ask again. Do you have any other board certifications?"

"No."

"Thank you. So, you are not board certified in hematology. Is that correct?"

"Yes, correct."

"But Mr. Jennings told the jury you have special training in hematology."

"I do."

"But you are not board certified in hematology?"

"Objection. Asked and answered."

"Sustained."

"Well, let me ask, are there board examinations in hematology?"

"Yes."

Rhonda Uft pulled away a few inches, her jaw sagging in utter disbelief. "Are you saying, Doctor, that there is an examination to be passed before a physician is allowed to claim they are a hematologist?" Shaking her head, she huffed, "In other words, any doctor can wake up one morning and just start practicing the very complicated specialty of hema...?"

"Objection, Counsel is testifying, and she is badgering the witness."

"Sustained. Move on, Counselor."

"Well, Your Honor, I believe the witness has not been forthcoming in her answer to my question about why she claims to have special training in hematology, but freely admits she is not board certified. You can be sure we are going to get to the reason why."

Jennings snapped, "Objection, inflammatory. And, furthermore, Counsel is flat wrong."

"Ms. Uft?"

Her face flushed. "Okay, I withdraw my last statement."

She turned back toward Khai, but the judge interrupted. "Ladies and Gentlemen of the jury, you are to disregard Defense Counsel's last two statements." He went on with a sharp note of caution in his voice. "Go on Ms. Uft."

She barked at Khai, "Is there an examination one must take before they can say they are a hematologist?"

"Yes."

Rhonda Uft heaved a grand sigh. "Okay, Doctor, did you take the subspecialty exam to be certified as a hematologist?"

"Yes."

"But you said you were not certified in hematology..."

Jennings was on his feet. "Objection. Is there a question somewhere in Counsel's remarks?"

"Sustained. Rephrase, Ms. Uft."

"Well, let me ask, how can a doctor take a certification exam in a subspecialty and not then be certified in that specialty?"

"I did a fellowship in hematology at M.D. Anderson but didn't pass the exam the first time." Her body wilted, a flower withering in time lapse. A second later, though, her face hardened, and after another moment, her shoulders squared as she locked Rhonda Uft's eyes. "I had just lo..."

Rhonda Uft interrupted, raising an index finger to wave in Khai's face. "I only asked how it was possible to take the medical subspecialty exams and not be certified. Not interested in excuses for failure."

Khai's face reddened, and her hand began to rise to slap away Rhonda Uft's finger, but she caught herself as Harrison Jennings jumped to his feet. "Objection. We will get to this later, and Counsel is, once again, badgering the witness."

"Sustained. Ms. Uft, Dr. Weathersby appears to be answering your questions precisely and honestly. Move on."

"Okay, Your Honor, I'm trying not to waste the court's time or that of the jury. I would ask the court remind the witness she is to answer only the posed question, not editorialize."

Galanter's head dropped a few centimeters. "Very commendable, Counselor, your consideration for the court's time. I would remind the witness to answer Ms. Uft's questions without additional comment." Khai nodded deferentially. "Thank you, Doctor. Please go on Ms. Uft."

"Now, Doctor, we have established that you failed your certification examination for hematology."

"Objection. Asked and answered and, once again, badgering." Jennings shook his head and, with a very gentle but confident smile, snuck in, "The jury can be assured we will get to the bottom of this on redirect."

Galanter sighed, "Sustained."

Rhonda Uft barely paused before asking, "If a patient is having a stroke, what specialty is called to care for that person?"

"Internal medicine or neurology."

"Doctor, are you telling the court you wouldn't call a neurologist immediately if you had a patient in the hospital undergoing what you believed to be a stroke?"

"I would do the immediate evaluation and treatment, and when the patient was stable, ask for a neurology consult."

"Doctor, do you have any training in neurology?"

"Of course. All internal medicine specialists do."

Rhonda Uft glanced at the judge, but when he stared back at her, she went on. "Have you earned a board or other certificate in neurology?"

"No."

"Did you lecture us on strokes?"

"I answered Mr. Jennings' questions about strokes. I hope I wasn't lecturing."

"But you are not board certified in neurology, are you?"

"No."

"And how long is a neurology residency?" She lifted a palm in Khai's face. "Let me rephrase. How long a period of training in just neurology is required before you are even allowed to take the board exam to call yourself a neurologist?"

"Four years."

"And please remind the court just how long your plain internal medicine residency lasted."

"Three years."

"Would you agree that a neurologist, that is a stroke specialist, is far more highly trained in strokes than you are?"

Khai grimaced. "Yes."

"You mentioned the plaintiff's psychiatric problems. Let me ask, are you board certified in psychiatry?"

"No."

"Yet you spoke to us about complex psychiatric problems the plaintiff claims she is suddenly suffering from. Is that correct."

"Is what correct?"

"That you lectured the court in regard to a complex claim of psychiatric disease."

"I read the letters to the court I was asked to and gave my professional evaluation of Dr. Maddingly's psychiatric state before and after the stroke at Mitchie-Sterling Hospital."

"Do you consider yourself an expert witness in regard to psychiatric disease?"

"I am knowledgeable."

"No. I am not asking that. I am asking if you are an expert in the sense of a doctor who does psychiatry exclusively and is board certified in psychiatry."

"No, I am not."

"Oh, and by the way, how long is a psychiatry residency?"

"Four years."

"Would you agree that a psychiatrist is more familiar with diseases of the mind than is an internist?"

"I do not agree. If the problem is simple depression, an internist is as capable of handling the early treatment as well as a board-certified psychiatrist. And I did not treat Dr. Maddingly for her depression. A psychiatrist, many psychiatrists, did."

"So, in other words, Doctor, you are not an," she made quotes with her fingers, "an expert in anything."

"Objection. Argumentative and demeaning."

"Sustained."

"Let me rephrase. So, in other words, Doctor, you are not a," up came the fingers, "a board-certified specialist in anything we've discussed today. Is that correct?"

"No, it is not. I am competent in all of the specialties we have discussed today. That's what being board certified in internal medicine means."

"We'll see about that. Now, you have testified that plaintiff's depression is quite complicated, haven't you?"

"Yes."

"So, it follows that you have testified about a level of psychiatric disease beyond your training. Is that true?"

"No. I understand the level of complexity of her problem, though I don't treat that level. That is because the medications and the procedures are complicated, not the concepts."

"Okay, so, does that mean if the defense puts a board-certified psychiatrist on the stand, you would feel comfortable disagreeing with their opinion regarding the plaintiff's level of psychiatric disease."

"I certainly might. Especially if it is clear that there are questionable motives behind that doctor's opinion. Don't care who he is."

"Are you suggesting, yes or no, please, that this defense team would seek to color the opinion of an expert physician?"

"Frankly, yes."

Rhonda Uft blurted, "Your Honor, that is so prejudicial, I don't know how to stop this other than excusing the witness and redacting her testimony to just her findings on the night of November 25th."

Galanter looked down at Khai. "Doctor, this is a court of law. Every word uttered within these walls has the potential to affect the jury. In the end, that can lead to an incorrect decision on their part. That is a disaster. Our whole system is based on teasing facts from the morass of assumptions, mistakes, and lies. We are here to bring factual evidence, not our personal opinions, before the jury. Unless you can substantiate your opinions, they are not facts, and I will not tolerate their introduction in my courtroom. Are we clear?"

"I guess so, sir, but I have been called as a witness for the defense in several cases, and I was briefed on what to and what not to say."

"Well, Doctor, we have no facts to indicate that is the case here. The jury is to disregard the witness's non-medical opinion that lawyers tell expert doctors what to say in court. Don't do that again. Continue, Ms. Uft."

"Thank you, Your Honor. Now, Doctor, we have established that you are not board certified in neurology or psychiatry. Is that correct?"

"Objection. Asked and answered."

Rhonda Uft snapped at the judge, "Well, I have a right to recap for the jury after a substantial delay. I didn't cause this waste of the jury's time."

"Sustained."

"Doctor, last housekeeping question. Are you board certified in obstetrics, I mean the specialty that has to do with childbirth?"

"No."

"Is there a board certification for that specialty?"

"Yes."

"How long, I mean how many years, is the most basic obstetric residency program before a young doctor may take the boards and call themselves an obstetrician?"

"Four to five years."

"Would you argue with the opinion of a board-certified obstetrician regarding the proper handling of a patient with a tubal pregnancy?"

"I would argue if that so-called expert just quoted the textbook."

"Textbook. Okay. Are you familiar with Williams Obstetrics?"

"Yes."

"Is it well-respected?"

"Yes, of course."

"When was it first published?"

"I haven't the slightest."

"Nineteen-thirty. So, if we have a board-certified obstetrician testify regarding the proper treatment of a tubal pregnancy, and they quoted Williams Obstetrics, you would testify that you knew more than the textbook and the obstetrician?"

"The obstetrician wasn't there that night. I was. I am sure if you read the book closely, you will find the part where Dr. Williams refers to the attending physician's need to use his or her best judgement."

"Please tell me exactly which page and which paragraph and to which of the eleven editions you are referring."

"I can't, but it is definitely in there. That sentiment is in every textbook of medicine."

"Have you read all of the eleven editions?"

"No, nobody has."

"Have you read as much as a board-certified obstetrician?"

"No."

"But you say you would dispute the testimony of a board-certified obstetrician?"

"Yes, depending what the obstetrician said. Just reading a textbook does not mean you can't make mistakes. That's why there are malpractice cases. Doctors do make mistakes."

Rhonda Uft took a deep breath to appeal to the judge but calmed and turned back to Khai. Okay, doctor, let's move on. Just a few more questions.

"Please tell us, on the night of November 25th, the first time you met the plaintiff, did you make a diagnosis on why the plaintiff had abdominal pain?"

"No."

Rhonda Uft again pulled her head away in mock surprise. "I seem to remember you testified that you felt the plaintiff suffered from a tubal pregnancy. Was that not your testimony?"

"My testimony was that I feared she might have a tubal pregnancy. That is not a diagnosis. I sent her to the hospital for a diagnosis. Had I had a diagnosis, I would not have bothered to get the tests to prove it."

"Are you referring to the tests Plaintiff underwent that night you ordered her to go to the emergency room?"

"Correct."

"Do you think, on a more probable than not basis, that a board-certified obstetrician would have diagnosed a tubal pregnancy without wasting time getting those tests?"

"I have no idea, but I cannot imagine a decent doctor guessing about a diagnosis of that magnitude. We just don't go opening up people's bodies without some objective evidence in advance."

"Well, is it possible that the time spent on those tests contributed to the plaintiff's internal bleeding?"

"The delay brought her closer to the point of rupture. There was still plenty of time…"

Up came Rhonda Uft's palm in Khai's face. "Would you agree that if the plaintiff had been seen an hour earlier at the hospital, she would have had a greater chance of this just having been a small surgical procedure without the possibility of low blood pressure?"

"If she had been seen an hour earlier when she walked into the ER."

"That's not what I asked. Had she been on the Mitchie-Sterling campus an hour earlier, would there have been an hour more for the ER to follow their usual procedures and see her in turn? Yes or no?"

"Yes."

"Well, let me ask." She went back to her desk and pulled a sheet of paper from a three-ring binder. "This is Exhibit A-6." She handed it to the bailiff, who handed it to the judge, who perused it and handed it back down until it eventually got to Khai. Rhonda Uft smiled at the judge. "Your Honor, I would like to project this document on the screen."

"You may."

Her assistant placed the form on an overhead projector. The screen flashed with a document.

AGAINST MEDICAL ADVICE (AMA FORM)

This is to certify that I, Michael Maddingly, for Sabrina Friday Maddingly, my wife and a patient at the Evanston Medical Center, am refusing care for my wife at my own insistence and without the authority of, and against the advice of, my attending physician, Khai Weathersby, M.D. I am requesting to leave against medical advice. The medical risks/benefits have been explained to me by a member of the medical staff and I understand those risks.

I hereby release the medical center, its administration, personnel, and my attending physician(s) from any responsibility for all consequences which may result by my leaving under these circumstances.

MEDICAL RISKS:
- Death
- Additional pain and/or suffering
- Risks to unborn fetus,
- Permanent disability/disfigurement
- Other:_____

MEDICAL BENEFITS:
- CAT scan
- X-rays:
- Ultrasound (sonogram)
- Laboratory testing
- Potential hospital admission and/or follow-up
- Medications as indicated for infection, pain, blood pressure,

etc.

Other: Life-saving surgery

Please return at any time for further testing or treatment.

Patient Signature: Michael Maddingly
Date: November 25th/2048 hrs.

Physician Signature: K. Weathersby, M.D.

Date: November 25th/2048 hrs.

Witness: S Fritzer, R.N.
Date: November 25th/2048 hrs.

"Doctor, would you tell the jury what this form is used for?"

"When a patient does not wish to follow a doctor's advice, there is no law that says they have to. The attending doctor, though, has a duty to inform the patient of the potential for problems if they refuse the recommended care."

"Let me stop you there. Have you ever used one of these forms?"

"Yes."

"How often?"

"A few times."

"I believe you said in your deposition that you have used this four times in the past ten years. Is that a correct characterization of your testimony during your deposition for this litigation?"

"Yes."

"And you testified to having seen how many patients over the past ten years?"

"Many thousands."

"So, would you agree it is very rare to have a patient refuse care?"

"Yes."

"And didn't you testify during your deposition that the three other times were when you were a resident, and the patients in question were end-stage alcoholics from the streets of Boston?"

"Yes."

"So, it is truly remarkable when a reasonable patient chooses to leave a medical facility while a doctor is essentially begging them to stay. Is that correct?"

"Yes."

"Would you please look up at the document on the screen." She played a laser pointer over the signatures and asked Khai if they were what they appeared to be. She allowed they were. "And, as a good military person, you even included the time the document was signed. Is that notation of the time correct?"

"Yes."

"What time does it say?"

"Twenty-forty-eight hours."

"What is that in civilian time?"

"Eight-forty-eight P.M."

Rhonda Uft bristled over to the desk, pulled another document from the binder, and had it perused by the judge and Harrison Jennings. She placed it on the overhead. "What is this, Doctor?"

"That is the laboratory report of Dr. Maddingly's pregnancy test."

"What time does it say the test was performed?"

"The test was completed at twenty-three-hundred hours."

"In English, please?"

"Eleven P.M."

"So, essentially two and some hours went by between the time you informed the patient she might die and the time her husband got her into the hospital for the battery of tests?"

"No. They did not leave the clinic immediately after signing the AMA form. I went over it again with them. And the drive takes twenty-plus minutes, it takes half an hour to check in, and the test itself takes nearly an hour. That's nearly two hours."

"Your Honor, yet again, I object to the witness's babbling."

Harrison Jennings was on his feet. "Your Honor, this is not a hostile witness, far from it. I think what she told us is a reasonable answer to the way Ms. Uft phrased her question."

"Objection overridden."

Rhonda Uft's mouth twisted in contempt. "Now, Doctor, I know you are not an expert in obstetrics, so we will wait until we have a board-certified obstetrician on the stand to establish how long it takes for a young woman to bleed nearly to death from a burst tubal pregnancy. Would you, though, agree, yes or no, the time required is measured in minutes, not hours?"

"No. Minutes count only after it has burst. A tubal can go on for weeks, usually does, even under a doctor's watchful eyes. And in this case, she hadn't bled until she reached the..."

The palm was back in Khai's face. "Again, Your Honor, I didn't ask for explanations."

Galanter sighed. "Doctor, I remind you again to answer the question asked, not to offer a clarification unless Ms. Uft asks an open-ended question.

Mr. Jennings will have the opportunity to ask for an expansion of your answers on redirect." Khai nodded.

Rhonda Uft continued. "Doctor, do you know where the Plaintiffs spent that time?"

"I know what they told me."

"What did they tell you?"

"They told me Dr. Maddingly was much better, so they put her to bed, but half an hour later, she worsened."

"Okay, Dr. Weathersby, at some point before 9 P.M. that Thanksgiving Eve, when you made them sign the Against Medical Advice form, were you worried, yes or no, that the plaintiff might die if she didn't go directly to the hospital?"

"Yes."

"So, yes or no, would we be here today if the plaintiff's husband had taken his precious wife to the hospital, as strongly urged by a board-certified medical doctor?"

"Don't know."

"Yes, you do." Harrison Jennings started to rise, but Rhonda Uft smiled at the jury, "Withdrawn. Now, Doctor, how long have you been practicing in the Northwest at this point?"

"Sixteen months."

"Have you joined the County Medical Society?"

"No"

"Have you joined the State Medical Society?"

"No."

Have you joined the American Medical Association?"

"No."

"Do most doctors in good standing join these organizations?"

"I have no idea how many doctors join the good-ole-boy clubs."

"Are you accusing these organizations of being nothing more than a bunch of cigar-smoking, bourbon-guzzling, rich doctors?"

"I don't know. I don't join clubs."

"So, the legislation they support on behalf of patients is not part of their good works. Yes or no, are you saying that?"

"Again, I have no idea what they represent. All I know..." She stopped and glanced cautiously at the judge, who stared down at her.

Rhonda Uft interjected, "I have no further questions for this witness, Your Honor."

As she took her seat, the static began to seep from the room.

Galanter turned to Jennings. "Counsel, I imagine you will want to do a redirect."

"Yes, Your Honor."

"Well, we've been at it for some time today. It might be time to adjourn. Do you have a problem waiting until morning to redirect?"

"Respectfully, Your Honor, if we postpone until tomorrow, I won't have the opportunity to address some of the problems that have come up during cross-examination. I want to nip them in the bud, sir."

"Ms. Uft?"

"It seems to me there isn't much to cover on redirect. I think the facts have been laid out, and it's time to let the jury go home, relax, and absorb what they've heard."

Jennings growled, "Excuse me, sir, but I would like to do my redirect right now."

Galanter turned to the jury and polled them by watching their body language. Mostly, there were nods, and one old man in the back row lifted a thumb. Galanter smiled. "So be it. I trust, though, Mr. Jennings, that we will not be here until midnight."

"No, sir. Quick and dirty, not a minute past 11:45."

There were giggles from the jury, though Rhonda Uft remained poker-faced until Galanter chortled. A milli-second later, an on-demand smile warped Rhonda Uft's lips. She nodded to Galanter.

Harrison Jennings approached the witness stand. "Dr. Weathersby, let's quickly go over a few points. First, you studied for and took the certification examination for hematology, did you not?"

"Yes."

"When was that exam given?"

"On Tuesday, March 28th, 2009."

"You seem to remember the date very well. Why is that?"

Khai's face tightened to the point that some of the jurors' shoulders tensed. She hissed through clenched teeth, "It was two days after I was notified...No, I will maintain my privacy. I failed the exam. I have no excuse."

"I'm sorry, Doctor, I have to be honest and say I don't know what happened, and if you wish, we will leave that alone."

"Thank you."

Judge Galanter asked softly, "Do you want to take a break, Doctor?"

"No way, sir," she growled.

Jennings went on. "Okay, when did you arrive in Chicago from Boston to take the exam?"

"An hour before starting time."

"What time was the exam?"

"Zero-nine-hundred."

"Nine o'clock in the morning? So, you must have flown all night?"

"Yes."

"And, last question about the exam, does everyone pass the first time they take it?"

"Not at all."

"Oh, and please tell us, what was your class standing when you graduated from medical school at Yale?

"Six."

"Out of?"

"About one hundred."

"Now, in regard to your description of a tubal pregnancy: Dr. Weathersby, would you ever try to treat a tubal pregnancy?"

"Of course not."

"Why?"

"It takes years to learn the skill set to do the surgery. I know what to do, but my hands are not trained to do it."

"So, you feel comfortable telling us you were concerned that Dr. Maddingly was suffering signs of a tubal pregnancy, but also felt there had not yet been bleeding when, in the end, she left your clinic and went directly to the hospital. Is that true?"

Rhonda Uft jumped to her feet. Her assistant pulled the chair away before it could fly backwards. "Objection. Leading question. Compound question. Counsel's trying to confuse the jury, *and* he's testifying."

"Mr. Jennings, please restate as a single question."

"Yes, Your Honor. Dr. Weathersby, were you trained sufficiently in your residency to recognize a tubal pregnancy?"

"Yes."

"As a board-certified internist, are you able to recognize when someone is severely bleeding internally."

"Of course. It is one of the most important skills an internist must perfect."

"In your professional opinion, on a more probable than not basis, was Dr. Weathersby bleeding significantly when she left your clinic and went to the hospital?"

"No, she was not."

"In your professional opinion, on a more probable than not basis, was Dr. Weathersby bleeding significantly when she left the ultrasound examination at the hospital that night and walked, unaided, to the emergency room?"

"No, she was not bleeding significantly."

"In your professional opinion, on a more probable than not basis, was Dr. Weathersby bleeding significantly while she was sitting in the emergency room for the first hour?"

"No."

A shrill, "Objection!," echoed off the dull green walls of the courtroom. "The witness has no idea what was going on in the ER while the plaintiff waited to be seen."

"Sustained."

Harrison Jennings nodded. "Withdrawn. I guess we'll have to wait to establish how long it took before Dr. Maddingly was seen and, more importantly, what was going on in the emergency room while Dr. Maddingly was sitting there. I have no further questions for Dr. Weathersby."

"Ms. Uft, do you wish to re-cross?"

She glanced furtively at the jury. Eyes were rolling. "No, Your Honor."

While she seethed, Galanter thanked Khai and dismissed her as a witness. Court was adjourned for the day.

CHAPTER FORTY-THREE

H arp phoned Rhonda Uft late that afternoon. He asked, without offering a greeting, if there had been any startling revelations after he'd left the courtroom. She answered cautiously, "Don't worry, I took very good care of that doctor from Evanston. She's not going to be a problem. I do think, though, that they are going to beat the ultrasound report to death."

"I thought we were out of the woods on that one."

"Depends. I don't think they can afford much in the way of professional witnesses, so forensic experts are probably out of the question. And I still don't think that the case hinges on that report. They *are* going to be able to convince the jury that the bleeding took place in the emergency room. What we need to do is prove that Cardozo was never informed on the phone by Weathersby that the situation was dire, and that the husband didn't even check in properly. Another one of the husband's critical mistakes. And we are going to beat the previous medical problems to death. Lot of directions to come from."

"Rhonda, I thought juries don't like holding patients responsible for minor lapses in judgement."

"True, but his actions were more than just a lapse. As far as I'm concerned, he's going to carry the load of the delay himself. And it is going to be clear she was defective the moment she was conceived. At least, that's what the jury is going to believe."

"All while preserving her dignity?"

She was so startled by Harp's question, she could not speak for a moment. Finally, "Hers, yes. But don't you worry; when we get done with Mr.

Maddingly, you might expect our sad little plaintiff to start divorce proceedings. There's an attorney in my firm who specializes in untidy marital cases like these."

Harp snorted, "Soup to nuts, huh?" He was quiet for a long moment. "Well, certainly seems you have things under control, but we also have to keep in mind the level of publicity. That whole Agent Orange thing could be a trap. People don't hate Viet Nam vets so much anymore. What they hate on this cycle of idiocy are government and corporations, like us. Morons don't understand how many jobs we create. We're feeding the worker bees, and they sting our fingers." There was another silence then, "Whatever, we have to be careful."

"I certainly understand, Norman, and we will tailor our attack to your needs. The corporation comes first." Her voice trailed off, and Harp felt a disquiet building on her end of the line. He was not surprised when she took a deep breath before continuing. "You know, Norman, the other side is going to be calling your Dr. Gauthé to the stand pretty soon."

He waited for the other shoe to drop, but when she said nothing, he muttered stiffly, "Is he going to be a problem? Poor man's finally back from his time out. Should be relaxed, easy to manipulate."

"You know, Norman, I'm not sure how he's going to come across in court. I haven't shared this with anyone yet, but I saw that Dr. Weathersby getting out of his car early this morning. I am not sure what it means, but I have an..."

She stopped abruptly to force a response. It was, as she had predicted, edgy. "You think he's going to side with her, turn on us?"

"I have no idea. You've known him for years. I had three hours with him during a deposition. He's smart, answered every question with a response that could go either way. Not sure where he's coming from. I was hoping you might know."

"Well, I don't, but I'm sure you can sculpt whatever you want out of his testimony. You're very good."

"Thank you, Norman. I work hard at it, but there's something that bothers me about him. One of our new attorneys, my assistant at the depositions, is a young woman. I'll be honest, she's striking, but even the fat old men in the office know when to stop staring at her tits and get back to work. Your Dr. Gauthé was riveted on her. At lunch, he cornered her, though I don't think she minded. He's that kind of man."

"Rhonda, I value your input, but Gauthé is apparently having troubles at home, like most of us. This is not the 1950s. He's free to do what he wants."

"Agreed, but I felt it important to alert you about the Weathersby connection. He may be thinking with the wrong head. Not the first doctor over at the hospital to suffer from that malady."

"Thank you for your observation. Let me mull it over. You free to talk in the morning?"

"Have to be up very early. One of the ER nurses is being called to the stand, first witness of the day. I'll be at it all night, cooking up excuses for what will certainly be a cavalcade of incompetence she'll shriek at the top of her lungs. She's the one who quit that night."

"Because Cardozo screamed the F word at her? That the one?"

"The very one. I'm sure you remember; her husband came to the ER the next night and threatened to bust Cardozo in the nose. Cost him Thanksgiving weekend in the city lockup, and a couple of thousand in legal fees before you so graciously dropped the charges. From what I heard, they're going to use the trial as a sounding board then file a suit against the hospital if the jury seems sympathetic. I understand their lawyer's going to be in the Peanut Gallery. So, I have to work on impeaching her testimony for both cases."

"And, Norman, did you read Cardozo's deposition?"

"Yes, carefully."

"Then you saw how he made a fool of Jennings."

"I saw that. Was surprised. Thought it might be a prelude to an out-of-court settlement."

"Well, it's an old trick. You don't try your case in the deposition. You feel around and see what kind of witness you're dealing with. Let them have the upper hand, and when the trial comes, you eat 'im alive. I had Cardozo in for a little prep, but he won't listen. Convinced he's smarter than all of us put together. Mark my words. By the time Jennings is done with him, I'd have an easier time defending Dr. Mengele. Maybe you could have a chat with him."

"Ah, and therein lies the problem. I have no control over him. It's a separate corporation, sort of. All of the specialties are going that way. I've chatted with the administrator over there, but she hates us, and just yesterday she told me that if I didn't like Cardozo, then I could fire the whole group."

Rhonda Uft laughed. "She may think she's got you over a barrel, that they're the only game in town, but if Cardozo loses this case, he won't be able to buy insurance, and everyone in the group'll see their rates double. That will be the third malpractice action for their group in as many years. He's a liability for them in a lot of ways."

Harp asked, "I imagine it doesn't matter that the first two were nuisance cases, settled for a song to save attorney fees?"

"Maybe the first one got settled for a song. Malpractice carrier may forgive that one, but after the second, no matter the outcome, the insurance company's antennae are a mile high. And with this one, if he takes the stand, and they lose because of his testimony, Cardozo will be lucky to find work in the U.S; maybe get a walk-in clinic job in Uganda.

"But Norman, you can lean on him and have his malpractice insurance company's in-house lawyers lean on him. If that doesn't work, there'll be a lot of saber rattling from the insurance company execs, and his pals in the ER corporation will fold like a cheap suit. They'll take him out into the woods for a little persuasion, insurance company may join in."

"Maybe we will, too. Just between us, he's a piece of work, but have you ever tried to fire a doctor? Easier to get rid of a postal employee." Harp paused for several seconds then began again conspiratorially. "Rhonda, wait a minute. In the transcript, do you remember when he admitted to growing pot?"

"Yeah, I do. Sorry to tell ya, but that's not a big deal anymore. Seattle City Council has virtually legalized heroin and coke and meth. Become sort of a badge of honor to be one of the dregs of society around here—move your bowels in the street, beat up people who won't give you cash."

Harp hissed, "But when he filled out the application for a medical license in Washington State, it was still illegal, and he must have sworn he'd never been involved in drugs. Is that correct?"

"Norman, I guess so. But we aren't going to win our case on the grounds that he smoked the Devil's lettuce when he was a kid. Comes with the territory of having grown up in the 60s and 70s, and the 8os and 90s, on and on ad nauseum."

Harp smirked, "Not for me."

"Well, Norman, I'm quite impressed, but I don't think a 21st Century jury is going to give a hoot, either way. Anyway, I'm going to spend some time thinking about what to do with him. Still, maybe a word to the wise from the Grand Puba? And, again, maybe one for your Dr. Gauthé as well."

"I'll do it, but as far as I can see, nothing Cardozo did beyond growing cannabis is actionable."

"Norman, everything is actionable."

After he put the phone down, Harp sat in his office for a half-an-hour staring at Mt. Rainier from the windows of his corner office. At five-thirty, he called the surgical floor and asked if Chris Gauthé was done with his cases for the day. The clerk cooed, "Oh, yes, Mr. Harp, he's just finishing up in Six. Did you want to speak to him, sir?"

"No, no. I'll catch him some other time. Please don't bother him." He dropped the receiver and descended the stairs to the surgery floor, where he stood pretending to be gazing out the window into an old parking lot, scribbling notes and a clumsy sketch of a building. He looked up sneakily when Chris pushed head down, shoulders slumped, through the swinging doors into the hospital proper. Harp brightened and chuckled, "That you, Chris?"

Gauthé looked up and smiled weakly, "I think it's me. What are you doing slumming down here?"

"Just reviewing plans for the new annex. Wanted to get an idea of what it's going to do the view from the surgical recovery area. Nurses gotta have a scenic vista or they grumble, threaten slowdowns. And the patients—all of a sudden, good food and good care isn't enough. Patients want a view from their hotel room. Nothing's easy anymore." Harp put the pad in his jacket pocket and murmured, "Well, now that I got you here, why don't you walk with me? Something I want to bounce off you anyway."

Gauthé nodded resignedly. "Lotta stuff goin' on around here. Your plate's pretty full, isn't it?"

Harp forced an insincere smile. "Indeed, it is. But right now, one of the biggest challenges is resolving the Maddingly lawsuit without us getting our heads handed to us. That's what I wanted to visit with you about."

"Uh huh. Well, let's visit. How can I help?"

Harp muttered, "Let's wait until we get up to my office." Gauthé followed until they stopped in the empty area outside Harp's door. He looked around and spoke softly. "This is fine. Let me ask, Chris, how's things at home?"

"Hey, Norman, that's a whole 'nother topic. Doesn't concern the hospital."

"Well, I'm just asking because, you know, I keep my nose pretty close to the ground around here. Just wondering if you're on the market."

"Norman, I'm not sure I like where this is going."

"Look, Doctor, let me be right up front. You know hospital policy. You can't be involved with the staff. Terrible for business. Never turns out well."

Gauthé's face reddened. "Like I said, I'm not sure I like where this is headed. This is the twenty-first century. I mean, sexual harassment's a no-no, but half the docs around here are getting some on the side from the nurses, and the boy nurses, I might add. Some of it's going on right here in the patient rooms, even the bathrooms—before work, after work, and I know of at least one little tryst during work. You might not want to open that Pandora's box—no pun intended."

Harp snorted a laugh. "I hear ya, but what I'm concerned about, I mean right here, right now, just between us, is that lady doctor from Evanston."

"Norman, don't tell me. She's the newest member of the staff?"

"Chris, please. I have one job in this world for which my bosses, you and the rest of the doctors, pay me well, thank you, and that is to protect the corporation. How can I justify that salary if I see something in the vapors that has the potential of really hurting the hospital, and I don't at least try to examine the prospective damage?"

"Understood."

"Okay, Chris. Let me be direct. I don't give a shit if you are banging every doctor and nurse in the county, just as long as they don't work here. What concerns me is the possibility that your testimony might not be clearly pro-hospital if feelings are involved. It's also not going to look so slick if word gets out to your wife, and there's another messy divorce. Think of Rockham and his crazed ex-tuna; lady running through the halls of the hospital screaming that he's a scumbag. I think she said, 'He's infected with AIDS and hepatitis C and syphilis.' You have to admit, that's not great for business."

"Norman, I understand where you're coming from, and I respect your concern. I assure you; I know where my bread is buttered. I hope that's good enough. I trust you will be judicious in regard to keeping this conversation limited to two people—you and me."

"The conversation will, but I have to tell you, that bitch from Evanston was spotted getting out of your car this morning."

"By whom?"

"Chris, let's say I will speak to the party concerned and insure, as a quid pro quo, discretion on our part."

Gauthé snapped, "Our, Norman?"

Harp nodded to Chris and heeled around into his office.

CHAPTER FORTY-FOUR

Thelma Tharker's name was called by the bailiff at 9:00 the next morning. Rhonda Uft watched the faces of the jury as the woman hitched up to the witness stand, her lips tensed, not so much by the pain coming from her hip, but from the fact that the only other words she had ever uttered before an audience were on the day she graduated from nursing school, chanting with her class a promise to uphold the finest traditions of medicine. The band of defense attorneys rolled their eyes as the woman sat, pale and shaking, waiting to be sworn. Her, "I do," was so nearly inaudible, Galanter looked down and smiled, "Ma'am, if you could speak up so our jury and the court reporter can hear you. Thank you." She bobbed her head, but her eyes clouded, and several of the jurors looked away.

Galanter nodded at Harrison Jennings, who stepped toward the stand, a broad smile aimed at his witness. He, though, left a fifteen-foot gap between himself and the woman. "Now, Mrs. Tharker," he spoke softly, "thank you very much for agreeing to speak to us this morning." A few tears coursed along her ghost-white, chipmunk cheeks. "This is really very easy. As you know, I will ask simple questions about your time working at Mitchie-Sterling Hospital. You only have to answer yes or no, if that makes you more comfortable. If you do not understand a question, please ask me to restate it. Is that okay?"

Her head jiggled again. The judge spoke a bit more forcefully. "Madam, you'll have to speak your answers. You see, we have a court reporter recording every word of the trial, and she has to be able to hear you. Thank you."

"Yes," she blurted.

Jennings smiled and nodded. "Did you answer 'yes' to my question asking if you understood my instructions?"

"Yes."

"Great. Now, we are just going to ask about your position at Mitchie-Sterling Hospital. First, what was your title there?" She said nothing, and Jennings smiled. "Okay, I understand that you wish to answer my questions with a yes or no, just as we agreed."

"Yes."

"Then let me ask, did you earn a bachelor of science degree in nursing from Seattle University in 1981?"

"Yes."

"Okay, were you hired immediately by Mitchie-Sterling Hospital as a registered nurse after your graduation?"

"Yes."

"So, you have worked for Mitchie-Sterling Hospital for more than two decades?"

"Yes."

"Did you take off any time during your employment by Mitchie-Sterling Hospital?"

"No."

"Not even when you had children?"

"No."

"You were very dedicated to the hospital, weren't you?"

"Yes."

"Did you work in the emergency room at Mitchie-Sterling Hospital for eighteen of those years?"

"Yes."

And so the testimony ground for the next ten minutes, punctuated with grunts of, "Yes, I was," or, "No, I didn't," until the other shoe dropped, and Harrison Jennings asked quietly, "Are you aware of a Dr. Peter G. Cardozo?" The woman's face twisted like a piece of balled up aluminum foil. The pallor fled, replaced by the scarlet of a pre-cancerous sunburn. She reached into her purse for a tissue to wipe her brow.

"Now, Mrs. Tharker, were you on duty on Thanksgiving Eve, the night of November 25th two years ago?"

"I was," she snarled.

Rhonda Uft rolled her eyes again, this time directly at the jury. There were a few snickers, but the judge glowered, and a tense solemnity, as thick as an asbestos curtain, fell upon the jurors' faces.

As Jennings spoke, setting the scene, several jurors crept closer to the edge of their seats. He finally took a deep breath and locked his witness's gaze. "Mrs. Tharker, do you still work for Mitchie-Sterling Hospital?"

"No, I resigned in protest."

"Protest? But you are a very kind, quiet, respectful..."

Rhonda Uft was on her feet. "Objection. Counsel is testifying."

"Sustained."

"What were you protesting, Mrs. Tharker?"

"That Godless man." She looked about the courtroom, expecting Cardozo to be smirking back at her, as Jennings had presaged, but the man was not there.

"Who?"

"Cardozo."

"What did he do?"

"He blasphemed!"

"Blasphemed! How did he do that?"

"He took the Lord's name in vain, and he used a word of filth in the same sentence."

"What did he say?"

"You can put me to death, but I will not answer that question."

Rhonda Uft stirred as if she was about to stand and object but nodded to herself, then to the jury, and settled back in her seat.

Jennings smiled at his witness. "Don't worry, no one will make you say anything that obscene in public."

"Or private," she hissed.

"Or private. Could you tell us, though, what the situation was in the emergency treatment room when he acted so unprofessionally?"

"Objection. Leading, and we have not established that anyone committed or uttered a single unprofessional word. Now Counsel wants the jury to guess at what was said. And a guess should be good enough to convict a good man, a competent man, and ruin his life? I move to strike all of the testimony regarding these supposed acts on the grounds that the witness is not emotionally competent to testify before a duly constituted jury. She is wasting the court's time."

"I will sustain the objection regarding the unprofessional language and acts, but let's give Mr. Jennings a chance to expand the witness's testimony. I will warn, though, that I will strike the totality of the witness's testimony if she is unwilling to provide the court with specifics that can be challenged on cross-examination. The jury is to ignore Defense Counsel's characterization of Dr. Cardozo's professionalism." He turned to Jennings. "Counsel, proceed—cautiously."

Before Harrison Jennings could turn back toward Thelma Tharker, the woman shrieked, "Jesus Fucking Christ. Fuck! Goddamn you..." The overwhelming, shocked silence was so thick, Galanter did not expend the energy to lift his gavel. He did, though, glare down as he demanded, "Explain yourself, madam."

"That was the filth he screamed at me and the rest of the ER staff. Now put me in jail, but he will not get away with his behavior. He's always like that..."

The gavel flew. "That is enough, madam. You may not just start talking in a court of law. You may only answer questions posed by one of the attorneys."

She harrumphed, "He asked me, and I told him."

Galanter's shoulders sagged. "Let us take a break. Mr. Jennings, please meet with the witness and explain the rules. One more outburst, and I will hold you both in contempt. Am I clear?"

Jennings nodded, "Yes, Your Honor. I will explain the proper way to get a valid, factual point across in court."

Rhonda Uft grunted, "Objection, yet again. We have not established anything this witness has said as factual."

"Sustained."

During the break, Jennings met with Thelma Tharker in a conference room off the legal library. "Is he going to put me in jail? My husband told me it wasn't terrible, just boring. I'm not afraid."

"Thelma, listen to me. We both want to see Cardozo punished for his terrible behavior. But you have to understand that in our free society there has got to be a place where we can sit down and calmly tell our side of the story, then let the jury determine if it is factual. Right? And we know that everything you have to say is factual. Right? So, please let me ask the questions, and if you want to answer with a yes or no, fine, and if you wish to answer more fully, just say, 'I would like to answer that question.' Okay?"

"I'm sorry, Mr. Jennings. But he must be punished for his blasphemy."

"I know. And he will be, mark my words, but please accept that the jury needs to hear how he did not do his job correctly. They may not be as properly upset with his foul words as we are. It's not against the law to say the things he did..."

She muttered, "Should be."

"Of course, it should be. But you are a professional, and you know that Cardozo's first duty is to the patient. Yes?"

"Yes."

"Well, let's get back up on the stand and tell the jury how he failed to do just that; how he cost this good Christian woman her life, essentially. Are you with me?"

"Okay, but he also has to be reprimanded publicly for his wickedness before the Lord."

"Thelma, don't you think God is going to do that for us, that it's His job?"

"That's what I pray every day."

When court reconvened, Judge Galanter spoke to the jury. "You are to ignore the witness's outburst before the break. Testimony in this court, in any court, is only allowed in response to a question from an attorney or the judge. Continue, Mr. Jennings."

"Thank you, Your Honor. Now, Mrs. Tharker, let's start from the moment Dr. Maddingly was wheeled into the treatment room. Are you willing to tell us what happened to make Dr. Cardozo say that to you? She was silent. "Do you want me to repeat the question, ma'am?"

"No."

"Well, let's start."

As Galanter shifted about in his chair, the defense counsel's shoulders tensed, her fingers drumming faster and louder as the silence deepened. Jennings, though, stood poker-faced for another full minute, right up until the thunderclap of Rhonda Uft exploding from her chair. "I move to have this witness dismissed. She is wasting the court's time."

Jennings was very subdued as he queried, "Your Honor, I would like to meet with my witness for a moment, if it pleases the court."

"It does not please the court, but I will allow one more interruption in order for you to get this case back on its wheels. Five-minute break."

Several of the jurors rolled their eyes as they had seen Rhonda Uft emote just seconds before. It was not lost on Harrison Jennings.

They spoke in the hall. "Thelma, tell me right now, yes or no, if you want to testify on behalf of Dr. Maddingly."

"Yes."

"Yes, what?"

"I want to sink that Cardozo and Mitchie-Sterling Hospital, too."

"Well, then why are you refusing to answer in a way that will help us?"

"I'm afraid I'll just burst out again."

"Can't you control that? You've been a top-notch nurse for two decades. A true professional. I talked to a lot of people at the hospital and your church before I asked you to be a witness, to join our case, our team, against those horrible people. Everybody respects you, and they love you. They want to sink Cardozo, but they don't have the opportunity. Only you do. Everyone's counting on you."

She was quiet for a moment, and her eyes dropped, but her lips tightened, and her shoulders snapped into attention. "I will testify."

On the stand, Jennings asked, "What happened when Dr. Maddingly was wheeled into the treatment room?"

"Someone took a blood pressure."

"Was the blood pressure high or low?"

"Very low."

"Have you seen this before."

"Yes."

"Is this common?"

"Yes."

"What is the usual treatment for this problem?"

"Start large bore IVs in the arms, and if that is not possible in the subclavian vein."

"Is it critical that the IV be introduced quickly?"

"Yes."

"How quickly?"

"Seconds."

"Why?"

"The patient is losing blood, and they will bleed out if you don't replace that blood."

"Objection. Beyond the scope of the witness's training."

Jennings growled, "The witness has been an ER nurse for two decades. I would suggest she knows more about emergency resuscitation than many a new doctor; maybe even most of the old ones."

Galanter monotoned, "Overridden."

Jennings asked, "Did Dr. Cardozo do that?"

"Do what?"

"Put the IV in within seconds?"

"No."

"How long did it take him?"

"He never got it in."

"Please tell the jury why he failed."

"He is incompetent."

"Objection. Stating facts not in evidence, yet again. I move to have this witness excused. She is clearly not able to provide probative testimony."

As the judge lifted his eyes to consider the motion, Nurse Tharker sucked in a grand breath to fuel a discourse of Hitlerian calumny. "He is no doctor, that Cardozo. All he does all shift is take the Lord's name in vain. His Jew lips spew the filth, the defilement, the desecration. That's all that big-nose Jew knows how to do. And I'll tell you, they're all the same. It turns my stomach."

"Objection. Argumentative and contemptuous."

"Sustained." Galanter paused until the scarlet in his face faded to crimson. "Madam, I am holding you in contempt of court. You are excused as a witness, and you will pay five hundred dollars to the Clerk of Court before you leave, or you will be held in the city lockup until you do so. Bailiff, please escort the witness to the Clerk's office. Court is adjourned for the morning. Counsel, my chambers."

Galanter dropped into his chair with a bang. He did not motion for the two lawyers to sit. "Jennings, you get what you wanted? I mean masterful, and on so many levels. Martyrdom for a witness. You know damn well this is a very conservative, lily-white, blue-collar constituency. Lot of white supremacist leanings. That kind of anti-Semitic trash talk plays nicely in these parts. You also fashioned a tale of deep dissention in the hospital ranks. Cardozo's a hero or his reputation is in the street, depending on which way you lean, all based on a madwoman's outburst. He isn't even a Jew. And, best of all, since I am a Jew, anything I do from here on that's not positive for your case, or for the defense, is just more fodder for an appeal. Judge is ruling for the anti-Semites because he wants to hide that he's a Jew, or he's ruling against anti-sematic witnesses because he's got that big chip on his shoulder, want's to show everybody that even though he's just one of those Jews, he tries to be like us, real Americans. This BS should not have ever percolated to the surface. You should have known what was on that moron's mind..."

"Listen, Your Honor," Harrison Jennings hissed in interruption, "you are not going to hold me responsible for some fanatical witch's ravings. We take our clients and witnesses as we get them. Or, have you been on the bench for so long you've forgotten?"

"Mr. Jennings you're skating on thin ice, sir."

"Well, Your Honor, you might remember that my kids are Jewish because my wife was, of course, only until she was...So, maybe there are crazies out there with hate in their hearts, but some of us believe in right and wrong; some of us fools live to right the inequalities that we've seen pass for justice in this very building."

Rhonda Uft sniffed deeply. Galanter ignored her. "Listen, Mr. Jennings, I know very well what happened. We will never be free of the tarnish one of our colleagues foisted on this Superior Court."

"And the son of a bitch still wields a gavel—right down the hall."

"That, Counselor, did not happen in my courtroom, and never will. You know that, sir.

"And, Ms. Uft, you are in my purview now. Your Seattle ways don't go over so well with these folks. You need to cool your jets." She nodded and let her head drop, but her lips tightened and quivered as if she was muttering. Galanter went on. "That is all. I want to see the deposition transcript for your next witness, Mr. Jennings. And within five minutes. If this is another wacko, I will make sure the witness never sees the light of my courtroom."

Jennings' next witness was, in fact, Chris Gauthé. He was scheduled to testify the next morning, as Jennings had assumed Thelma Tharker would take up the full day—most of it with his questioning—and just an hour on Rhonda Uft's end, for he knew Uft would impeach her on cross-examination into a sobbing puddle of helpless Jell-O within thirty minutes, and that would adjourn court for the day.

Chris Gauthé, though, had not scheduled the afternoon off and was deep into a bowel resection when Jennings' call filtered its way into the operating suite. Galanter dismissed the jury for the afternoon, growling his apology for the lack of planning on the part of Plaintiff's Counsel. Jennings went to his car and wrote a word-for-word transcript of the morning's discussion with the judge.

CHAPTER FORTY-FIVE

The older women of the jury watched with locked stares as Christopher René Gauthé took the witness stand. The crease in the pants of his Armani suit was as razor-sharp as a scalpel's edge, his shoes shined to a fare-thee-well. After being sworn in, he pulled rimless glasses out of a pocket and carefully wound the temples about his ears.

Harrison Jennings moved smoothly through the surgeon's credentials, dwelling on his appointment at the University of Washington as a researcher. Jennings established that the man had never been a defendant in a lawsuit, even the one this jury was hearing. He had never had more than a parking ticket or two and was even an elder in his church.

The meat of the examination began gently enough: "Let's get the big picture of what you did on the night in question, then we'll get down to specifics. Is that plan satisfactory?"

"Yes."

"In your capacity as a medical doctor, have you treated Dr. Maddingly?"

"Yes."

"When did you first treat Dr. Maddingly?"

"On the night of the 25th and the early morning of the 26th of November, two years ago."

"Where did you first treat Dr. Maddingly?"

"In the emergency room at Mitchie-Sterling Hospital."

"Generally, where do you practice medicine in the hospital?"

"In my office, in the operating room, and in the emergency room."

300

"How do you determine which of those three locations you might go to?"

"I see patients for preoperative and postoperative care in my office. I operate on them in the surgical suite, and I get called to the emergency room if I am needed there."

"How do you know if you are needed in the emergency room?"

"I get a call."

"Did you get a call on the night of November 25th?"

"No, I did not."

"Well, how did you find yourself treating Dr. Maddingly in the Mitchie-Sterling Hospital Emergency Room on the night of 25th November?"

"My nurse."

"Could you explain what you mean by 'my nurse'?"

"My nurse told me."

"What did she tell you, sir?"

He answered coldly. "I was needed in the ER."

"Where were you when she told you?"

"In the operating room."

"What were you doing?"

He hissed, "Operating."

"Let me ask, how does a nurse usually get a message to you during surgery? Slip a note into your hand?"

Gauthé growled, "I already said she told me."

Harrison Jennings took a step back and rested his chin in his hand. A moment later, he looked up at the judge and spoke softly. "Your Honor, this is quite unusual, but to save the court's time, I move to have Dr. Gauthé declared a hostile witness."

Galanter thought for a moment. "I'm not going to grant that, Mr. Jennings. Not at this time. Though, Dr. Gauthé, please respond to Mr. Jennings' questions a bit less aggressively."

"Yes, sir."

"So, Dr. Gauthé, what phase of the surgery were you in when your nurse told you that you were needed in the ER?"

"I was finishing."

"Could you explain that to the jury? I mean, what steps are taken to finish the surgery?"

He rolled his eyes and snipped. "You close the various layers of tissue, then you place a bandage over the wound."

"Did you actually do the final steps of the surgery?"

"I finished my part of the surgery."

"Where did you leave the process?"

"As usual, I left the closure of the skin and the application of the dressing to the assistant surgeon."

"Did you leave the patient before the final stitch was placed?"

"As usual, yes, when I was sure the patient was stable and safe."

"What did you do when you left the operating room?"

"My nurse and I went down to the emergency room."

"What nurse is that, sir."

"My personal nurse."

"What was her duty that night in that surgery?"

Gauthé's jaw dropped, his head shook, and his palms opened in disbelief. "She was my scrub nurse."

"Please tell the jury what that means."

"She hands me the instruments I call for."

"But you said she left *with* you. Who did that function when she left the operating room?"

"Obviously, another scrub nurse took over."

"Is that the standard procedure at the end of a surgery, I mean for the scrub nurse to leave when the main surgeon does?"

"Well, if we have another case coming up, she needs to get to the next room to set up."

"Did you have another case that night?"

"No."

"Can you tell us why she left with you?"

"It was a very long night. I needed someone I could trust to go along and help me in the ER."

"That is understandable." He turned away but over his shoulder asked, "Oh, does that mean you don't trust the nurses in the emergency room?"

"Objection. Leading."

"Sustained."

"Withdrawn. Let's go over just how you were given word that your presence was requested in the ER. You said your nurse was handing you instruments. So, she was in the room with you. Is that true?"

"Yes."

"How did the message get to her?"

"Someone told her."

"Do you know who that was?"

"No."

"I don't understand. You were standing a foot away from your scrub nurse, and someone came up to her and whispered in her ear. Were you so engrossed in the surgery that you simply didn't see?"

Before Rhonda Uft could object, Gauthé cracked, "I saw someone. They had a mask on. I don't know who it was, and I didn't pay attention. Could have been someone telling my scrub nurse that it would be another two minutes before the next tray of instruments was out of the sterilizer."

"Do you remember who told her to tell your scrub nurse?"

"I don't know who did."

"Do you know if the call come by telephone, or did a runner fly up three flights of stairs to get you?"

"I don't know."

"Well, Doctor, how long was it between the message to your scrub nurse and moment you left the ER?"

"Thirty seconds."

"What did you tell your assistant surgeon?"

"I don't remember the exact words. I probably told him we were asked to come to the ER to lend a hand, and for him to close. We do it all the time."

Jennings thought for a second then went on. "Okay, what did you do then?"

"Went to the ER."

"How did you get down there? Stairs, or did you wait for an elevator?"

"We used the stairs."

"Was it faster to use the stairs?"

"Yes."

"Did you rush down to the ER?"

"I'm not sure what you mean by rush."

"Well, it seems you were out of the operating room quickly; you said thirty seconds. I imagine you used the fastest method to get to the ER. Is that correct?"

"Yes."

"How long would you say it took from the time you got the message from your scrub nurse until you were in the treatment room in which Dr. Maddingly was on a gurney?"

"No more than two minutes."

"So, it seems it took less than two and a half minutes to gather your thoughts, move from the middle of an emergency surgery on Thanksgiving Eve to the stairwell, down three flights of stairs, along the two-hundred-foot hallway to the ER, then through two sets of closed doors, and find the treatment room in which Dr. Maddingly was waiting for you. Is that correct?"

"Yes."

"Were you running?"

"We moved quickly?"

"Please tell the jury if you were concerned at this point that a patient was in trouble."

"I don't know about trouble, but we were asked to help out."

"Well, do you normally run through the hospital pants on fire?"

"Objection."

"Sustained."

"Do you normally run through the hospital?"

"When I have to."

"When was the last time you had to?"

"I don't remember."

"Are you testifying, Doctor, under oath, that to this day you do not know who summoned you to the ER?"

Gauthé's lips tightened, and he paused a fraction of a second longer than he had planned. "I do not know. And it makes no difference. The patient was treated appropriately."

"Well, that remains to be seen." When Jennings saw Rhonda Uft lifting her frame from the chair, he turned to the judge. "Withdrawn. So, let's just recap for the jury. You were in the operating suite, and somehow a message came by carrier pigeon or GPS to your..."

There were giggles from the jury.

"Objection. Argumentative and leading."

"Sustained. Mr. Jennings, keep it professional."

"Yes, Your Honor. So, Doctor, when you were in the operating suite and got word through your nurse that your presence was needed in the ER, did you sense this was an emergency?"

"My sense was that I needed to lend a hand to a colleague who had called for assistance."

"I thought you said you didn't know who summoned you."

"I imagine it was not Dr. Cardozo, himself, who picked up the telephone. He was too busy saving a life."

"But, do you believe that it was Dr. Cardozo who initiated the call to you, that it was he who asked for your immediate presence?"

"I told you: I just don't know."

"Okay, let's change gears. When you entered Dr. Maddingly's treatment room, did you recognize that she was suffering from a serious medical problem?"

"Yes, many serious problems."

Harrison Jennings quickly turned his face away from the jury to hide his surprise, but he hoped not from his witness. "Well, at that moment, what did you feel was the most important problem?"

"Hypotension."

"What is that, sir?"

"Low blood pressure."

"How did you know that?"

"My nurse told me."

"And you say you don't know who told her of so important an emergency?"

"Objection. Asked and answered."

"Sustained."

"So, was the blood pressure already low when you were summoned to the emergency room?"

"Yes."

Rhonda Uft took a breath, and her lips tightened, but she quickly let her shoulders relax and said nothing.

"What procedure did you carry out in the emergency room?"

"I placed a central line in her subclavian vein and had the nursing staff replace the blood the patient was apparently losing."

"Excuse me, Doctor, how did you know she had lost blood?"

"Her blood pressure was low."

"How did you know so quickly that it wasn't from another cause, let's say septic shock?"

"Dr. Cardozo said it was a ruptured ectopic pregnancy."

"How could he have known if there had not yet been surgery?"

"I imagine he made the diagnosis on the information he had received."

"Objection. Calls for facts not in evidence."

"Sustained."

Harrison Jennings startled, and not theatrically. "Wait a minute. There is no mention on the ultrasound report that the radiologist advised the ER that there was a patient on the way down there that had a life-threatening bleed. How could they possibly have known?"

"I don't know; I wasn't called until after all that."

"Were you aware of the positive pregnancy test?"

Gauthé's eyes tightened as he deliberated. "I don't remember."

"Was Dr. Maddingly's blood pressure dangerously low?"

Rhonda Uft was on her feet. "Objection. Calls for a conclusion not in evidence."

"Sustained."

"Okay, Dr. Gauthé, how low was her blood pressure when you first laid eyes on her?"

"We could barely measure it."

"Does that mean it was below 70?"

"Yes."

"Wait a minute. This is the first time we have heard it was below 70. That is not in the records we have. It is not even in your operative note. Why not?"

"I do not even remember dictating the note; it was such a harrowing night."

"'Harrowing night.' Ostensibly, you do this sort of work on a daily basis. Is that correct?"

"This was exceptionally challenging, redeeming a life so far gone."

"'Redeeming a life so far gone?'" His voice had risen, the tremulous warp frightening even Rhonda Uft. "Thirty minutes before, she was walking and talking, a respected doctor at the University of Washington. There was no intervening trauma. How could this have happened, sir?"

Rhonda Uft recovered sufficiently to hiss weakly, "Objection. Badgering his own witness. And further, Dr. Gauthé...."

"Sustained. Let's just take a minute to let things cool."

"Your Honor, I do not need a minute for anything. I want an answer."

"Well, Counsel, we're going to take a five-minute break. Perhaps you can meet with your witness."

Jennings used the time to exit the building and walk a couple hundred yards in the cold mist. His color had brightened by the time court resumed. He was quiet and steady when he addressed Gauthé. "We have established that Dr. Maddingly's blood pressure was below 70 for some period of time. Is that correct, Doctor?"

"Yes."

"Is that sufficiently low to lead to a stroke or brain injury?"

"Depends."

Harrison Jennings looked toward the jury. "Below 70. Okay. Oh, and by the way, were you the first to treat her that night?"

"No."

"Who was, Doctor?"

"A doctor in Evanston."

"What was the last blood pressure taken by the doctor in Evanston?"

"I don't remember."

"Was it normal?"

"I think it was."

"Well, if you're not sure, we can have you look at the records again. You did review the records before this testimony, didn't you, Doctor?"

"I'm pretty sure it was normal."

"Were you the first to treat her in the emergency room at Mitchie-Sterling Hospital?"

"No."

"Could you tell us who was."

"An emergency room doctor."

"Who was that?"

"I believe it was Dr. Cardozo."

"You just believe, sir?"

"I believe it was Dr. Cardozo."

"Well, do you know of any other doctors who treated Dr. Maddingly in the emergency room before you stepped in?"

"Objection. Asked and answered, and Counsel is, once again, badgering his own witness."

"Sustained."

Jennings' body tightened. "Dr. Gauthé, please tell us why you were called to the emergency room to place an IV in Dr. Maddingly when there was already an emergency room doctor there."

"Surgeons are routinely called to the ER to do emergency surgical procedures."

"Had Dr. Cardozo tried to start the IV?"

"That was the report I was given."

"How many times had he tried to start the IV?"

"I don't know. That was not in the records."

"Do you know why that was not in the record?"

"No."

"Again, let me ask, do you know why Dr. Cardozo had failed to start the IV?"

"You'll have to ask him."

"Well, were you able to start the IV on your first try?"

"Yes."

"How is it that you were able to start the IV in short order, and Dr. Cardozo, by the timeline in the medical record of that night, failed after nearly half an hour of repeated attempts?"

"You know, sometimes, dumb luck is on your side."

"'Dumb luck,' in a hospital emergency room...? Withdrawn. Let me ask. Is starting a central line a common procedure for a general surgeon to do?"

"Can be."

"Is it a common practice for general surgeons at Mitchie-Sterling Hospital to start IVs down in the ER?"

"It certainly happens."

"When was the last time you placed a central line in the ER?"

"Which ER?"

"Mitchie-Sterling Hospital."

"I do not remember."

"In fact, at your deposition for this case, how long did you tell us it had been since you did the last one in the ER?"

"I don't remember my testimony. It is a common surgical procedure. That's like asking me how many sutures I have placed in the past year. You do IVs, and you move on. It's not like it's a heart transplant."

"Okay, but could you please tell us, in the past two years, how many central line IVs have you started?"

"I have no idea."

"Do you remember a single one that we could look up in a hospital chart to confirm?"

"No."

Jennings stopped and let his eyes drift upward in thought. "Well, Doctor, is there a certain amount of skill required to be able to place a central line?"

"Yes."

"Does it follow that the more lines a doctor places, the better that doctor gets at them?

"It's hard to argue against that."

"I take that as a yes."

"Yes, it follows."

"In the emergency room, is it very common for central lines to be placed for emergency fluid resuscitation?"

"I don't know if it is very common, but it is not unusual."

"Do board-certified emergency room physicians start central lines on essentially all patients who need an emergency central line in the ER?"

"Not in all cases."

"Please give us a case in which an emergency room physician may not be able to start a central line."

"When a patient is obese."

"How about another?"

"When the patient won't sit still."

"Do either of these problems apply to Dr. Maddingly?"

"I wasn't there when Dr. Cardozo was faced with the placing of a central line in Dr. Maddingly."

"Well, was Dr. Maddingly a quite thin woman when you placed the central line in her?"

"Yes."

"Was Dr. Maddingly awake and moving around when you flew into the emergency room to save her?"

"Objection. Flew? More hyperbole and stating facts not in evidence."

"Sustained."

"Okay, was Dr. Maddingly conscious when you stood above her and placed the central line?"

"No."

"On a more probable than not basis, was Dr. Maddingly conscious in the ten minutes before you arrived in the ER?"

"I can't answer that."

"Certainly, you received a status report from Dr. Cardozo before you touched Dr. Maddingly. What did he report her blood pressure had been?"

"I don't remember exactly." He quickly rethought his answer. "But it was definitely low enough to require a central line."

Jennings pulled a binder from his desk. "Doctor, is this Book I of Dr. Maddingly's hospital chart for the admission of the night in question?

"If you say so."

"Your Honor, would you instruct the witness to answer my question?"

"Dr. Gauthé, please, sir. This is a court of law, not a sitcom. Please answer Counsel's questions to the best of your ability. Thank you."

Gauthé nodded and spoke sharply. "Yes, these appear to be the notes from that night."

"Doctor, do you see the notation that, 'Dr. Gauthé has entered the treatment room'?"

"Yes."

"What is the systolic pressure noted at that moment?"

"Seventy."

"What was the pressure two minutes before you got there?" Gauthé looked at the chart for longer than he should have. Jennings queried, "Doctor?"

"Eighty."

"Was the pressure dropping?"

"Yes, obviously."

"Is a blood pressure of seventy enough to keep a patient alive?"

"Apparently, it is. Dr. Maddingly was and is, thankfully, still with us."

A grunt issued from one of the older male jurors. Jennings turned toward him and nodded knowingly then said harshly. "If you had not started the central line on the first try, would your patient have died?"

"It is a possibility."

"Would, strike that, could her bleeding have suddenly stopped at that moment if you had done nothing?"

"I can't say for sure."

"Then, why did you take her to surgery?"

"To save her life."

"So, she would have died."

"Objection. Counsel is testifying."

"Sustained."

"Withdrawn. Did you feel it was appropriate for you to try and start the central line?"

"Yes."

"Now, when you walked into the ER treatment room itself, how many patients were in there?"

"Just one."

"Who was that?"

"Mrs. Maddingly."

"Ah, are you referring to Dr. Maddingly."

"Yes, of course; I apologize, Dr. Maddingly."

"Was Dr. Maddingly conscious?"

"No."

"Was there blood on the floor?"

"Yes. There often is."

"Was it a lot of blood?"

"Depends what you mean by a lot of blood."

"Was there enough blood on the floor that your scrub nurse slipped and fell to the floor and had to be helped up?"

"Yes."

"Had you ever seen a hospital employee fall to the ground as a result of blood on the floor of the ER?"

"I imagine I have."

"When?"

"Ah, I guess the last time was in my residency."

"How long ago was that?"

"Twenty years."

Jennings stopped, his eyes toward the ceiling, his lips pulsing as if calculating. He smiled and looked back at Gauthé. "So, in those twenty years, have you spent thousands of hours, no, tens of thousands of hours, in operating rooms?"

"I can't tell you how many hours."

"Would you say you spend twenty hours per week in the operating room?"

Gauthé snickered, "At a bare minimum."

"Twenty hours times fifty weeks, that's a thousand hours per year for twenty years. Twenty thousand total hours! Very impressive. But you've only seen that much blood on a floor once?"

"Objection. Asked and answered."

"Sustained."

"Well, let me ask, when you got to the ER, was there blood on the walls?"

"Some. There often is."

"Often blood on the walls? Is that your testimony?" Jennings shook his head angrily and walked to the plaintiff's table. He took a sip of water. The jury's eyes were locked on him, their faces tensing with the seconds. He slowly turned and walked back toward his witness."

"Was this the patient's blood, or blood bank blood?"

"I do not know."

"Did you see any source of bleeding coming from the patient?"

"Yes, around the site at which attempts had been made to start a central line."

"How can any more than a drop or two from starting an IV get on the floor and the walls?

"I don't know. I wasn't there."

"How much blood did you actually see with your own eyes at the failed IV site?"

"I don't know."

"Was it less than one quart?"

"Yes."

"Was it more than a tablespoon or two?"

"Probable not."

"Then where did all the blood come from that soaked the floor and the walls?"

"Objection. There is no testimony that defines the amount of blood in the treatment room."

"Sustained."

Jennings shook his head. "Thank you, Your Honor. But, isn't it true, Doctor, that your nurse slipped and fell because of the blood on the floor?"

"I don't know if it was the blood."

"Was she drunk?"

"Objection."

"Sustained."

"Withdrawn. Doctor, you are a consummate professional, a master surgeon, by all accounts. Please help us understand where that much blood could have come from."

"I was not there when it happened."

"When what happened?"

"When the blood got on the floor."

"And the walls. Doctor, what was the first thing you did when you saw Dr. Maddingly on the table?"

"I grabbed a central line and placed it."

"You mean you just ran into a room, and, without any information, did a surgical procedure?"

"No, of course not."

"What did you do first, then?"

"I asked for a report from the attending physician."

"Was the attending physician Dr. Peter Cardozo?"

"Yes. I already told you that."

"Did Dr. Cardozo advise about the number of times he had tried and failed to start an IV?"

"No."

"Do you know about how many times?"

"No."

"Was it more than two times?"

"I don't know."

Rhonda Uft bellowed, "Badgering. The witness answered long ago that he didn't know."

"Withdrawn. Let's take a look at Dr. Maddingly's hospital bill for her emergency care that night." Jennings had that document introduced into evidence and handed it to Gauthé. "How many central line catheter kits was she charged for that night?"

"Six."

"Six at one-hundred-and-nine dollars per kit. And how many did you use?"

"One."

"Did anyone else besides Dr. Cardozo try and start a central line before you arrived?"

"I don't know."

"Have you ever been told that another physician, besides Dr. Cardozo, had attended Dr. Maddingly that night?"

"No."

"Do nurses put in central lines? Strike that. Do nurses put in central lines at Mitchie-Sterling Hospital?"

"No."

"So, let's cut to the chase. Did Dr. Cardozo use five central line kits? Yes or no, please."

"I have no way of knowing if some of those kits were opened by nurses and wound up on the floor. Happens when you're trying to save a life."

"Fine. So, how long did it take you to place the central line?"

"I don't recall."

Jennings snapped. "Was it five minutes?"

"No."

A millisecond after Gauthé's answer, Jennings spit, "Was it five seconds?"

"Not that fas..."

The next question was barked before Gauthé finished. "Was it less than thirty seconds before the blood was flowing into the patient that was now dying in front of your eyes?"

"Objection. Foundation. And this is not some melodrama; it is a court of law. No facts have been presented to substantiate that the plaintiff was dying."

Jennings sucked in a deep breath to explode, but the judge, who had, like the jury, been rivetted by the testimony, looked up, and it was several seconds before he reoriented himself and mumbled, "Overruled. We already know the plaintiff's blood pressure was far below normal and was falling. Go on, Counsel."

"Thank you, Your Honor. Now, isn't it a fact, Doctor, you were so scared that Dr. Maddingly was about to die that you told the x-ray technician not to take a film to prove the tip of the central line was where it was supposed to be?"

Gauthé hesitated. "Yes."

"In fact, you physically struck the x-ray tech in the chest to move her out of the way, didn't you, Doctor."

"I certainly don't remember that."

"Do we need to have you read her deposition testimony to refresh your memory, Doctor?"

"It was the heat of battle. That's all I'm going to say."

"So, in the heat of battle, it's okay for a large man to assault a one hundred-and-five-pound Asian woman?"

"I did not assault her!"

"Was she about to do harm to your patient?"

"Not harm, but we didn't have time for her."

"No time for her so you hit her? Withdrawn. Let me ask, have you ever, ever, done that before when things were not going your way in the operating room?"

"I am sure I have."

"When?"

"I can't remember."

"I didn't think you could. Withdrawn. Back to your medical activities that night. Is that an unusual step, to start introducing pressurized fluid through a tube deep inside the body when you are not absolutely positive where that fluid is going? Is that correct, yes or no?"

"We usually wait for an x-ray to see the tip of the catheter."

As an incensed Jennings bristled closer to the witness stand, he paled, and his pace slowed. He grabbed the edge of the judge's bench for support. Rhonda Uft rolled her eyes and shook her head skeptically, but Jennings wobbled back to his table and took a seat. He sipped at his water as the judge, wide-eyed, spoke in nearly a whisper, "Counsel, are you okay?" When there was no answer, Galanter turned to the bailiff and asked him to summon the medics.

The judge's command was, though, sufficiently loud that Jennings looked up and smiled. "Your Honor, sorry, had a bit of cramp—stomach. You know, cafeteria food. I'm fine. Let's continue. No need to call our medical friends. Just a twinge. Gone now."

Galanter looked at him askance, but Jennings came to his feet and moved toward the witness stand. The judge nodded. "Okay, Counsel, but if you want to take a break, that will be fine."

Jennings stopped and his eyes rose to the ceiling. "Your Honor, I can go on, but I'm not sure that would be in the best interest of Dr. Maddingly. May I respectfully, with apologies to the jury and the witness, ask the court for a recess until morning?

Galanter's gavel tapped lightly, and the jury was excused.

Harrison Jennings visited his doctor that afternoon. A migraine headache was diagnosed. The treatment was simple: the man was urged to take a couple of weeks off. Jennings agreed readily and walked slowly from the office. The instant he got into his car, he phoned the Maddinglys and then the courthouse, assuring both he'd been cleared to return to work the next day.

Galanter saw both attorneys in chambers early the next morning. Rhonda Uft eyed her adversary, but Jennings smiled at both of them and declared he was ready to continue.

"No more stunts, huh?" Uft hissed under her breath, but loud enough for Galanter to hear.

The judge shook his head. "And I was hoping we could get off on a new and peaceable foot."

Rhonda Uft snarled, "I'd like nothing better, but please remember, Judge, this is costing my clients an arm and a leg, to say nothing of delayed justice."

Jennings whispered under his breath, "Like it cost my client an arm and a leg."

Galanter suppressed a grin. "Thank you, Ms. Uft, for reminding me of my judicial responsibilities. But be assured I would offer you the same courtesy if you became ill."

"And thank you, Your Honor, but I manage to isolate my personal matters far from the courtroom."

Galanter's head drooped a fraction, but he sucked in a deep breath and spoke quietly, "Well, let's get the wheels of justice aturnin'."

Jennings reminded the jury that he had been asking the witness how long it had taken him to start the IV. Gauthé finally conceded it had been less than two minutes.

"Good. What did you do next?"

"I had the nurses run the next bag of blood."

"Run the blood, sir? What does that mean?"

"Have the blood sent through the IV into the patient."

"You say next, but there was no previous blood introduced into Dr. Maddingly, was there?"

"Not to my knowledge."

"Where did this extra blood come from?"

"The blood bank."

"Could the first unit of that blood have been the source of the blood all over the floor and walls?"

"I don't know. I wasn't..."

Before he could finish, Rhonda Uft was on her feet. "Objection. Calls for speculation, and we've been over this several times."

"Sustained."

"What happened to Dr. Maddingly's blood pressure when the blood was introduced?"

"Her blood pressure rose for a while..."

"How long?"

"A minute."

"Then what happened?"

"It began to drop again."

"Why?"

"The blood was leaking out of her ruptured ectopic pregnancy just as fast as we were pouring it in."

"Does that mean the tear in her fallopian tube was getting bigger?"

"Probably not."

"Does that mean that once the final rupture took place, it stayed the same size and just bled and bled?"

"The process is so complex, I can't answer your question."

"Yes, you can."

"Objection. Badgering his own witness—yet again."

"Sustained. The witness said he cannot answer the question. We have to accept that."

"Thank you, Your Honor. Let me ask, what causes the rupture of the wall of the fallopian tube?"

"Many things."

"Name one."

"I am not an obstetrician."

"Well, in this case, were you able to determine, when you did obstetrical surgery on Dr. Maddingly to stop the bleeding, what caused the rupture."

"It might have been the fetus had grown to the point the fallopian tube could no longer contain it. Perhaps there are other factors. As I said, I am not an obstetrician, but I'm good at saving lives."

Jennings paused to stare at Gauthé. The corners of his mouth curled down, transmuting his kindly face into an ireful mask. "Good at saving lives, but not so good..." He stopped himself abruptly and spit, "Strike that." There was another pause, but his face soon relaxed, and he asked without emotion, "Doctor, what else could have caused the tube to rupture?"

"I don't know."

"Well, if the fetus was that large, how would it have escaped notice by the radiologist?"

"Objection. Calls for speculation."

"Sustained."

"Let me ask, then, looking back from surgery, would you agree that by the time you placed the central line the bleeding was at a maximum?"

"I can only say that it was heavy enough to render the patient unconscious."

"And how much blood did Dr. Maddingly have to bleed into her pelvis to become unconscious?"

"Depends upon her red blood cell count before the rupture. If she had been anemic for a long period, she may have only needed to lose a small amount of blood to push her over the edge into unconsciousness."

"Are you suggesting that Dr. Maddingly was one of many women, who, before the change in life—menopause, at around age fifty—have low blood counts due to blood loss during their periods?"

"Might be. Might also be a low blood count as a result of her exposure to Agent Orange."

"Well, sir, what would be the usual blood count for a young woman who was healthy, but had the usual slight anemia associated with blood loss from monthly periods?"

"From thirty-eight to, say, forty-four. Probably the lower range if she had a history of heavy periods."

"We have testimony in the court record that three months before the night in question, Dr. Maddingly had a physical at the University of Washington in anticipation of her new position as a staff psychologist. Were you aware of that, sir?"

"No. And it made no difference that night."

"Well, did you just testify that she might have been anemic, you know, have a low red blood cell count?"

"I just said, 'might'."

"And did you testify that a low blood count might have had an effect on her health on the night in question?"

"Yes."

"Would you be surprised to learn that she had a totally normal red blood cell count during that physical?"

"I don't know her medical status prior to the surgery I performed."

"Did you know that Dr. Maddingly had a hematocrit of 42, and a hemoglobin of 13.6, on her physical exam three months before?"

"No. Wasn't important that night."

"But if it was 42, would you say she was not anemic for any reason? In fact, it was just the opposite."

"No. Not at all. She could have had hemoconcentration on that physical exam at the U. due to being dehydrated."

"How does a doctor tell, on a general physical exam, if a patient is dehydrated?"

"There are many tests."

"Is one of those tests a urinalysis?"

"Yes."

"How can a urinalysis test for dehydration?"

"One can test the specific gravity of the urine to see if the urine is especially thick. If it is thick, that means there is less water in the body. If there's less water in the body, there's less water in the bloodstream, and the red blood cells are floating in less water. That makes it appear their number is higher, falsely high."

"If we give you her urine specific gravity the day of her employment physical, would you be able to interpret her state of hydration?"

"I can try, but let me warn you, I'm not an internist."

Jennings snorted and handed Gauthé the medical record from the University Hospital. "Sir, what was her specific gravity on that physical three months before the night in question?"

"One-point-oh-one."

"Was she well hydrated?"

"Yes. All those numbers appear normal, but Dr. Maddingly could have an abnormality in her blood production due to her exposure to Agent Orange that finally showed up when her body was stressed by the pregnancy. Could be just like the other abnormalities I found when I did surgery on her."

"What if I told you that she had not had even a cold while working at the University over those three months..."

"Objection. Stating facts not in evidence."

"Withdrawn. Can you think of any plausible reason why she would have presented on the night in question with a low blood count other than, of course, bleeding from her ectopic pregnancy?"

"Objection. Calls for speculation. The witness is not a hematologist."

"Sustained."

Jennings tightened for a moment. "Well, let's talk about her ability to produce red blood cells. In the period after surgery, were you treating her for the blood loss?"

"I was one of the many doctors."

"Did you tell the family that you wanted to slowly raise her blood count back toward normal?"

"Yes."

"What was your goal for her blood count?"

"Forty-two or three."

"Did her blood count rise as it would in a normal patient?"

"Slowly."

"Did it rise any slower than you would have expected?"

"No."

"How high did it finally get?"

"I guess 44."

"Please don't guess. It's right here in the hospital records. Could you read this for us."

"Forty-five."

"Is that better than expected in a woman of her age?"

"It's a normal hematocrit."

"Do you have any experience treating patients who are one-generation removed from Agent Orange exposure?"

"No."

"So, Dr. Maddingly was the first?"

"Yes, as far as I know."

"Since she was your patient, and you had no experience with a patient of this nature, did you exercise due diligence and read up in the medical journals about the possibilities of Agent Orange exposure?"

"Yes, of course."

"So, you read widely on the subject?"

"I read enough to carry out my responsibilities to my patient."

"Could you name for the jury the scholarly articles or textbooks that made mention of Agent Orange's side effects in the children of American soldiers who served in Viet Nam?"

"I don't remember specifically. I simply went to the NIH website and read selected articles."

"Could you name for the jury even one of the scholarly articles or textbooks that made mention of Agent Orange's side effects in the children of American soldiers who served in Viet Nam?"

"I will tell you again, I did not memorize the authors' names, and there are usually many for each paper, but I did learn what I needed to treat my patient appropriately."

"Did you come across a single article on the subject of a low red count due to Agent Orange?"

"Yes. Several."

"Did those articles say that anemia was a direct result of Agent Orange exposure?"

"Yes."

"Or, sir, did those articles really say that the anemia they found in some of these patients was caused by the leukemia they had from Agent Orange exposure?"

"I'm not sure I can answer that."

"Why?"

"I do not know if Dr. Maddingly has an underlying leukemia from her exposure to Agent Orange. It is entirely possible."

"Did you do complete blood counts on Dr. Maddingly?"

"Yes."

"How many?"

"Many."

"Three, ten, twenty?"

"Around six, but I'm not sure."

"Okay, Dr. Gauthé, just to let you know, it was actually twenty-one, but what would you see on a complete blood count that would lead you to diagnose leukemia?"

"You may see an elevated white blood count."

"May?"

"It could be a low red count or even low platelets."

"But is an elevated white count the most common presentation?"

"I can't answer that. As we know, I'm not a hematologist."

"But you were treating this woman for a hematologic problem, weren't you, Doctor?"

"Yes."

"If a patient with leukemia has an elevated white count, would you say that high white count was most likely due to the leukemia?"

"That is often the cause of an elevated white count."

"Can you also see an elevated white count in an infection?"

"Yes."

"Did you ever see an elevated white count in Dr. Maddingly?"

"Yes."

"When you saw that elevated white count, did you think it might be leukemia, or did you know in your heart that it was due to the infection she contracted during the surgery you did on her."

The screeched "Objection," rattled the windows. "Foundation!"

"Sustained."

"Did Dr. Maddingly suffer a surgical infection after you operated on her?"

"Yes, but you can't tell if that was from the surgery or the post-surgical care."

"How many days after the surgery did the infection begin?"

"A day and a half."

"Doctor, how long does it take for an infection to make itself known after surgery?"

"Depends."

"Is a day and a half unusual?"

"Depends."

"Is six hours normal for an infection to show up?"

"Depends."

Jennings hissed, "Your Honor, the witness is clearly non-responsive. I would ask you have him stop wasting the court's time."

Rhonda Uft squealed, "Once again, Counsel is getting belligerent because the witness is not spitting back the answers he wants to hear."

"Approach." With Jennings and Rhonda Uft glaring at each other a foot from the bench, Galanter scolded, "Counselor, he doesn't want to answer your questions, at least as you've framed them. That is your problem. And, Ms. Uft, I want you to stop shrieking in my courtroom. Is that clear? You're giving me a migraine. Now, step back."

Jennings turned to his witness and asked quietly, "But there was an infection, Doctor. Is that your testimony?"

"Objection. Asked and answered."

"Sustained."

Gauthé blurted, "Surgical infections are just part of the risk of doing emergency surgery to save a young life."

Jennings turned to the judge and spread his hands. Galanter leaned toward Gauthé. "Doctor, please do not make statements unless they are in answer to a question from the attorneys. Thank you."

Jennings continued. "And, back to the white blood count. Did it ever return to normal?"

"Yes."

"How long did it take?"

"Three days."

"Does leukemia get better in three days if you simply give a patient antibiotics?"

"Depends."

"Given what you have just told the jury, is it reasonable to conclude that

Dr. Maddingly did not suffer from leukemia, at least during her hospitalization for the ectopic pregnancy?"

"Yes."

"Was there any indication that her blood count rose under your able care differently than a normal patient's?"

"No."

"Are there any other reasons to suggest that she came into the hospital that night suffering from a subnormal amount of red blood?"

"There might be."

"What are they."

"At the moment, I can't think of any, though I warn you, there are other possibilities."

"You warn me? We owe it to the jury to give them all of the information they need to determine if Dr. Maddingly had an abnormal amount of red blood that night. So, what are the other reasons?"

"Objection. Asked and answered."

"Withdrawn."

"Well, does it follow, Dr. Gauthé, that her low red count was simply from bleeding, and that she recovered her blood count normally?"

"First, I want to apologize for the comment about warning. This is very stressful. Surgery's easy by comparison." He laughed. The jury, though, remained without expression.

"Very good. But I still have to ask, on a more probable than not basis, was her low red count simply from bleeding?"

"It is a fair guess."

"This is a court of law, sir. Guessing's not allowed. Was her low red count more likely than not from bleeding?"

"Probably."

"And, more likely than not, did she recover her blood count normally?"

"Yes."

"Thank you. That did not need to take nearly an hour to come to the same conclusion. Withdrawn. Now, Doctor, let's go back to the central line placement. Please give us the reason you really believe Dr. Cardozo was unable to start the lifesaving central line."

"I hope I have made it clear that I was not there to see his technique."

"Apparently, you had the right technique. Is that correct?"

"Perhaps it was just dumb luck."

"Well, here we go with luck in an emergency room again. I certainly hope it isn't just dumb luck when you see one of these jurors' kids for an emergency surgery. Withdrawn. I have just a few more questions for this witness." He walked to his desk and retrieved a loose-leaf binder. "Doctor, would you look at this document? Please tell us what it is."

"It appears to be the discharge summary for Dr. Maddingly's stay at Mitchie-Sterling Hospital."

"Would you turn to the last page, please? Who signed it?'

"Harvey Klat, M.D."

"Please remind the jury who Dr. Klat happens to be."

"He is our medical director."

"Did Dr. Klat treat Dr. Maddingly at any time during her stay at Mitchie-Sterling Hospital?"

"I don't really know. There were so many consults. We pulled all the stops to save Dr. Maddingly."

"We have testimony from another medical doctor that Dr. Klat's name was not mentioned in the treatment portion of the summary. Please save us yet another hour going through the records to prove Dr. Klat did not treat Dr. Maddingly."

"I do not remember."

"Well, for argument's sake, say Dr. Klat did a consult on the patient. When was the last time you saw you a peripheral doctor on a case write the discharge summary?"

"I don't remember."

"Does the medical director usually do the discharge summary?"

"Not generally."

"Can you think of any reason why the medical director wrote the discharge summary in this case?"

"Yes. It was a particularly complicated case in a young woman who got a rotten deal because her father went to Viet Nam and was exposed to Agent Orange. Like I said, we all worked a lot of extra hours to save her."

"Are you suggesting that her father is responsible because he was drafted and went to Viet Nam?"

"I am not suggesting anything. I am stating a fact."

"Are you aware, sir, that her father earned the Medal of Honor in Viet

Nam? Do you know how many lives he saved?"

"Objection! Foundation, leading, and of no probative value."

Before Galanter could speak, Jennings hissed. "Withdrawn. No further questions for this witness."

Judge Galanter had taken a deep breath to sustain the defense's objection, but Rhonda Uft had flown out of her chair, the yellow legal pad fluttering in the wind as she charged the witness. "Dr. Gauthé, let's correct the record on certain points. First, is there any medical test that can be done at this juncture to determine if the plaintiff began to bleed significantly before or after she came to Mitchie-Sterling Hospital?"

"No. Never was."

The judge banged his gavel. "Excuse me, Ms. Uft. I did not invite you to start your cross-examination. I think it's time for lunch, don't you?"

"Your Honor, there is so much misleading testimony to correct."

Jennings had not had time to take his seat at the plaintiff's table, but heeled around and called out, "Objection. I object to Counsel's characterization of Dr. Gauthé's answers as misleading. They came from his own mouth."

"Sustained, but we will continue after lunch." The gavel banged, marking the termination of the morning's testimony.

CHAPTER FORTY-SIX

Rhonda Uft squirreled in her chair waiting for the judge to call the court to order. With the thirteen triers of fact in their seats, Galanter looked toward her, but before the judge decreed that counsel could approach the witness to start her cross-examination, she lunged toward Gauthé.

"Doctor, thank you for agreeing to help us finally sort this matter out for the jury. Let me start by asking you some very direct questions. Drawing on your expertise, would you say that bleeding was already present when the plaintiff presented to Dr. Weathersby?"

Harrison Jennings leapt to his feet. "Objection. He is not an expert in obstetrics. He told us so. Over and over."

"Sustained."

"Sir, we have heard testimony that the plaintiff had an ultrasound of her pelvis that night. Is that your understanding?"

"Yes."

"Are you familiar with the findings on that ultrasound?"

"Yes, very."

"Did you review the ultrasound yourself?"

"Yes."

"Was that just the report, or the images as well?"

"All the available images."

"How, sir, would you explain the massive amount of blood seen on the ultrasound?"

Jennings rose. "Objection. Stating facts not in evidence. No one has ever shown it was blood."

"Sustained."

"What else could that fluid have reasonably been?"

"It couldn't have been anything else."

"Objection. I thought the witness wasn't a radiologist."

"Sustained."

"When you were given the report in the emergency room as you stepped up to treat the plaintiff, what did you believe that fluid was?"

"Blood."

"Objection. Foundation. I do not believe the witness ever swore under oath that he had any information regarding the ultrasound before he treated Dr. Maddingly."

"Sustained."

"Well, then, Doctor, did you see the ultrasound or the ultrasound report before you treated the plaintiff?"

"No."

Rhonda Uft's lips tightened as she stared into his eyes. "Were you told in the report given by Dr. Cardozo that an ultrasound of the plaintiff's pelvis had been done?"

"I believe so, but I just don't remember. I've said that from the beginning. I will not perjure myself."

She hesitated for several seconds. "No, no, of course not. The ultrasound report, what did it mean to you?"

Gauthé paused, confused. "The ultrasound did not matter. If it had shown the patient had four ovaries, it wouldn't have made a bit of difference. Her blood pressure was low, and she needed a central line immediately, and it had fallen upon me to get it done." Rhonda Uft had suddenly begun nodding at the testimony, the bobbing of her head going on mechanically, metronomically, even when Gauthé stopped speaking to take a sip of water. He looked at her curiously for a moment, flushed, but went on, his voice hardened and direct. "My vision and mind were fixated on Dr. Maddingly's neck and where it would be best, safest, and fastest to place the line. The only thing that mattered was the blood pressure."

Rhonda Uft's torso sagged, and she spoke softly. "Your Honor, I'm sorry, but may I take a short break?"

Before Galanter could open his mouth, Rhonda Uft suddenly

straightened her shoulders and croaked, "After you placed the line, what did you do?"

Galanter said nothing. Gauthé's face twisted in surprise, but he answered in a tense monotone, "Had the blood run, ah, introduced."

"We have heard that her pressure went up but right back down. What does a surgeon do under those circumstances?"

"Open the patient, find the source of bleeding, and clamp it off as fast as your hands can fly."

"Did you do that?"

"Yes."

"What did you do then?"

"Had additional blood products introduced."

"What happened?"

"The blood pressure went up."

"What did you do then?"

"Sighed in relief."

Both he and Rhonda Uft looked to the jury, but they remained poker-faced.

"Then what?"

"I examined the patient's organs."

"What did you find?"

"I found an ectopic pregnancy."

"Had it burst through the wall of the fallopian tube?"

"Yes."

"Was that the source of the bleeding?"

"Yes."

"What else did you find? Strike that. Let's save the jury's time. What did you find in regard to the ovary and fallopian tube?"

"They did not look normal."

"Objection. The witness is not an obstetrician. He has no idea of all the normal variations of the human ovary and fallopian tube. That can come only from an OB, and only one trained, specifically, in all the anatomic variations seen in all body types. And, further, he failed to take pictures of the anatomy, so we only have the witness's description, and he is, per his own testimony this morning, far from an expert."

"Sustained."

Rhonda Uft now turned her glare toward Jennings but spoke over her shoulder. "Dr. Gauthé, what did you do after that?"

"I thought for a moment about removing Dr. Maddingly's left ovary. But I chose to leave that to a GYN surgeon, if they felt it was necessary."

"Smart of you. Did you close at that point?"

"I cleaned up the tissue that no longer had a blood supply and did my best to seal off all the bleeders. Then I closed."

"Let's go back to the malformed anatomy."

"Objection. The tube may have been damaged, but we have no evidence on the record of a, so-called, malformation. That term makes one think of a malformation from birth. That is not the case here, and it will not be until there is evidence that Dr. Maddingly's reported anatomy was anything other than a common, very normal variation."

"Sustained. The jury will not consider that Dr. Maddingly had a malformation. Continue, Ms. Uft."

"Thank you, Your Honor. Doctor, please describe exactly what you saw when you examined the fallopian tube."

"The tube took a hard dogleg just as it left the fimbria."

"English, please."

"The tube that carries the egg showed a hard dogleg as it left the ovary area.

"Why did that catch your attention?"

"I had never seen that."

"Or heard of it?"

"Or heard of it."

"Objection, and I want to make this a standing objection, that this witness is not qualified to lecture the jury on a medical subject for which he admits he is not a specialist, and, in fact, had not done a single obstetrical operation in twenty-years."

"Sustained, but only the portion of the question when the witness testifies he has never heard of a certain anatomic finding. He may certainly comment on what he saw. He may not, though, draw medical conclusions regarding the normality, or abnormality, or cause of that gynecologic anatomy."

Rhonda Uft smiled gracelessly. "Thank you, Your Honor. Well, Dr. Gauthé, are you qualified—as a board-certified general surgeon who has, I might add, operated on many, many thousands of patients—to comment on how a particular body part looks."

"I am."

"What are tubes, like the fallopian tube, used for in the body?"

"The same thing they are used for in regular life. They allow transport of something from one place to another."

"Can you give us an example?"

"Blood vessels are tubes that carry blood from the heart to the organs of the body. The intestine is a tube that moves food from one end of the body to the other."

"Are you aware of any tube in the body that, in its normal form, makes a dogleg turn?"

"No."

"Why is that so?"

"If there is a very sharp turn, whatever is supposed to be moving through the tube will get stuck."

"What is the function of the fallopian tube?"

"To allow the egg to move easily from the ovary to the uterus."

"Considering basic medicine, basic anatomy, would a kink in the tube hinder that process?"

"Yes."

"Could that kink cause an egg to get stuck?"

"Yes."

"On a more probable than not basis, Doctor, considering basic medicine, basic anatomy, medical school pathology, and common sense, would a kink in the tube hinder the process of normal fetal development?

"Yes."

"On a more probable than not basis, Doctor, considering basic medicine, basic anatomy, medical school pathology, and common sense, would a kink in the tube likely have a part in causing the ectopic pregnancy?"

"Yes."

"Had the plaintiff not had the tubal pregnancy, would she have had the episode of bleeding that night?"

"No."

"And, just to make sure we are clear, is it your testimony, on a medically more probable than not basis, that it is impossible to say for certain when the bleeding you discovered at surgery began?"

"Yes."

"Thank you. No more questions for this witness."

CHAPTER FORTY-SEVEN

Jennings walked forward slowly to begin his redirect. He kept a bit more distance from the witness than he had earlier. "Doctor, when you operated on Dr. Maddingly, you testified you removed some tissue, 'just to clean things up.' I think that was the gist of the remark. Let me ask, did you remove the fallopian tube?"

"Some of it."

"What part?"

"The fimbriae..."

"What is that, Doctor?"

"That's what catches the egg when the woman ovulates. It is essentially a funnel."

"Why did you remove it?"

"I had to remove most of the fallopian tube. It had burst open, and in stopping the bleeding, I had to tie off the blood vessels to it. The tube would have died in a day or so, and, essentially, rotted inside the patient. You don't leave dead tissue behind."

"Doctor, it's very clear you did right. But, with the removal of the fimbriae—the funnel—and the tube, is there any x-ray, or MRI, or ultrasound that would show the deformity you described?"

Gauthé paused and thought. "No. It's all been removed."

"Were there any x-rays, MRIs, or ultrasounds taken the night of the surgery, before the surgery?"

"Why, yes, there is the ultrasound of the fallopian tube taken when the

333

patient first arrived at the hospital."

"Did it show the kink you described?"

"First of all, the tube is so small, it would be hard to be positive you were looking at it. And, in this case, I could not have seen it had I examined the ultrasound beforehand because there was some clouding of that area due to the blood in the pelvis."

"How did the radiologist see it then and declare there was thickening of the fallopian tube?"

"He was a specialist."

"So, all we have is your verbal description. Is that correct?"

"No, it is not. I drew a sketch of the anatomy. I gave it to Ms. Uft."

"That's very nice, but we apparently do not have a medically acceptable, objective test to show the jury, other than the ultrasound, which didn't show it, and your drawing, which did. Is that correct?"

"Objection. Since when is a drawing by a highly trained, experienced surgeon not as good as a medical test? Dr. Gauthé saw the deformed fallopian tube with his own, expert eyes."

Jennings took a step toward the bench. Galanter looked down. "Counsel?"

Jennings started counting on his fingers. "To start with, this is the first time we have heard of any drawing. Why was it not provided to the plaintiff as part of our demand for production of documents?"

Rhonda Uft snarled, "Work product privilege. We have not introduced it as evidence because it was produced by a non-attorney. Fed. r. civ. p. 26(b)(3)(a). A party may not discover documents and tangible things that are prepared in anticipation of litigation or for trial by or for another party or its representative, including the other party's attorney, consultant, surety, on and on."

The judge sighed, "Ms. Uft, thank you for your second-year law school lecture. Bailiff, please escort the jury into their deliberation room. Ladies and Gentlemen of the jury, we will make this as short as we can."

When they were gone and the door to their room shut, Galanter sent Gauthé into the hallway. As he passed Sabrina and Mike, they turned their faces away from him. His shoulders sagged, and he walked from the courtroom head down. With the whoosh of the swinging doors, the judge droned, "Mr. Jennings?"

Jennings nodded. "Very clever, Ms. Uft. But you're going to need to come up with the date that Dr. Gauthé made the drawing. And he's going to have to swear to it under oath, and so will you. If it's before you got involved, in other words, if he made a sketch of the anatomy before there was talk of a lawsuit, it is discoverable and part of the record; and if it is discoverable, I will seek sanctions against you. And, Your Honor, when will I be able to see this work of art? When the trial's over?"

The judge thought for a moment. "He's got a point, Ms. Uft. But, on the other hand, Mr. Jennings, you have an opportunity on this redirect to elicit that information from Dr. Gauthé."

Jennings locked the judge's eyes. "If you'll allow it, sir."

Galanter ignored him and called the jury back in and then the witness.

Jennings went on. "Looking back now, besides the fallopian tube, what did you find when you operated on the plaintiff?"

"Blood."

"Was it fresh blood?"

"Can only say it wasn't days old."

"Was it in the pelvis?"

"Yes."

"How much?"

"Several units."

"Was it fresh blood, I mean uncoagulated?"

"Yes."

"Was there, though, some coagulated blood?"

"Yes."

"How much?"

"I can't tell you how much. Some."

"One tablespoon?"

"More."

"Five units?"

"Less."

"One unit?"

"Maybe."

"How long had it been there?"

"There is no way to tell. It was more than fifteen minutes. That's how long it takes blood to clot."

335

"Doctor, do you remember when Ms. Uft asked you if a kink in the tube would alter the egg's ability to move through the fallopian tube?"

"Yes."

"Let me ask, was the kink located above or below the ectopic pregnancy?"

"Above"

"Does that mean the egg had, in fact, already moved through the so-called dogleg?"

"Yes, but we don't know what effect that malformation had on the rest of the tube."

Jennings clenched his fists. "Your Honor, I respectfully ask you to remind the witness, yet again, that he does not have the training to call the so-called dogleg, that apparently isn't a roadblock at all, a malformation."

Galanter glared down. "Doctor, please, I don't want to have to warn you again. The jury is to disregard that word." He nodded to Jennings.

"Thank you, Your Honor. Doctor, did you send the tube you removed off to a lab to be examined by a board-certified medical doctor called a pathologist?"

"Yes."

"What do pathologists do?"

"They look at the tissue under a microscope and determine if a disease process has taken place."

Jennings went to his desk and pulled a sheet of paper from the mammoth binder. "Doctor, what is this?"

"It appears to be a pathology report."

"Dated when?"

"November 30th."

"Who is it addressed to?"

"Me."

"What tissue is it referring to?"

"The surgical tissue I removed from Dr. Maddingly."

"What does it say about the fallopian tube, only, not the contents?"

"It says the tissue appears to be a fallopian tube."

"And?"

"The fallopian tube is torn longitudinally. The edges are ragged. There is also a fet..."

"Jennings growled. "Stop there. I asked only about the fallopian tube. We do not need to be discussing the private aspects of the report and harming Dr. Maddingly any more than she has already been. Please do not do that again."

Rhonda Uft started to rise to object to Jennings' usurpation of the judge's prerogative but glanced furtively at the jury and saw the concern in the women's eyes. She surreptitiously slipped down into her seat. Galanter also held his tongue.

"Doctor," Jennings spoke a bit more softly, "then there is no objective, microscopic, evidence of a problem in the tube itself. Is that correct?"

"Yes."

"But we do have objective evidence that the egg passed the part you testified was impassable, and then entered a tube you told us might be damaged, but the pathologist did not say it was. Is that correct?"

"The pathologist did not say it was normal."

"No, he did not. He did not comment. Do medical professionals typically waste time commenting on what is normal?"

"In this case, he couldn't tell. There was too much damage."

"Is that what he said?"

"It is implied."

"Implied? What else is implied?"

"I can't tell you."

"I know, I know, you're not a pathologist. Withdrawn. So, in fact, the only doctor making a direct statement that can be used in a court of law regarding disease in that fallopian tube, before the night in question, is you. Is that correct?"

Gauthé paused for a moment, his lips tight, mind roiling for an escape route. He finally droned, "Yes."

"Thank you. I am almost done, so please bear with me for a few more minutes. Doctor, this morning you stated you had made a drawing of the so-called dogleg in Dr. Maddingly's fallopian tube. Is that true?"

"Yes."

"Did you ever meet Ms. Uft, or any attorney or staff in her law firm, before this case arose?"

"No."

"Have you met anyone in Ms. Uft's law firm prior to this morning?"

"Yes, but only at the deposition."

"Did you speak privately to them at that time?"

"No."

"Well, how did Ms. Uft come into possession of your diagram?"

"I do not know."

"Did you give the diagram to anyone prior to this morning?"

"Yes."

"Who?"

"Dr. Klat."

"Remind us again just who he is."

"He's the medical director of Mitchie-Sterling Hospital."

"When did he ask you for the diagram?"

"I do not remember the date?"

"Was it two years ago?"

"No."

"Three months ago?"

"No."

"Last night?"

"No."

"Two weeks ago?"

"Approximately."

"What did he say to you?"

"He asked if I had any recollection of the patient's pelvic anatomy."

"What did you answer?"

"Yes."

"What did he say next?"

"He asked me to make a detailed drawing of that anatomy."

"Did he tell you why he wanted it?"

"He said he wanted to think about what had happened in this case."

"What did you understand that to mean?"

"I imagined he was preparing our defense in this case."

"What was your intention in doing the drawing?"

"To fulfill a request of my boss..." He paused and thought, "and to refresh my memory of the pathology."

"What do you mean by pathology?"

"The medical problem."

"But I thought you were not a gynecological surgeon and could not be certain that it was truly abnormal."

"I am not, but I am a surgeon with thousands of patients under my belt. I know pathology when I see it."

"Very interesting. Let me ask, did you happen to see Dr. Maddingly's other ovary and fallopian tube?"

"No."

"Why not?"

"A surgeon only makes the smallest incision to resolve the issue. I would never extend a surgical field a single millimeter out of personal curiosity."

"In your reading, did you see reference to a problem of this nature happening on both sides?"

"No."

"Did you see any diagrams that even remotely looked like what you say you saw that night."

"No."

"Then, it looks like you have made a new finding that should be submitted for a journal article. They might even call it Gauthé's Kink."

"Objection. Is there a question in there?"

"Sustained."

"Thank you, Your Honor. Dr. Gauthé, did you submit your diagram to a medical journal?"

"No."

"Why not?"

"I thought about it, but I was just too busy."

"Just too busy..." Jennings let that sink in for a few seconds. "So, you are testifying that you made no diagram of the anatomy to show others?"

"I made a rough sketch and showed an obstetrician."

"What did they say?"

"Something about it being interesting."

"Did they make a statement about it being a malformation?"

"No."

"How big was the pregnancy in the tube?"

"As big as my thumb."

"How big is the normal tube?"

"I do not know the exact dimensions."

"Well, it is between a quarter and half-an-inch across. And it is very delicate. Do you think it is possible that the actual ectopic pregnancy might have pulled on the tube and changed its shape?"

"I do not know that much about it. That is not what I saw in my study."

"Okay, Doctor, would you please stand up and, using the easel, make a drawing that is as identical as you can of the drawing you provided to Ms. Uft."

Gauthé looked to her. She nodded, but Jennings shot, "You can save us all a lot of time and nonsense if you will just provide the court with that drawing."

Rhonda Uft jumped to her feet. "Objection. Work product privilege."

Galanter thought for a minute. "Mr. Jennings, since you have established when the witness did the drawing, and when he gave it to Defense Counsel, I am going to rule in Ms. Uft's favor. At this point, the drawing, in the form provided to Ms. Uft, remains non-discoverable. That is, Ladies and Gentlemen of the jury, neither Dr. Gauthé nor Ms. Uft has to make that document available to the plaintiffs or to the court. This is not my decision—it is the law. That does not mean, however, that Dr. Gauthé is excused from making a drawing at this juncture in the trial. Mr. Jennings?"

Jennings nodded in accordance. "Thank you, Your Honor. Doctor, please do the drawing."

Rhonda Uft spoke to the bench. "I renew my objection."

Galanter nodded. "So noted and overridden. Doctor, please do as Mr. Jennings has requested."

Gauthé put on his wire-rimmed glasses and bristled to the easel. He made a few strokes using only the black Magic Marker. The details were no more specific than a pair of stick figures drawn by a four-year-old. As he dropped back into his seat, Jennings asked, "Are you comfortable again, Doctor?"

"Yes."

"Well, let me ask, is that drawing similar in detail to the document you provided Ms. Uft?"

He opened his mouth to speak, but Rhonda Uft bellowed, "Objection. Given the doctrine of Work Product Privilege, which Your Honor just upheld, my witness cannot be forced to produce that document or its facsimile."

"Overruled. Yes, Mr. Jennings may not force the witness to produce a facsimile, but he can answer a question regarding its fidelity."

Harrison Jennings nodded. "Thank you, Your Honor. Doctor, please tell us if that drawing is a facsimile of the drawing you provided Ms. Uft."

"As far as I can remember, it was a very basic sketch. I am not an artist."

"Yes, you've mentioned your limited skills on any number of occasions in this trial."

Before Rhonda Uft could respond, Judge Galanter banged his gavel. "Mr. Jennings, you are on the cusp, yet again, sir."

"Yes, Your Honor. Last questions. When you operated on Dr. Maddingly, did you see any previous surgical abdominal or pelvic scars?"

"No."

"Did you see any evidence of internal surgical intervention?"

"No."

"Did you see all the normal organs?"

"As many as are in plain sight. I did not want to keep the patient under anesthesia for a second longer than absolutely necessary to look around."

"Of course not. Thank you. No further," he paused and looked up at the ceiling, "ah, one last question. Did you call Dr. Cardozo and his emergency room crew 'Keystone Cops' when you saw the situation in the ER that night?"

Rhonda Uft started to rise but withdrew into her seat.

"I have no recollection of making that statement, and it would have been questionably professional to say something like that."

"Indeed, it would. Thank you. Your Honor, I have no further questions for this witness."

"Ms. Uft, do you wish to recross-examine?"

She growled, "No, Your Honor."

And so ended Christopher Gauthé's testimony.

CHAPTER FORTY-EIGHT

It had been Khai's day off, and she'd thought about sitting in the back of the courtroom to hear Chris testify. In the end, she had the gnawing feeling it would come back to nip her, so she stayed home and spent the day catching up on charts.

Chris called at 7 P.M. His voice was flat and weak. "Hey, how ya doin'?"

"Okay, okay. How'd it go?"

"So, you haven't heard?"

"No. Are you in jail for contempt of court for telling that horrible lawyer to go to hell?"

"Actually, it's sort of the opposite. You're going to hear, so you might as well hear it directly from the horse's mouth."

"Okay, but I guess I don't understand."

"Well, I'd rather tell you face to face, sort of horse to princess."

"What's going on, Chris?"

"Well, I guess I wasn't the hottest witness for the prosecution. Things got a bit muddled. Got a little tripped up. Are you free Saturday? I could meet you in Seattle. Better not too close to home."

"Your home, you mean. But, okay."

"I have a short procedure on Saturday morning at the U. Should be done around ten. How about eleven?"

"Okay. I'll meet you in front of the University Book Store. Picking up a new copy of Harrison's."

"Oh, my lord, no one really reads that stuff, do they? Thought that was

342

strictly for an internal medicine residency, mental masturbation and that sort of thing, fodder to pimp your fellow residents on rounds. To kill them. Am I wrong?"

"Chris, you're such a professional! At least our mistakes don't die on the table an hour after we first meet them. Takes us weeks."

He laughed. "Hey, Khai, if you hear what a wimpy witness I was before the weekend, please hold judgment until you let the man talk. Then you can hang 'im."

"I'm afraid to hear."

"Not that big a deal. Just not so good in court."

Khai ended the call warily and scrolled through her contact list for Harrison Jennings' cell phone. She was about to push the talk button when it dawned upon her that Jennings would surely ask how she had learned so soon. She put the phone down and went back to her charts.

On Saturday morning, she left her tiny apartment early to beat the oppressive Seattle traffic and find a bookstore where she could sit and think. She couldn't clear her mind of the night she'd spent at his condo in Soundview, how he'd gotten up in the middle of the night to go to the bathroom, and how he'd stumbled back to bed, unable to answer when she asked if he was okay. Yet, by morning, he was moving around the condo easily. She asked again what had happened during the night, but he laughed that he was a sleepwalker.

Khai thought back to the morning after they'd first slept together. Before they left the condo for her cross-examination, she had opened the refrigerator, hoping for half-and-half with which to lace her coffee. There was no cream or milk, but on the very bottom rack, in a far corner, was a container of yogurt. Initially, she laughed, remembering how Chris had made ugly faces when she'd bought a Yoplait months before. He'd groaned, "Yuk, girlie food."

Khai pulled the little container out and read the label. It was a few days after the pull date. She shrugged as she placed it back and, five minutes later, forgot about the mystery of the stale yogurt, not giving it another thought until the morning she was to meet Chris in Seattle.

Khai parked just east of Pike Place Market, planning to get her workout over early by power walking the hills of Seattle. After the third hump, she took a break, walked down Yesler toward Pioneer Square, and stopped at the Safeway. As she grabbed a can of club soda from the cooler, her eye caught the piles of yogurt on the next shelf. She pulled one free and looked at the best-by date. It was almost a month in the future. So, the cup in Chris's refrigerator had been purchased before he'd gone on his sabbatical. She had no idea what it meant.

Khai drove back up to the University Bookstore, paid her two hundred some dollars for Harrison's Textbook of Medicine, and stood outside waiting until Chris pulled up. A block later, he took her hand, but she flinched almost imperceptibly, and Chris slowly pulled away. Without looking at her, he muttered, "I see you've already heard."

"Heard what?"

"You know darn well know what. My performance at the trial."

"Chris, I have not heard a word about the trial. So, maybe you need to tell me."

"Well, if it's not the trial, what is it?"

"What is what?"

"There's something wrong. I may be a surgeon, but I'm not devoid of all sensitivity."

"Okay. Yogurt," she laughed mockingly."

"Hate the stuff. Can't make my mouth close down on it. Yuk. Girlie food. Why?"

"Straight up, Chris, I found a cup of the stuff in your fridge."

"Didn't know it was there. Maybe been in there a year or more."

"Yeah, well, it was dated not all that long ago."

He flushed but came back quickly, "Uh, that was from my daughter. She spends the weekends with me sometimes. Tell me you haven't seen orange Pringles dust all over the place, Madame Detective."

"Wow. Well played, Doctor." She stared straight ahead for a moment then smiled curiously. "So, tell me about the trial."

"Okay. You belted in?"

"Fire away."

"So, the day before the trial, I got a little visit from Norman Harp. You remember him, our CEO. A real Mother Theresa. Threatened to go to the local medical society and tell them about my dissolving marriage."

"And? That's the situation for a good ninety percent of the people working for him."

"Yeah, but he knows about the condo in Soundview."

"Okay, now we're down to seventy-five percent of the moral paragons practicing at Mitchie-Sterling."

"Maybe, but as long as it isn't made public, it's cool. Don't ask, don't tell. You get away with anything and everything in medicine as long as someone doesn't file a complaint. And, anyone who files a complaint, if it's another doctor, they're next in line for the hatchet."

"Okay, he threatened you, and you had no choice but do what?"

"Okay, maybe I wasn't the witness that lawyer, Jennings, wanted, or should I say, expected. But that's not the whole story."

Khai did not speak for a moment. "What is...the whole story?"

"In my own defense, I didn't come across as very believable, kind of a confused doctor, not really sure what the hell happened that night. On the surface, I appeared hostile to the Maddinglys. But not really. May still cost me my behind at work. Have to wait and see."

Khai shook her head. "How come they don't tell you all this before you put in six years getting into medical school? And how 'bout ten more before you rise to the rank of peon?"

"It stinks, but it's a living. I'm sure no different than any of the professions, and better than working in the non-professions."

"If you say so." She paused. "I'm sorry you had to listen to their threats. Then I give you a hard time about yogurt. Sorry."

"No problem. Yogurt's a touchy subject—girlie food's a touchy subject. I like to touchy you."

"Just keep your eyes on the road."

"How 'bout my hands?"

CHAPTER FORTY-NINE

Peter G. Cardozo's arms just didn't swing quite right as he sought a swagger along the center aisle of the courtroom. Harrison Jennings tried not to shake his head as he started his direct examination.

"Dr. Cardozo, let's get some housekeeping out of the way. It is very unusual that you agreed to testify on your own behalf in this trial. Please tell the jury why."

Cardozo snarled, "I have done nothing wrong. I saved a woman's life that night. I am not responsible for birth defects patients drag into my emergency room. I want my name cleared."

Jennings stared at his witness for a moment then mumbled, "You will have that chance, sir." He went on to have Cardozo list his credentials without interruption until Cardozo offered, "I completed my residency at the University of Idaho Health Center."

Jennings held up a hand and took a few steps closer to the witness stand. "Doctor, please tell us what type of residency that was."

"It was a full residency."

"No, I mean, sir, was it in transplant surgery, maybe neurosurgery?"

"No."

"Doctor, what was it in?"

"Family medicine."

"I don't understand. Do you have a family practice office?"

"No."

"In fact, the only place you work in the Mitchie-Sterling Hospital is in

346

the emergency room. Is that correct?"

"Yes."

"Well, tell us, is there such a thing as an emergency medicine residency?"

"There is now."

"Are you suggesting that there was no specific emergency medicine residency when you did your family practice training."

"There were very few of them."

"But there were some? Is that your testimony?"

"Yes."

"Are there any doctors in your emergency medicine group who did residencies specifically in emergency medicine?"

"Yes."

"Were any of them at Mitchie-Sterling Hospital when you got there?"

"I'm not sure."

"Is Emergency Partners West the name of the corporation to which you belong?"

"Yes."

"Does Emergency Partners West have the exclusive contract with Mitchie-Sterling Hospital to provide emergency room services for the hospitals owned by Mitchie-Sterling Hospital?"

"Yes."

"Doctor, who is the medical director of Emergency Partners West?"

"Molly Morningstar."

"Is she a medical doctor?"

"Well, she's a D.O."

"Is that a doctor?"

"I don't want to say anything politically incorrect."

"Sir, this is a court of law. We are interested in the truth here, not social fashion."

"Well, she went to a Doctor of Osteopathy school."

"How is that different than a Doctor of Medicine school."

"The truth?"

Jennings' shoulders drooped. "If you don't mind, Doctor."

"Much easier to get into the D.O. schools."

"Are D.O.s considered lesser doctors?"

"All I can say is that they don't have to climb the same mountain we do to become medical doctors."

"Was this doctor working at Mitchie-Sterling Hospital before you started there in the ER?"

"Yes."

"Where did she do her residency?"

"I don't know, to be honest. It was a D.O. residency."

"Do you know if that was a proper emergency medicine residency?"

"I don't know what you mean by proper."

"Did she do an emergency medicine residency?"

"Acts like she did, but I don't believe she did."

"Doctor, did any physician in your emergency room do an emergency medicine residency?"

"I'm not sure."

Jennings walked to his desk and pulled a sheet of paper from a loose-leaf binder. "Dr. Mary Mirkovich. Did she come to the practice before you?"

"Yes."

"Did she complete an emergency medicine residency?"

"I don't know."

"Well, she did." Jennings had the paper in his hand introduced into evidence. It was a Mitchie-Sterling advertisement that listed Dr. Mirkovich as having completed an emergency medicine residency in the 1970s. "So, we know of one person, at least, who you work with who did an emergency medicine residency in the old days. Is that so?"

"If you say so. I do not know that for sure."

Jennings' shoulders drooped again. "Now, Doctor, what is the mission of an emergency medicine residency?"

"To train a doctor to carry out emergency medicine."

"And, what is the mission of the family medicine residency?"

"To train family doctors."

"Are the two specialties the same?"

"There is a lot of overlap."

"What are some of the common problems seen in the ER?"

"Coughs, colds..."

"Doctor, please, tell us why an emergency medicine doctor gets paid far more than most family physicians."

"It's what the insurance companies decide."

"Well, does emergency medicine handle more than coughs and colds?"

"Yes."

"Can you handle a heart attack?"

"Yes."

"Do you do that frequently?"

"Yes."

"Does a family doctor handle heart attacks, or do they, at least here in a metropolitan area, send the patient directly to the ER?"

"Yes."

"Yes, what?"

"They send them to us as fast as they can."

"Do you see patients frequently who need resuscitation?"

"Yes."

"Routinely?"

"Yes."

"Can you handle that?"

His lips twisted arrogantly. "Of course."

"Do family doctors see patients routinely who need resuscitation?

"They can."

"Do first responders coming upon a patient who needs resuscitation take that patient to a family doctor."

"No."

"So, in both cases, the heart attack and the patient in need of resuscitation, how are you different than a family doctor?"

"I have the skills to do what is needed to serve these patients."

"Are these skills things like putting a tube into a throat to set up an airway?"

"Yes."

"How about using complex chemical algorithms to treat a patient with a deadly arrhythmia who has already been shocked in the field and hasn't responded?"

"Yes."

"Do family doctors do those resuscitations?"

"They can."

Jennings raised his voice. "Do they routinely even have the medicines and catheters in their offices to do those resuscitations?"

"No."

"So, would you agree there are many physical procedures you have to learn to do to be a minimally effective emergency medical doctor?"

"Yes."

"Is that why an emergency medicine residency is three or four years?"

"It isn't the only way to learn the skills."

"Are you suggesting that these skills can be perfected OTJ, on the job?"

"Yes."

"What about the poor patients who you learn on?"

"It is the same as in a residency. You have to learn somewhere?"

"Yes, but even in an emergency medicine residency, are you ever, ever, all by yourself with a dying patient without a trained emergency medicine physician just a minute away?"

"Probably not."

"So, was there always an experienced EM doctor available when you made the jump from family medicine to the emergency room?"

"At first there was."

"For four years!?"

"No, of course not."

"For how long?"

"Oh, I can't tell you."

"Was it a week?"

"No, of course not."

"How about two years."

"Not that long."

"Was it a couple of months?"

"Probably."

"So, you learned in sixty days what it takes the average doctor three or four years to learn. Is that what you are telling us?"

"I am telling you I learned enough to be safe and serve my patients. Look, I learned a lot in my residency. A family medicine residency isn't just coughs and low back pain. I had a lot of exposure to the ER. And I have put in years of study, years since I got into emergency medicine."

"In other words, by reading books you are getting the same training as in a full emergency medicine residency?"

Rhonda Uft was on her feet. "Objection. He is clearly badgering his own witness."

Galanter thought for a second. "I don't think so, Ms. Uft. Counsel has the obligation to impeach the credentials of a defendant. Overruled. Carry on, Mr. Jennings."

"Thank you, Your Honor. Doctor, is one of the skills you learn in residency the placing of central lines?"

Cardozo grinned. "I wondered how long it would take you to start screwin' with me."

Jennings looked up at Judge Galanter, who spoke in a monotone. "Doctor, this isn't a friendly conversation we're having here over a couple of beers. You are on trial for a serious matter, an incredibly serious matter. Keep your comments to yourself. Go on, Mr. Jennings."

Well, Doctor, let me ask again, is one of the skills you learn in residency the placing of central lines?"

"Yes."

"How many did you do in your residency?"

"I have no idea."

"I thought you residents keep a list of all the more complex procedures, even things like baby deliveries, that you carry out over the years, and that is how you are judged competent to do these techniques after residency. Is that true?"

"Yes."

"Well, where is your little book?"

"That was nearly twenty years ago. I didn't keep it, as far as I can remember."

"Okay. So, let's get down to brass tacks. You have testified that you were on duty in the Mitchie-Sterling Hospital Emergency Room on the night of 25th November and the early morning of 26th November? Were you alone that night? I mean the only ER doctor?"

"Yes."

"In the course of your normal duties as the emergency medicine doctor in the hot seat, do you field telephone calls from outlying doctors who have emergency medicine-type questions?"

"Yes."

"Did you take the Hippocratic Oath at the end of medical school?"

"Yes. Some form of it."

"Some form? Do you remember which form?"

"It's always changing."

"Always changing. Well, would you take look at this? It is the version to which you swore the day of your graduation from medical school."

Cardozo perused it quickly. "I cannot say this is the oath I took."

"Well, sir, we received it from the dean of your medical school. Would you like to see the letter she sent along with it?"

"No, I believe you."

Jennings said nothing in reply and entered the document in the record.

"Doctor, would you read the paragraph I highlighted in yellow, please."

Cardozo rolled his eyes and began. "I will respect the hard-won scientific gains of those physicians in whose steps I walk, and gladly share such knowledge as is mine with those who are to follow."

Jennings nodded and repeated, "'And gladly share such knowledge as is mine with those who are to follow.' On the night of 25th November, did the Mitchie-Sterling Hospital ER receive a call from Dr. Khai Weathersby?"

"Yes."

"Did you know if she had to call several times before she was put through to you?"

"I don't know. I don't answer phones. I save lives."

"Is it your policy, when you are the physician on duty, to have your secretarial staff tell medical doctors who are declaring a medical emergency to, 'Cool your jets?'"

"Objection. More prejudicial than probative."

"Sustained."

"Did you finally speak to Dr. Khai Weathersby?"

"Yes. I guess that was her name."

"Did she identify herself as a medical doctor?"

"I don't remember the conversation."

"Did Dr. Weathersby inform you that she had sent a young woman with a probable ectopic pregnancy to sit in your waiting room?"

"I told you, I don't remember the conversation."

"So, you don't remember the part of the conversation in which you screamed at Dr. Weathersby, 'What the hell do you want me to do with her?'"

"I told you..."

Rhonda Uft blurted, "Objection. Badgering. Dr. Cardozo said he did not recall the conversation—period."

"Sustained."

"That's fine. We'll move on to your actions in the treatment room. Oh, but first, do you happen to know how long Dr. Maddingly sat in your waiting room before she saw a doctor."

"I do not."

Jennings had Cardozo read through Sabrina's chart, noting the time the ultrasound machine was used that evening, and then the time her first low blood pressure was noted in the ER treatment bay.

"Now, Doctor, at what time was Dr. Maddingly logged out of the ultrasound department that night?"

"Twenty-one-twenty."

"In civilian time please."

"Eleven-twenty P.M."

"Thank you. Now what time was the first note regarding her in the treatment area of the ER?"

"Zero-zero-forty-nine."

"English, please."

"Twelve-forty-nine A.M."

"How about the first time a blood pressure was taken?"

"Twelve-fifty-two."

"That's a gap of over one and a half hours given it took a few minutes to go from the ultrasound department to the ER. How do you explain that?"

"Simple, the family was so, so, shall we say, disorderly, they never signed in. And they never signed in because that doctor in Evanston told them to just sit there. That's not the way it's done."

"But, did Dr. Weathersby tell you the emergency patient was there?"

"I told you, I don't remember what she told me."

"Hypothetically, Doctor, if she did tell you Dr. Maddingly was there and was a possible unstable patient with an ectopic pregnancy, would you have alerted your staff?"

He paused and thought. "Not unless they signed in."

"So, are you saying that if the paramedics call and tell you they're bringing in a woman with an ectopic pregnancy, you would not alert your staff to be waiting?"

"I trust them."

"Who, the medics?"

He paused for a moment to consider the consequences of an answer. "Yes."

"So, you did not trust Dr. Weathersby?"

"I don't know her."

"But she identified herself as a medical doctor, and she told you she had a very sick patient. Why would you doubt her?"

"I didn't know her, and she told me she worked at that Doc in a Box up in Evanston."

"Oh, so, suddenly, some of that conversation with Dr. Weathersby has been restored in your mind. Is that true?"

"I don't remember the conversation, just that I got a call from a doctor in Evanston."

"Well, let's see if we can refresh your memory a bit more. Perhaps you remember saying, and I quote, 'You know, goddamnit, I'm so tired of you quacks up in Evanston ripping off patients, and then sending them down to me to patch up your mistakes.' Do you remember saying that?"

"Absolutely not."

"No, you don't remember, or you never said that?"

"I never said that."

"Well, then, what did you say?"

"I told you, I don't remember."

"Okay, but you remember what you didn't say. Is that correct?"

"Yes."

"Is it possible that Dr. Weathersby said to you, 'Look doctor, we'll take care of your attitude in the morning with the state medical society, but for right now, you've got a sick patient in your ER. I didn't ask you for anything. Just called to tell you, you have a ticking time bomb thirty feet away from where you're standing.'?"

"I do not remember any doctor telling me that."

"Okay, do you remember your reply, 'You can go to hell?'"

"I never said that."

"Did you verbalize, under your breath, a profane word referring to Dr. Weathersby's sexual organs?"

"Never."

"Did you say to her, 'If you want to talk to someone here, call my

354

secretary?'"

"I never said that."

"Do you remember slamming the phone down?"

"I do not remember ever doing that to a fellow physician."

"So, the only thing you remember of that conversation was that it was with a doctor from a walk-in clinic. Is that a true statement?"

"Yes."

"You really hate doctors who work at walk-in clinics, don't you?"

"I don't hate them. I have no respect for them."

"Why is that?"

"They're basically quacks."

"What evidence do you have to make that statement in a court of law?"

"Evidence? I don't need evidence. I have to clean up after them every day."

"What do you mean by 'clean up'?"

"Undo their mistakes."

"Would that include their inability to do basic medical procedures? Strike that. Please give us an example."

"I had one of those quacks miss an inflamed appendix."

"Ah, yes. We'll get to that case in just a minute. And how about the doctor from a walk-in clinic who sent you a little girl who had had a near leg amputation. She didn't even start a usual IV. Just another walk-in quack?"

"Yes, another quack. And I know what you're getting at."

"What am I getting at, Doctor?"

"You're going to have me tell the jury I didn't start the IV in Mrs. Maddingly."

"Excuse me, Dr. Cardozo, but that's Dr. Maddingly."

Cardozo smirked, though Jennings ignored him and went on. "Let me ask, sir, did you know she was a doctor?"

"She's not a doctor. She's a psychologist."

"I will not dignify that with a correction. Let's go back a step to the patient you told us was sent to you, the little girl who nearly lost her leg, and the quack doctor in Evanston hadn't started an IV. Please tell us the reason the doctor at the walk-in clinic wasn't able to start an IV in that child.

"The excuse was the child had bled so much, the veins had collapsed."

"How was that different than your failure to start an IV in Dr.

Maddingly?"

"All you need to know is that an IV was started. That's why I say walk-in clinics are dangerous. We have surgical backup in a decent hospital. Bottom line: job got done on my watch."

"That's a fair point, but could you tell the jury what sort of procedure the doctor in the walk-in clinic did to get fluid into the little girl with the amputated leg? You know, the procedure that kept her alive long enough to reach a surgeon at your hospital?"

"She stuck an IV needle into her abdomen. It was barbaric."

"Excuse me. Did it get the job done?"

"Some fluids were getting into the child."

"Was the child's blood pressure maintained?"

"Yes, but..."

"Yes, but what?"

"It was barbaric."

"Do you know where the doctor learned that technique?"

"At a zoo?"

"Your Honor, I'm losing patience with this witness. I submit that he is demonstrating contempt for this court."

The judge exhaled through pursed lips. "Doctor, this is my last warning. We are here to gather facts about an incident that left a woman maimed. Snide remarks are not helpful, nor will they be tolerated. Is that crystal clear?"

"Yes."

Rhonda Uft stood. "Your Honor, this man has been under incredible stress as a result of this lawsuit, and has been for nearly a year. It has affected his wife and children. In fact, his life is essentially changed forever over something for which he not responsible. I believe to my core he did nothing to bring him to this courtroom. That is why I am defending him. He knows nothing of courtroom etiquette. He is protecting himself from this unfair attack the best he knows how. Anyone who was as innocent as he is would act in the same fashion."

"Very eloquent, Ms. Uft. A wonderful summation. I am going to grant a short recess, one sufficiently long, I trust, for you to give Dr. Cardozo a crash course in how one acts in front of his peers. We will reconvene in ten minutes. Bailiff, please escort the jury to their room."

When court resumed, Cardozo sat in the witness chair blank-expressioned. Jennings approached him slowly. "Dr. Cardozo, let's turn the page and start anew. Is that satisfactory?"

"Yes."

"I do want to ask again, though, if you were aware that it was Dr. Weathersby who placed the needle in that girl's abdomen?"

"No, I didn't, but I am not sur..." He stopped abruptly as Galanter peered down at him.

"Do you know where Dr. Weathersby learned the technique of placing a needle directly in the abdomen of a patient who was is so dehydrated that the blood vessels had collapsed?"

"I do not know how she learned that, but it sure isn't in any of the textbooks we use here in America."

"Well, she learned it treating dying children in Afghanistan—after the earthquake in 2009. Surely you remember that catastrophe? That's after she served as a decorated helicopter pilot in the First Gulf War, before she became a doctor."

"Yes, of course."

"Let me ask, in your fifteen years of practice, have you volunteered for service in disaster areas?"

"I have a family. I can't leave the U.S. But I help out where I can."

"And where is that?"

"I don't run up the bill on the poor."

"So, you run up the bill on the rest of us?"

"Of course not."

"I'm relieved to hear it. Withdrawn. Now, I do want to go over what happened when Dr. Maddingly first entered the treatment area. Were you watching as she was brought in?"

"No. I had two men with heart attacks in separate rooms."

"Do you know if she walked into the treatment area or was brought in in a wheelchair?"

"I honestly do not know."

"When was the first time you saw her?"

"She was in the treatment room on a table."

"What were you told, and by whom?"

"I remember only that she was identified as a thirty-something white woman who had been sitting in the in the waiting area."

"Did you have any idea why they brought her back?"

"Someone said she looked pale."

"Was Dr. Maddingly conscious at the time?"

"I don't remember."

"Here are the ER intake notes from that night. Please read the highlighted section."

"It's in cursive. Very hard to read."

"Well, it's your staff's handwriting. Please give it a try."

He paused, removed his glasses, brought the page an inch from his eyes, and squinted. "Patient needs help to get on exam table. Reports C/C possible ectopic pregnancy."

"What is C/C?"

"Chief complaint."

"What does chief complaint mean?"

"It's what the patient has come to have examined."

"Okay, so, it looks like she was able to do some of the work of getting on the exam table. Is that true?"

"I can't tell you. I wasn't there."

"Was that written by a Mitchie-Sterling Hospital nurse?"

"Apparently."

"Apparently? Strike that." Jennings read stiffly. "'Reports C/C possible ectopic pregnancy.' Does that mean the patient, herself, spoke those words?"

"I don't know. I would have to make an assumption, and I have been instructed not to."

"Fair enough. But that is what is written. Yes?"

"Yes."

"So, it seems clear Dr. Maddingly either walked into the treatment area and then into the examination room on her own steam, or, if she was in a wheelchair, she was able to get out of the wheelchair and needed help to lift herself onto the exam table. Is that correct?"

"I wasn't there yet."

"Were you called into the treatment room at that point?"

"I don't know how long it was before they came and got me."

"Do you remember the first thing a nurse told you about Dr. Maddingly?"

"It wasn't a nurse, if I remember correctly. It was the unit clerk."

"How do you remember that?"

"It was unusual for a clerk to get involved in patient care."

"What did she tell you?"

"As far as I can remember, it was something about a lady in Two who looked terrible."

"Did you leave what you were doing immediately?"

"Yes."

"Why."

"The clerk seemed upset, and I assumed the woman was in trouble, probably bleeding."

"When someone doesn't look well, do you immediately think of a bleeding problem?"

"No, but in this case, that was the most likely diagnosis."

"Wait. You knew nothing about this patient. She was just sitting in the waiting area. Is that correct?"

"I assumed it was the woman the doctor in Evanston had sent down."

"So, you were aware of this woman?"

"Barely."

"Were you surprised the patient had arrived in your ER?"

"No. She had nowhere else to go."

"Then, if you knew very well she was going to present herself asking for help, why didn't you alert the waiting room staff to the strong possibility of a very sick patient showing up on your doorstep?"

"I was overwhelmed with two heart attacks."

"For an hour and a half?"

"That is correct."

"In retrospect, Doctor, who turned out to be the sickest patient?"

"You want me to say Dr. Maddingly, but if you ask one of the guys with the heart attack, I wager they would say themselves."

"Who, though, was left with the greatest deficit?"

"Using the retrospectoscope, that's easy: your client."

"Using the what, Doctor?"

"Retrospectoscope. That's doctor talk for sort of using one of our scopes to look at something in retrospect. You know, Monday morning quarterbacking."

"Thank you. But I guess my question remains; had Dr. Maddingly been seen earlier, would we be sitting here today?"

"Again, using the retrospectoscope, that's easy. The answer is no. But, let me know after you've done a few thousand emergency room shifts if you have a crystal ball in your armamentarium."

"Armamentarium?"

"That's doctor talk for our bag of tools; our armaments against disease."

"I guess we're all going to have to go to medical school to make sense of your testimony." Jennings heard Rhonda Uft draw in a grand breath. "Withdrawn. Now, Dr. Cardozo, when you eventually showed up in her treatment room, what was the first thing you did?"

"I don't remember, but I imagine it was to ask for vital signs."

"Please tell us, what are vital signs?"

"You know, the signs vital for life. Blood pressure, heart rate, breathing rate, and let's see, temperature."

"Did you ask what was going on before you started your doctoring?"

"Well, yes, of course."

"What were you told?"

"That she was an ectopic."

"She was an 'ectopic'?"

"You know what I mean. That was her diagnosis."

"Did you get a report from one of the nurses about the pregnancy test?"

"Yes."

"Did you get a report from one of the nurses about the ultrasound?"

"Yes."

"Do you remember what you were told about that ultrasound?"

"Some."

"Did you actually see the report, or just a description from a nurse?"

"I don't remember."

"Did you see the actual ultrasound image?"

"I don't remember, but I am sure I looked at it to orient myself."

"Have you looked at the image since that night?"

"Yes."

"Please tell us what you remember of it."

"Actually, I would need to look at the report."

"So, you are saying that you do not have independent recollection of that ultrasound?"

"I do not?"

"Didn't you prepare for this testimony?"

"Of course I did?"

"But you don't remember one of the most important elements of this case?"

"Objection. Badgering."

"Sustained."

"Okay, here's the report. Please refresh your memory."

Cardozo read for a minute. Jennings inquired, "What does it say about the presence of free fluid in the pelvis."

"It just says there is free fluid in the pelvis."

"Does it say how much?"

"No."

"Do radiologists generally give you the dimensions of abnormal findings?"

"Sometimes."

"Sometimes? Withdrawn. The ultrasound machine has a function that measures things on the screen in centimeters. Is that correct?"

"Yes."

"So, it is easy for the radiologist to use his mouse and draw a line around the pocket of fluid and let the machine do the math to figure just how much, in this case blood, is present. Is that correct?"

"Sometimes they do, and sometimes they don't."

"Can you think of a single reason why the radiologist did not provide you with the most important detail on the ultrasound, and maybe the most important detail in the life of your patient?"

"You'd have to ask him."

"Was that meant as a joke, sir?"

"What do you want me to say? I have no idea."

"Okay. Well, then, were you surprised that he did not make a notation of how much blood was in the pelvis?"

"To be honest, I was far too busy trying to save my patient's life to critique an ultrasound report."

Jennings walked to his desk, hit a few keys on his computer, and an electronic image of an ultrasound flashed on the screen. "It isn't terribly clear but is this the ultrasound of Dr. Maddingly that you saw the night of 25th November."

Cardozo squinted at the screen. "Yes."

"Please come over here, if you would, Doctor, and point out the fluid about the which the report speaks."

As Cardozo walked to the screen, Jennings handed him a long wooden pointer. Cardozo stared at the screen for a moment and tapped a dark area of the image. "There it is."

"How much fluid is that?"

"I'm not a radiologist."

"Yes, but you made life and death decisions that night based on what you saw in this image that night. Is that correct?"

"It was just one of the tools we used."

"Okay, thank you. But you ordered whole blood from the blood bank, did you not?"

"I did."

"How much?"

"I don't remember."

"Upon what would you base that decision?"

"On the blood pressure, on the size of the patient, and on the amount of blood you see in the pelvis."

"What would you guess, just guess, is the amount of the fluid in this ultrasound image?"

He took the pointer and made imaginary lines, circumscribing a half sphere. He asked, "May I sit down and do some calculations?"

"Did you sit down and do calculations that night?"

"I'm sure not, but this is a court of law. I want to be precise."

"Oh, yes, of course. A court of law. Please take your seat."

Cardozo scratched on a piece of paper for a minute. "I would say nearly four units."

"And you ordered five units of blood that night according to the blood bank and emergency room records. Is that correct?"

"If you...if that's what the record says."

"Thank you. Now, I would like to enter into the record this ultrasound report signed by Dr. Childress. Do you know Dr. Childress?"

"'Yes."

"Is he respected?"

"Yes."

Rhonda Uft was on her feet. "Objection. This is a ruse, Your Honor. This is not the ultrasound regarding the plaintiff. It is of a different patient. The name of this patient is blacked out and the date is not that of the evening in question."

"Mr. Jennings?"

"That is true, Your Honor. And Ms. Uft is stepping in to testify to save her client further embarrassment. On the other hand, Dr. Cardozo seems to think this is the ultrasound in question. In fact, this image was provided to Ms. Uft labeled, 'Image for Comparison.'" Jennings pointed to those words printed in the lower left corner of the film. No ruse there."

Galanter spoke without expression. "Is that correct, Ms. Uft?"

"Yes."

"Well, then what is your objection?"

"My objection is that Mr. Jennings' case is being built on deception. It is a ruse."

"Ms. Uft, you've had the document for nigh on a year. Objection overruled. Mr. Jennings."

"Thank you, Your Honor. Dr. Cardozo, did you read the legend on this image before you came to a factual conclusion about it?"

"I trusted you to act professionally and not try to harm me."

"Well, Doctor, let's see if I can restore my professionalism in your discerning eyes. Are there mix-ups in the hospital when it comes to lab tests?"

"Sadly, yes."

"Doctor, are there mix-ups in the hospital when it comes to x-rays?"

"Sadly, yes."

"How do you prevent them?"

"Due diligence."

"Did you do due diligence in reviewing this image for the jury?"

"I don't have to; this isn't the emergency room."

"Oh, so this doesn't count. Withdrawn. Doctor, would you be surprised to know that there is no fluid on this image. That is, however, the image of an ectopic pregnancy."

"Yeah, well, I was told there was free fluid in the patient's pelvis that night, and I acted in accordance with accepted emergency protocol."

"Again, who told you?"

"I don't remember."

Jennings nodded without expression then smiled. "Your Honor, I'd like to ask that we take our lunch break at this point. It's been a full morning, and I would like everyone to feel comfortable before we embark on the most critical testimony."

"Ms. Uft, is that acceptable?"

"I don't know what he means by, 'the most critical testimony,' but I have no objection to a break."

This time, Mike wheeled Sabrina out feet first. Though he didn't smile, his eyes were bright. Jennings rode with them in the elevator and then into the cafeteria. Rhonda Uft was sitting with Cardozo, his back in a corner. Though they could not see Rhonda Uft's face, the look on Cardozo's was sufficient for Jennings to smile, "How'd you like to be in his shoes right about now?" Both Sabrina and Mike smiled as they nodded. Cardozo looked up at that very moment and saw them. He began to smile back in reflex, but his lips quickly twisted into a smirk.

Jennings explained that Cardozo had fallen into a hole from which he couldn't dig himself free. The damage had been done. "But don't you gloat. He could be the worst doctor in the world, and he might be, but Rhonda Uft had to know that I let him do well in his deposition, stoke his hubris, and that I was going to deep-fry him during the trial. They don't care what he says. They wrote him off months before the trial. He'll be gone from the stand soon and quickly forgotten. They are building their case around Sabrina's medical history."

Mike interjected, "Which is a red herring..."

"Well, nothing is if the right lawyer gets her hands on it."

Sabrina asked, "Is there still time to hire an expert to look at the drawing our friend Dr. Gauthé made?"

"Yes and no. We can get a sworn statement for the court that it is absurd to base a major legal decision on some scratches made by a doctor who is terrified his professional life hangs in the balance. But the other side will just come back with their hired gun and testify that there are no grounds to argue that a kink in a fallopian tube is normal. And another of their paid assassins will swear that where you see one congenital abnormality, you will always find another. Which may be true, but they have not proven the fallopian tube was one of those abnormalities, or even that it was defective. After all, you got pregnant, Sabrina."

Mike mused, "I still think something ain't kosher with the ultrasound image. Why did it take so long before they turned it over to us?"

"I don't know. Well, I do, but what we know to be the absolute, undeniable truth, and what we can prove, are worlds apart. I haven't stopped thinking about it. And any ideas you guys can come up...I'm all ears. And, by the way, our Dr. Weathersby told me she has a pal on the East Coast, apparently a guy she dated before she got married, who's a radiologist. She's thinking about opening a dialogue with him and asking for a favor: for him to pass the thing around and see if anyone can come up with fodder for our cannon."

Sabrina mused, "We got lucky with her...and with you, Harrison. We'll never forget you."

"Not so fast, case ain't over."

Mike smiled, "Doesn't matter."

Harrison Jennings gripped both their forearms.

CHAPTER FIFTY

For the rest of lunch, the Maddinglys sat quietly, picking at salads. Jennings finally looked up. "Okay, troops, time to remount. And remember, whether the jury hates him or loves Cardozo, our Ms. Uft is going to put on a good show to prove that regardless of who treated you, Sabrina, the Agent Orange thing trumps his miserable personality. And to be honest, it should. But I'm going to keep the truth about the ultrasound, which I still can't prove, floating around like a puff of skunk spray until the judge stops me. Believe me, that trumps Agent Orange. Even the lemmings in juries don't like to be lied to for a whole trial, only to be told the truth at the end. Now, chin up, and let's go back to work."

The afternoon's testimony began with a bang. Cardozo appeared with a thick medical text under his arm, though tripped on the step to the witness stand. The book slammed to the linoleum floor. Several of the jurors put their hands over their mouths to hide smiles their eyes could not veil.

Harrison Jennings nodded to Cardozo. "I hope you had a peaceful lunch, sir. Now, let's get back to that night in the emergency room. You have testified that you saw the ultrasound in question, evaluated it, and decided—using that as one piece of information—that Dr. Maddingly needed to be injected with blood. Is that correct?"

"Close enough."

"Well, if it isn't correct, please say so and correct the record."

"No, it's fine"

"So, are you agreeing that is what you testified in this court?"

Cardozo ground his teeth. "Yes."

"Good. On that night, sir, what was the first thing you did in terms of treating Dr. Maddingly?"

"I ordered blood."

"Yes, of course. How much?"

Rhonda Uft objected. "Asked and answered."

Jennings nodded. "Withdrawn. Yes, of course, five units. Did you feel, Doctor, that five units would be enough to resuscitate Dr. Maddingly?"

"Yes."

"I imagine that five units was more than she needed, but that it would cover any emergencies. Is that correct?

"Yes."

"So, emergencies occur when you have a very sick patient. Is that true?"

"It is a human endeavor. Of course there are mistakes."

"Could you tell us of the mistakes that happened with the blood that night?"

Rhonda Uft stood. "Objection. Leading. There is no evidence of a single mistake that evening."

"Sustained."

"Let me rephrase. Was a mistake made with the blood that night?"

Cardozo's pause elicited a round of headshaking among the jurors. He finally took a deep breath. "Yes."

"Please tell us what happened."

"An incompetent nurse tried to introduce the first unit of blood before I had established the central line."

"Okay, what did you say to the nurse?"

"I wasn't happy."

"I'm sure not. But my question was what did you say to her?"

"I don't remember."

"Did you say something that upset her?"

"Apparently. But she did something to upset me—like trying to kill one of my patients."

"How, in heaven's name, Doctor, did she try to kill a patient?"

"It is just an expression to note just how incompetent she was."

"So, it was all her fault?"

"Let's just say it caused a," he fashioned finger quotes, "problem."

"What, specifically, was the problem?"

"She wasted a unit of blood."

"What do you mean by 'wasted'?"

"It didn't get where it was supposed to get."

"Where was it supposed to get?"

"Into the patient."

"How was it supposed to get into the patient?"

Cardozo rolled his eyes. "Through an IV."

"What kind of IV?"

"A central line."

"Had you started a central line?"

"I was in the process. It takes more than twenty seconds, you know."

"How long? Twenty minutes?"

"Not that long."

"Two minutes?"

"Too short."

"What is a fair amount of time, Doctor? I would like an answer."

"It depends. In this case, the woman had bled so much, her veins were collapsed. And then I'm dealing with an incompetent who doesn't like me and takes it out on the patient. See it all the time."

"So, you are testifying that she, in some way, spilled the blood due to incompetence and to purposely harm you by placing a patient in mortal danger."

"Yes."

Harrison Jennings went back to the plaintiff's table and sat silently for a moment. He finally looked up to ask, "Please tell us what she did to spill the blood."

"She squeezed the bag of blood before I had connected the IV line to the central line."

"I thought you said you hadn't been able to get the line started. Is that correct?"

"As I said, I was in the process."

"What happened to the blood?"

"It spilled on the floor."

"How much spilled?"

"Some of it."

"Isn't it true it was most of it?"

"I don't know."

"Was there a puddle of blood on the floor?"

"I don't know if you would call it a puddle. There was some."

"Was there blood on the walls?"

"A bit."

"How much? A teaspoon?"

"Probably a bit more."

"How much more?"

"I'm sorry, but I don't remember."

"You were understandably upset. Is that true?"

"Objection. Asked and answered."

"Sustained."

"Did you use profanity?"

"I might have. I had every right."

"Why do you say you had a *right?*"

"I was mad as hell, to be honest. I was trying to save a life."

"Did your anger have an effect on your ability to do a technical procedure, that is, the placing of a central line?"

"Absolutely not. I remained professional."

"I see, by cursing."

"It was a few words; then it was over. These things happen in the heat of battle all of the time. There's hardly a single surgery that goes by without a word or two of profanity."

"Was any of your profanity of a religious nature?"

"For goodness sakes, it is a common term. It's used on TV."

"And what did you say, exactly?"

"I really don't remember. It was the heat of battle, I told you."

"Oh, on which TV program did you hear the religious slur you used that night, but also can't remember?"

"I can't tell you the specific program, but everyone knows that is not out of reason, to curse when the situation is so upsetting."

"Were you disciplined by the administration of Mitchie-Sterling Hospital for your language that night?"

"I don't know what you mean by disciplined."

"Did the medical director call you into his office and have a talk with you?"

During Cardozo's pause, Jennings went to his desk and pulled a slip of paper free. Cardozo head dropped. "Yes. All part of the new world of political correctness."

"Well, did the administration of Mitchie-Sterling Hospital place you on suspension?"

"No, of course not."

"Did they send you to an anger management class?"

"No!"

"I see. Do you know what became of the nurse who spilled the blood?"

"She was fired, I believe."

Both Harrison Jennings and Peter Cardozo looked toward Rhonda Uft, though her head was down, eyes hidden."

Jennings raised his piece of paper. "Well, I'll tell you, in case you were unaware; in fact, she resigned. I have the letter right here."

"I'm sorry to hear that. It was a minor mistake. These things happen."

Jennings nodded coldly. "Doctor, let's get back to the medical portion of the testimony. Did you start the central line right after that minor mistake?"

"I was in the process."

"For how long were you in the process?"

"I don't remember."

"How many times did you attempt to maneuver that six-inch needle into Dr. Maddingly's neck before the blood started into her body?"

"I don't remember."

"You do, indeed. It was..."

Rhonda Uft called out, "Objection. Badgering, and the doctor says he doesn't remember."

"Sustained."

"Well, we have testimony that the patient was charged for five IV sets while you attempted to start the central line. Does that mean you tried five times?"

"No."

"Why was Dr. Maddingly charged for five sets?"

"The first was wasted during the blood spill. A nurse dropped another needle as she was trying to hand it to me."

"Okay, that's two, and let's be clear, you did try to start the IV with the first needle. Then you had to open a new set. Is that when the next incompetent nurse caused the needle to be dropped?"

"I don't remember which one."

"So, that's two accounted for. Where did the other three go?"

"Just part of the process. You often don't hit the target on the first try in medicine. It's a fact of life in the emergency room."

"Or the second or third or fourth..."

"Objection. Badgering."

"Sustained."

"Did you ever consider calling for help when you weren't able to get the IV started on the second try?"

"Not at that point."

"For heaven's sake, why not?"

"I felt I could get the job done."

"Let me ask, and I want you to be a bit introspective; was your rage a factor in your failure to, as you say, 'hit the target'?"

"Absolutely not."

"What was, then?"

"First of all, she was fluid depleted. Her vasculature had collapsed."

"What do you mean by vasculature had collapsed?"

"There was no blood in her veins."

"Well, there must have been some. She was still alive."

"Not enough to start a central line."

"Doctor, please. Dr. Gauthé was able to start a central line on his first try. And that was half an hour, and a lot more blood loss, later."

"Objection. Counsel is testifying."

"Sustained."

"Dr. Cardozo, did Dr. Gauthé start the central line on the first attempt?"

"I don't know. I had to leave the room and tend to the backup of patients."

"Okay. Was that part of your decision to call for help, that there was a backlog of patients?"

"Yes."

"So, run from the one who's dying in front of your eyes and..."

"Objection. A more than adequate physician took over plaintiff's care. Plaintiff was never left alone."

"Sustained."

"Now, Dr. Cardozo, did Dr. Gauthé start the central line on the first attempt?"

"I don't know. I had to leave the room and tend to the backup of patients."

"How did you know there was a backlog of patients?"

"I don't remember."

"But you knew, apparently. Was that part of your decision to call for help, that there was a backlog of patients?"

"Once Gauthé was there, it probably was. The patient was being well cared for."

"How did you go about calling for help?"

"I certainly don't remember the specifics."

"But you did call for help?"

"Obviously, I did."

"Why do you say obviously?"

"He came to assist."

"Who came to assist?"

"Gauthé."

"Is it possible that another person called for help?"

"Well, do you mean, did I get on the phone and make the call?"

"No, I don't mean that at all. I mean did you, or did you not, initiate the call for help to Dr. Gauthé?"

"I have no recollection of the specifics."

"Is it possible that a staff member was so upset and concerned with your failure to do something to save Dr. Maddingly's life that she made the call on her own?"

"That is highly unlikely—no matter what some people may claim."

"What have you heard that some people claim?"

"Objection. Calls for hearsay."

Jennings blurted, "No. it doesn't, Your Honor. I'm asking what he heard with his own ears, not what someone told someone."

"Overruled."

"Doctor, what have you heard that some people claim?"

"That a clerk called Dr. Gauthé."

"Is that true? I mean that a clerk called Dr. Gauthé?"

372

Cardozo's complexion paled. "That's what I heard, yes, that she made the call. But you know, you believe half of what you see, and nothing of what you hear."

"Thank you for enlightening us on the rules of evidence. The question remains, did you initiate the call or not?"

"As I already told you, I do not remember. And neither does anyone else. There isn't a soul who was down there that night who remembers what the person next to them did or said. It was chaotic."

"So, you admit it was chaotic in the emergency room that night?"

"What I meant was that we were working so hard to save the patient's life, each one of us had a job, and they didn't stick their nose into someone else's assignment."

"So, let's sum up so far. You were aware that Dr. Maddingly was bleeding to death. Is that true?"

"She was in trouble."

Jennings's voice hardened. "Was, sir, she bleeding to death? Yes or no?"

"Yes."

"Did you ever get a central line started in Dr. Maddingly?

"No."

"Did Dr. Gauthé get a line started?

"Yes."

Jennings' head drooped, and he stood, forehead in his palm for a minute. He looked up at the judge. "Your Honor, I would like to move for a short break."

"How long, Mr. Jennings?"

"Ten minutes will be fine, Your Honor."

After the break, Jennings asked the judge if he could approach the witness then walked, head up, to Cardozo. "Do you like Dr. Gauthé?"

"Why do you ask?"

"Your Honor?"

"The witness shall answer the question."

"Actually, withdrawn, Your Honor." He returned to his desk to lift and set aside the top two binders from his pile. He opened the third and pulled a small rectangle of stiff paper from a pouch. "Your Honor, I would like to admit this greeting card into evidence."

When it was shown to Rhonda Uft, she harrumphed, "I've never seen this document."

Galanter looked down at Jennings. "Counsel, what about that?"

"Excuse me, Your Honor, this was given to the defendant's attorney as a Xerox copy on 2 February. It's right there on the date stamp."

Galanter peered at defense counsel. "Ms. Uft?"

"I'll have to look for it." She shoved a bear-sized, three ring binder roughly to her left, where a lesser attorney shoved it to his left, until it came to rest in front of a young woman at the end of the table. Her eyes dropped in a millisecond to start peeling madly through the hundreds and hundreds of pages in that binder.

Galanter sighed, "I'm going to allow Mr. Jennings to continue his examination of the defendant while you search. This could take an hour, and even if you don't find it, it doesn't mean it isn't in that morass of paper."

"I'm sorry, Your Honor, but I strongly object to the introduction of a document for which we have no basis to test its authenticity. Who knows who created this piece of work? It could be a forgery."

Galanter stared at her. "Chambers." He stood without an apology as the jury was led out. "Ms. Uft, if Mr. Jennings makes a statement that he forwarded it to you, I will accept that. I have no reason to disbelieve him."

Rhonda Uft looked up. "Nor do I, Your Honor, but I do, then, want a moment to review the document before it is introduced into evidence."

"You've had over a year, but I'll give you two more minutes to find it, madam. Go out and see if your assistant has had any luck. And you are not to read it until you are sitting in front of me. Is that clear?"

"Yes, Your Honor."

She returned a minute later, a sheet of paper in her hand. "You may look at it now," Galanter nodded.

As she read and wrote notes in the margins, her face reddened, and her shoulders tightened. She finally looked up. "Your Honor, this is a greeting card from Holly Cardozo, the witness's ex-wife. It appears to have been sent to Dr. Gauthé. It contains privileged information, and the contents are inflammatory, to say the least. This has no place in a medical malpractice case. It is simply an attempt by the plaintiff to further embarrass the witness. It has no probative value."

"Let me see it." Galanter snatched the paper from her. "Harrison, counsel has a point. This is pretty touchy stuff. I mean, here's a wife essentially begging to see Dr. Gauthé for obviously nefarious purposes."

"Well, Your Honor, it is indeed. But it certainly has probative value if you consider two things. First, it is my responsibility to impeach the moral and professional standards of my opponent. I'm sorry, but in this case, it is Mitchie-Sterling Hospital and its staff. And, God knows, there's a lot to impeach. It's an old boys' club, a fact about which I do not give a fig until it spills out of the board room onto the wards. They are out of control, and the administration exists strictly for profit, the original lofty ideals long buried, along with a hell of a lot of their patients."

Rhonda Uft sucked in a breath, though Jennings continued without pause. "And second, I believe the enmity between Drs. Gauthé and Cardozo played a significant role in the disaster that took place that night."

Rhonda Uft snorted, "Your Honor, I don't have to sit and listen to counsel's diatribe. He has a personal agenda, and he is using the judicial system to make trouble for a great institution."

Galanter raised his palm. "Okay, that's enough. Ms. Uft, I believe you have a point. I am not going to allow this document into evidence, but that does not prevent Mr. Jennings from asking pointed, and more pointed, questions about why the witness did not call for help. That's my last word on the subject. Back to the salt mines."

The jury was recalled, though not a word was directed toward them by the judge. The panel of fact finders quickly locked on Jennings' hand as he lifted the card from his desk but placed it slowly back into the binder from which it had emerged five minutes before. He moved toward the witness stand, apparently in deep thought. Finally, he spoke softly. "Dr. Cardozo, let me ask again. Do you like Dr. Gauthé?"

Rhonda Uft rose. "Objection. I still move to stop this line of questioning as not probative, but it is very inflammatory."

"Overruled. Continue, Mr. Jennings."

"Thank you, Your Honor. Dr. Cardozo?"

"You mean, do I like Dr. Gauthé?"

"Yes."

"He is a fine surgeon. I do not socialize with him outside the hospital."

"Oh, so you socialize with him in the hospital?"

"Of course not. We rarely run in to each other. We practice miles apart."

"Actually, Dr. Gauthé testified it took him only two minutes from the time he got word he was needed in the emergency room to break scrub, that is," he turned to the jury, "to leave the sterile confines of the operating table, and arrive at Dr. Maddingly's bedside in the emergency room."

"Objection. Is there a question in there?"

"Sustained."

Jennings pretended to think. "Are you married, Doctor?"

"Divorced."

"I'm sorry. Do you know if your ex-spouse dated Dr. Gauthé?"

"Certainly not!"

"How can you be so sure?"

"I just know."

"As a hypothetical, if your former spouse and Dr. Gauthé had an intimate relationship, would you be upset?"

Cardozo's face went from white to vermillion. "We are divorced. That is her business." It wasn't said clearly, and probably not heard by the jury, but Jennings was sure he muttered, "Bitch," under his breath.

Jennings pulled his head back in shock. "Would you be so good as to repeat what you said."

"I said we are divorced. Her personal life is her business."

"No, I mean after that."

"I said nothing. I think I cleared my throat." With that, he took a drink from the water bottle he'd carried into the courtroom.

"Well, if you don't know if they dated, do you know if your former spouse ever had written communication with Dr. Gauthé?"

"I have no idea."

"When you applied for a license in the State of Washington, did you read the application carefully?"

"Yes, of course."

"Was there a question about prior or present illicit drug use on that form?"

"I don't remember."

"Well, here's a copy of that application."

Cardozo belched, "Where the hell did you get that?"

"Freedom of Information Act. Now, did you deny illicit drug use in the past and present on this form?"

"Yes."

"Have you ever used illicit drugs?"

"I refuse to answer that. Fifth Amendment."

Rhonda Uft began to rise but thought for a moment and dropped quietly back into her chair.

"Your Honor? Would you explain the ramifications of that plea?"

Galanter nodded. "Doctor, this is not a criminal trial, and while you may invoke the 5th Amendment in a civil trial, pleading the 5th in a civil trial *does* allow a presumption of guilt, unlike in criminal court, where I would have to tell the jury that taking the 5th *does not* imply guilt. Do you understand the distinction?"

"Yes."

"Do you still want to invoke your 5th Amendment protection?"

"No. I think I grew some pot a long time ago. Didn't use it, though."

Jennings nodded, "So, you are telling the court that you were a drug producer?"

"It was one flowerpot's worth."

"Did you raise it for its natural beauty?"

"No."

"Well, you didn't use it, and it was of no horticultural interest, then it follows you raised it to sell, which means you are a nothing more than a drug runner."

Again, Harrison Jennings paused and braced for the burst, but Rhonda Uft kept her feelings to herself. Jennings was not sure then, or did he ever understand, why he suddenly turned the barrel away from Cardozo's head. He asked quietly, "So you just smoked a joint. Is that all?"

"Yes. I don't know a soul my age who hasn't."

"Please tell us, was that after you were working for Mitchie-Sterling?"

"I don't remember."

"Anyway, have you ever called for assistance from another doctor while you were on duty in the emergency room?"

"Yes, of course."

"How long do you usually wait before you call?"

"When the patient's welfare is in question, I don't hesitate."

"Are you telling this jury, after half an hour poking a patient with a steadily falling blood pressure, you did not feel it necessary to call for help?"

"Help came!"

"But we still do not have you swearing under oath that you requested that help! Withdrawn." Then he looked up at the judge and very softly purred, "I have no further questions for this witness.

It took a second for Rhonda Uft to shoot into seated attention. She turned to the left as if she had been hit upside the head by a two-by-four. The minions of assistants, though, were occupied, ostriches, heads buried in piles of documents. She flushed and grumbled, "Your Honor, may I ask for a short recess?"

He glanced quickly at Jennings. "Five minutes."

CHAPTER FIFTY-ONE

Rhonda Uft began her cross-examination with a forced smile. "Doctor, thank you for sitting through that interrogation so professionally. Now, we will hear the story of what really happened that night, and from the man who saved the Plaintiff's life." He nodded, and she paused again, waiting for Jennings to object. When Jennings dropped his head to search through one of the binders, she went on.

"Doctor, let's get a little housekeeping out of the way. Where did you go to college?"

"University of Idaho."

"And medical school?"

"University of Idaho."

"And your residency?"

"University of Idaho Health Center."

"Doctor, please tell us what type of residency you did."

"It was a full residency in family medicine, but after the first year, I got interested in emergency medicine and moonlighted in small ERs."

"Did you take extra courses in emergency medicine as a resident?"

"Yes, all my electives."

"How many years have you been employed at Mitchie-Sterling?"

"Sixteen or so."

"Now, we know that, as a doctor, being sued is very common. In all those years, have you ever been sued?"

Cardozo turned to Harrison Jennings and smirked. "Nope."

379

"Dr. Cardozo, what is your mission in the emergency room? Strike that. Is your mission in the emergency room to cure patients?"

"No."

"Please tell the jury why you come to work every day."

"My job, as a *board-certified* emergency medicine physician, is to stabilize patients to the best of my ability."

"Would you say that is to be done any way you can?"

"Yes, ma'am. Exactly. Doesn't have to be pretty. The only thing that counts is the life of the patient."

"So, does it matter to you who gets a patient back from the brink?"

"No."

"What was your mission the night you treated the plaintiff?"

"To save her life. Period."

"Was her life saved?"

"Yes."

"Though you got assistance from a surgeon who is trained specifically to do complex surgical procedures, what is the bottom line here?"

"The patient's life was spared on my watch?"

"No further questions, Your Honor."

"Mr. Jennings?"

"Just a couple of questions, Your Honor. Dr. Cardozo, you said you have worked for Mitchie-Sterling Hospital for sixteen years, but you finished your residency more than eighteen years ago. Where did you work for the two years before starting at Mitchie-Sterling?"

"Small ERs."

"Actually, they were walk-in clinics, just like the one Dr. Weathersby staffs. Is that correct?"

"Well, when I saw the quality of medicine being practiced there, I quit."

"It took two years to figure that out? I mean, you practiced substandard medicine, you compromised yourself, for two years?"

"I got out as soon as I could."

"You mean when Dr. Ezra Paull retired and there was finally an opening in the ER at Mitchie-Sterling? Strike that. Finally, when you said it doesn't have to be pretty as long as the outcome is the survival of the patient, were you referring to the devastating results you see before you? Is that what you meant by 'not pretty'?" He rolled his open palm toward Sabrina.

"She's alive. It is not my fault that she has underlying deformations and waited too long to come in. I am not God."

"One last question. Do any of the underlying deformations you claim in Dr. Maddingly happen to be in blood vessels"

"Who knows?"

"Is that the reason you were unable to start an IV in Dr. Maddingly?"

"I don't know."

Jennings let his head fall. The faces of several of the jury members tightened. Some shook their heads openly. It was not lost on Rhonda Uft or on the judge.

"No further questions, Your Honor."

"Ms. Uft?"

"No further questions, Your Honor."

CHAPTER FIFTY-TWO

Harrison Jennings called Alice Demdike to the stand. "Ma'am, thank you for helping us sort out just what happened on the night of 25th, 26th, November."

She nodded. "Now, let's introduce you to the jury. Please tell us, madame, how long have you been an employee of Mitchie-Sterling Hospital?"

"Twenty-three years."

"That's impressive in this day and age. And what is your position at the hospital?"

"Radiology Department Administrator."

"How did you get to be the department administrator?"

"I worked my way up in the radiology typing pool to dictation department head, then got certified as an ultrasound tech and worked very, very hard. Then I was made the radiology department administrator."

"Again, impressive. It sounds like you've experienced every level of work in a hospital imaging department."

"Yes."

"With that in mind, would you look at a document for us?"

"Yes."

Jennings called to Rhonda Uft, "Bates stamp 0249, Counselor." He paused until Rhonda Uft found the document. She snapped it out of her binder irritably. Jennings' shoulders shrugged in question, and he waited silently.

"Go ahead," Rhonda Uft grumbled.

"Thank you, Ms. Uft. Now, Ms. Demdike, what is this?"

"This appears to be a short consult from Dr. Evans."

"And who is Dr. Evans?"

"She was an OB-GYN. Somewhere else, now."

"Please read the part about the ultrasound." He pointed.

With hesitation, she looked up at Rhonda Uft, who nodded, and the witness read from the document. "Doctor Evans says, 'I would like to review the ultrasound of the patient's adnexa before commenting further about any underlying congenital or acquired malformations."

"What does adnexa mean?"

"That's the female organs inside, you know, the ovaries and uterus."

"This note from Dr. Evans was dated five days after the surgery. Yes?"

"Yes."

Harrison Jennings went to his desk and lifted another sheet of paper from the current binder. "Now, please look at this document." He turned to the defense table. "Ms. Uft, Bates 0336."

A minute later, both parties looked up. "Madame, what is this?"

"Another note from Dr. Evans."

"Please read the part I highlighted in yellow about the ultrasound."

"'I would still like to review the original ultrasound of the patient's adnexa. It has been promised by,'" she paused and flushed, "'by Alice Demdike, the department administrator, but not delivered. I reserve comment about the patient's pelvic anatomy until I peruse that imaging study.'"

"Does it appear to you that Dr. Evans is frustrated?"

"A bit. On the other hand, it is common for there to be delays in document delivery in the hospital. I'm afraid the wheels of medicine churn slowly, but not as slowly as your justice system."

Jennings looked up at the judge. "Objection. Non-responsive."

Galanter peered down. "Sustained. Please answer the questions without adding your opinion, madame."

Jennings stared at her for a moment before asking, "Ms. Demdike, do you have independent recollection of Dr. Evans calling you the first time?"

"Yes, she was very rude. She never learned our ways out here on the West Coast."

"What did she say to you that was so rude?"

"It's not what she said, but how she said it."

"I'll ask again, what did she say?"

"If I remember correctly, something like, 'Alice, please have that ultrasound image faxed to my office. Today, if you don't mind.'"

Jennings let his shoulders droop. "And that was upsetting because?"

"I don't run a department that drops everything every time there's a request for non-critical films."

"'Non-critical,' huh?" He paused. "I see. We'll talk about that in a few minutes. Now, Dr. Evans called again for the films on day eighteen of Dr. Maddingly's admission to your hospital. This doctor had asked for, and been promised, the pictures of the ultrasound, but nothing happened. It's your department. What was the reason for that discrepancy?"

"Objection. Calls for speculation."

Galanter thought for a moment. "Overridden. She's the boss. Buck stops with her. And I'm interested in where this is going. Mr. Jennings."

"Thank you. Now, in your long experience, have you ever seen a doctor or patient have to wait for the delivery of records from your department for nearly two weeks?"

"Yes."

Harrison Jennings paused to let the jury digest the answer. "Again, madame, please name the issue that caused the delay in this case."

"We are not perfect."

"That's not what I asked. Please tell us, specifically, what caused the delay in delivering the records to Dr. Evans."

"The films and the report were not available."

"Where were they?"

"I don't know. No one knew, and most importantly, the images were not critical to the patient's care at that point. She had been operated on, and the surgeon gave a much better description of the findings than could ever be seen on an ultrasound."

"Again, you hide behind the matter of the images not being critical."

"Objection, argumentative."

"Sustained. Rephrase."

"Well, let's move ahead. These images may not have been critical for you, but what if they had been images of your daughter or your husband? You have a consultant coming in, charging your family for two expensive medical visits on which nothing meaningful is done for the patient. Is that professional?"

"No, but I am not going to argue that hospitals or law offices have perfected logistics. We are pretty darn good, though." She smiled and snapped her head in solidarity with her statement.

"Well, let's see how good. First, let me ask, if your imaging department was ninety-nine-point-nine percent accurate in all its paperwork, would you consider your department exceptional?"

"Of course, but we strive to be perfect."

"Ms. Demdike, how many imaging studies a year does your department do?"

"Good gravy, it's so many, I have no idea."

"You don't?" Jennings' shoulders sagged again. "Withdrawn. Would you say one hundred studies?"

"Many, many more."

"A thousand."

"Many, many more."

"A million?"

"Oh, I don't think so."

"Well, madame, do you believe the number is proprietary? Is that why you don't seem to know it?"

"I'm sorry, can you repeat the question?"

"Of course. Is the number of imaging studies done by your department classified corporate information, open only to the administration?"

"I don't know, but I'm guessing it is."

"Well, according to your very public hospital brochure," he picked a document off the table and waved it at the jury, "over 100,000 studies per year. Does that surprise you?"

"Oh my, yes."

"Well, it shouldn't. Withdrawn. Madame, do you keep images on the hospital storage media for seven years?"

"Yes," she smiled smugly, "every single one. And in my department, it's for twelve years."

"Let me ask again, if ninety-nine-point-nine percent of those studies go perfectly–and every soul in this room knows darn well it's nowhere near that, nothing is–that still leaves a hundred missing at the end of the year, a hundred studies that got misplaced, misnamed, or just accidently erased—every year. That's two per week. Is it possible this is one of those?"

"No, because we have the images of the study."

"How many?"

"One."

"How many images are there in a typical ultrasound of the pelvis."

"I don't remember, and it varies."

"You told us that you were an ultrasound tech. Varies from what to what? Is it three to fifty?"

"No."

"Yes or no answer, madame. Isn't it usually around twenty or thirty?" He opened his binder

"Could be."

"Madame, where are the rest of the images."

"They've been lost."

"Could they have simply been thrown away by mistake?"

"No. All images these days are on the computer."

"Well, then, they must have been erased. Is that correct?"

"They don't know."

"Who doesn't know?"

"We had an army of IT people trying to find the rest of the images. They couldn't."

"Well, let me ask, would every image taken of Dr. Maddingly that night show three units of blood in the pelvis?"

"I imagine some would not."

"You imagine, or some would not, period?"

"Some would not."

"How is it the only image to survive is the one that so perfectly shows the blood in the pelvis?"

"Objection. Calls for speculation."

"Sustained."

"Again, please tell the jury a single reason a set of images could be lost."

"We don't know. The administration believes it was because the patient was so strange."

Jennings let his jaw drop. "What do you mean by strange?"

"Well, she was not sent by a real doctor." She hitched her head to the side. "That lady in Evanston."

"Who told you Dr. Weathersby wasn't a real doctor?"

"Everybody knows it, and Dr. Cardozo told us himself."

"Who is us?"

"The imaging department office. He said it to everybody in the room."

Jennings stopped again and stared at the floor. "He did. How professional of him. Withdrawn. How did Dr. Cardozo come to be in your office?"

"He was looking for the film himself."

"Why?"

"I don't know. I was told not to become involved."

"By whom?"

"The administration."

"Who in the administration told you that?"

She hesitated and looked toward Rhonda Uft, who nodded almost imperceptibly. "Dr. Klat."

"The medical director?"

"Yes."

"So, you did not have a lot of input or responsibility in finding out how the images were lost, did you?"

"No. I had a department to run. The administration was in charge of that problem. They didn't share much about it."

"When did the investigation begin?"

"Just a few days after the patient was admitted."

"How many days?"

The witness began to tremble. "I'm not at liberty to discuss that."

Jennings turned slowly toward the bench. "Your Honor," he asked calmly, "would you please instruct the witness to answer my questions?"

Galanter peered down stiffly and growled, "Madame, this is a court of law not a sales convention. You will answer the questions posed by plaintiff's counsel, or you will be held in contempt. Do you understand?"

She nodded and Galanter snapped, "Say 'yes' or 'no' for the court reporter."

She squeaked a tremulous, "Yes."

Jennings demanded, "When did the investigation begin?"

"I don't remember."

"Was it the day after she was admitted; what, three days later..."

Rhonda Uft hissed, "Asked and answered. Counsel is badgering the witness."

Galanter sighed, "Sustained."

"Ms. Demdike, were you prepped by Ms. Uft before your testimony?"

She shot a glance to Rhonda Uft, who simply blinked. The witness mumbled, "Yes."

"Were you prepped by any member of the Mitchie-Sterling administration?"

She looked again to Rhonda Uft, but this time the shake of the head was so faint, she had to lean forward to get her answer. Judge Galanter banged his gavel. "Ms. Demdike, do you remember swearing to tell the truth, and nothing but the truth, before your testimony began?"

Again, she nodded but quickly whispered, "Yes."

"Then tell the truth, not what defense counsel wants you to say. You are a department head in a large hospital. I hold you to high standards. You are getting dangerously close to being slapped with a contempt of court citation. That means a large monetary penalty and going to jail. Hospital may foot the bill, but they won't be doing the time for you. Last warning. Go ahead, Mr. Jennings."

"Thank you, Your Honor. Ms. Demdike, did Dr. Klat include you in any part of the investigation?"

"No."

"What did he tell you?"

"He told me they didn't want to waste my time on a simple clerical problem."

"Simple clerical problem. But you told the jury there was, I think you said, 'an army of IT people' looking for the images. Didn't that make you curious about what was so special regarding what you called a non-critical ultrasound?"

"No. I do my job and leave the big decisions to the administration."

"Big decisions. So, this was not your usual clerical problem, was it?"

"I don't know. They wouldn't tell me."

"Has that ever happened before in your years as a department head, that the administration came into your office and took over?"

"I don't remember."

"You don't remember. Okay, let's move on. Please look at the legend on this ultrasound." He handed her a printed copy of the image and called out to Rhonda Uft, "Bates 1,349," then asked his assistant to project the illustration on the courtroom screen. After a pause and a scowl, Rhonda Uft nodded. Jennings pointed to the upper left-hand corner of the exhibit. "We see Dr. Maddingly's name. Is that so?"

"Yes."

"Who is supposed to place that name on the film?"

"The tech."

"Is that done by typing it into a computer?"

"Yes."

"Thank you." Jennings handed her a second sheet of paper and announced to the defense table its place in the binders. "Now, madame, what is this document?"

"It appears to be a log of the ultrasound examinations done on the night of November 25th and 26th."

"Who enters names in the log?"

"Sometimes the tech."

Jennings walked to the other side of the bench, causing the witness to turn her head far to the right. That brought the judge into her peripheral vision. "Sometimes?" Jennings spat, "Who did it that night, madame?"

Without looking directly at Galanter, she blanched and nearly shouted, "The tech!"

"And how does the tech enter the name into the log?"

"The computer."

"Does the tech enter it twice? I mean once for the film and once for the log?"

She hesitated, but her hands began to tremble, and she jammed them between her legs. "No."

"No, what? Are there two entries made into the computer or just one?"

"Just one."

"So, let's recap. Patient comes in, hands the tech her papers, tech enters patient name in computer, and computer sends it to the log and, *and* the film at the same time. Is that correct?"

There was a tremulous, "Yes."

Jennings walked back to the other side of the witness. "How many exams are there on the log for that night?"

"Three."

"Is one of those names Maddingly?"

"Yes."

"Is it spelled on the log with one 'd' or two?"

"Two."

Jennings asked his assistant to flash the image of the actual film again. "How many d's on the film?"

"One."

"How is it possible, madame, that one entry in the computer gets spelled two different ways?"

Rhonda Uft objected. "This line of questioning goes beyond the scope of the witness's expertise. She isn't a forensic documents or computer specialist, and she wasn't there that night."

"Overruled. Presumably, the witness knows the procedure for inscribing a patient's name on an x-ray better than anyone in the hospital, or she should. Go on, Mr. Jennings."

"Thank you, Your Honor. Ms. Demdike, was there more than one tech on duty that night?"

"Probably not."

"Probably? Yes or no, was there more than one tech on duty on Thanksgiving Eve?"

"I don't think so."

"Your Honor..."

The woman squealed, "Yes."

Galanter shook his head subtly, "There was no question posed at the moment. Yes, what?"

"Yes, there was only one tech on duty that night."

Galanter spoke quietly, "Go on, Mr. Jennings."

"Again, how is it possible that the correct spelling was on the log but was wrong on the actual ultrasound film?"

Rhonda Uft was once more on her feet. "I object again on the same basis. This is a standing objection."

"Overruled, and so noted, Ms. Uft. Go on, Mr. Jennings."

The woman sat up, and her face tightened as she began to glare at Jennings. "I think we need to be reasonable and just assume that a simple clerical error was made. The films were lost because of a power outage, and who knows what the staff did on Thanksgiving Eve to correct all the technical issues that caused?"

"Power outage. This is the first we are hearing of a power outage. Was the ultrasound done before or after this power outage of yours?"

"I don't know."

Jennings called out three Bates Stamp numbers. When Rhonda Uft stopped grumbling, he asked his assistant to put the log of ultrasounds done that night back on the screen. "Ms. Demdike, three ultrasound studies were done that evening. Is that correct?"

"It seems so."

"What time was the first?"

"Nine-thirty."

"How many images are listed?"

"Twenty-two."

"The second?"

"Eleven-o-five."

"And whose name is listed there?"

"Maddingly."

"With two d's?"

"Yes."

"How many images?"

"Eighteen."

"And the third?"

"Four-thirty the next morning."

"How many images?"

"Nineteen."

Jennings asked for the next exhibit to be projected. "What does this appear to be, madame?"

"It says 'Report of Outage.'"

"What are the times and dates?"

"It says 2354 on 25November to 0152 on 26November."

"Is that 11:54 P.M. on the 25th until 1:52A.M. on the 26th?"

"Yes."

"Who is the issuing authority?"

"CUD."

"Who is CUD?"

"The electric company."

"Would you agree that the outage took place after the first two studies were done and before the third was completed?"

She hesitated but shot a glance at Galanter, who sat stone-faced waiting for her answer. "Yes."

"Is the first study, the one done at 9:30 present in the computer?"

"Yes."

"How is it possible that the only lost study was Dr. Maddingly's?"

"Objection. The witness is NOT a computer expert, nor is she an electrical engineer."

"Sustained."

Jennings smiled vaguely. "Is it possible that the ultrasound image of the blood in Dr. Maddingly's pelvis was actually that of another patient, and was accidently substituted for Dr. Maddingly's because the administration genuinely believed there was blood in Dr. Maddingly's pelvis when she had her ultrasound?"

"OBJECTION! Sidebar, Your Honor."

He waved them forward. "Your Honor, he's testifying, and he just poisoned the jury. I am calling for a mistrial."

"Mr. Jennings?"

"Counsel has a point, Your Honor. The only problem is, now this witness is changing her story and blaming the power outage when she testified it was a clerical error because the patient was so strange. The witness opened herself up to the question when she changed boats in the middle of the stream."

"Mr. Jennings, you have not yet shown to my satisfaction that the film is a forgery, certainly not to the point that allows you to make that statement, or even a hypothetical, to the jury." He snapped, "Step back," and turned to the jury. "You will ignore the suggestion that the ultrasound image you saw was not that of the plaintiff."

Rhonda Uft bristled back to her table, but before she turned to take her seat, she winked almost imperceptibly to Harp, who had recently come into the courtroom and squeezed his way into the first row.

Before Jennings could approach, Alice Demdike blurted, "No one at Mitchie-Sterling Hospital would ever do such a thing."

Judge Galanter banged his gavel. "Madame, again, there was no question posed. I am holding you in contempt of court. You will pay one hundred dollars to the clerk of court when you are dismissed as a witness."

When the mumbling in the courtroom settled, Jennings looked toward the bench. "No further questions, Your Honor."

The woman stood, gathered her purse, and started to take a step away from the witness chair. Galanter smashed his gavel as an undercurrent of giggling weaved through the courtroom. "Sit down, madame. The court is not done with you. Ms. Uft, cross-examination."

CHAPTER FIFTY-THREE

As Rhonda Uft approached her witness, the woman began to whimper. Rhonda Uft asked Galanter, "Your Honor, would you call a five-minute recess to allow Ms. Demdike to compose herself after counsel's inquisition?"

"Just five minutes." As he dismissed the jury, the woman ran from the witness chair. Rhonda Uft followed her into the ladies' room. A spectator reached the door the same moment Rhonda Uft pushed it open, so Uft used her hip to bump the other woman out of the way, then marched to stand outside the witness's stall.

"Alice, you're not helping the hospital, not one little bit. When I ask you questions, you sit up and answer like an adult. We'll pay the hundred dollars, but like the judge said, we can't do the time for you. That's the next step. And don't forget, when I'm done, Jennings will be able to ask some more questions. You answer 'yes' or 'no.' Do you understand?"

There came a sniveled, "Yes," from behind the stall door.

Rhonda Uft asked her first question on cross-examination. "Ms. Demdike, what is the usual procedure when a patient to arrives at the hospital with a request for an ultrasound?"

"The patient goes to the financial desk to check in, and that staff member looks up the requesting doctor's name and status."

"What do you mean by status?"

"If they are on our staff."

"Are you saying you would not do an x-ray for a doctor that wasn't on your list?"

"That is correct."

"How could you turn down a doctor?"

"How do we know it's a doctor? Can you imagine the chaos? Patients would be calling and making their own requests. No, we have to know who you are to use our facilities. You have to have been approved by the hospital board of directors. The liability would be unreasonable. Think of this: patient falls and his wife calls in, says she's Dr. A, a local physician, and asks for an x-ray of, what they fear, is a broken arm. They pick up the films saying they are taking them to so-called Dr. A, but look at the films themselves and don't see what turns out, actually, to be a serious, hidden fracture. So, they don't follow-up with a doctor. Three months later, arm heals cattywonkers, and they sue the hospital for not telling them the break was serious."

"Exactly. Now, was Dr. Weathersby's name on your list of staff members?"

"No, absolutely not."

"So, you had no idea where to send the results. Is that correct?"

"Yes."

"How did the ultrasound get done, then?"

"Again, that was Thanksgiving Eve. A long weekend. There was a terrible storm outside. That lady from Evanston was screaming bloody murder that the patient was going to die. She had the place in an uproar. The intake clerk told her supervisor she was scared that if she turned the patient away, she would have been sued."

Jennings was on his feet. "Objection. Hearsay and inflammatory. Dr. Weathersby spoke to three people at the hospital that night before the ultrasound, and only on the phone. And one of the people with whom she spoke was not the intake clerk. And there is no evidence she screamed at anybody, anytime, in fact, anytime in her career."

"Sustained."

Jennings added with a hiss, "And, once again, Doctor Khai Weathersby is not 'That lady from Evanston.' She is a board-certified medical doctor in good standing without a blemish on her record. I object to the witness's characterization. She had no right to say that."

"Again, sustained." Galanter peered down at the witness but only shook his head faintly and mumbled to Rhonda Uft, "Go on counsel."

"Thank you, Your Honor, but I think we've put this witness through enough today. I have no further questions."

"Mr. Jennings?"

"Just one, Your Honor. Madame, you said Dr. Weathersby had the place in an uproar, everyone scared to death. If that's the case, how the heck did Dr. Maddingly manage to sit, slowly dying, in a corner of your emergency room until a clerk just happened to see her and finally take action?" As Rhonda Uft leapt to her feet, Jennings shook his head and grunted, "Withdrawn. No further questions."

Galanter looked down at Rhonda Uft. She monotoned. "No further questions, Your Honor."

Jennings stood and spoke softly. "The plaintiff rests, Your Honor."

"Very well. We will hear the Defense's case in the morning. Court is adjourned for the day."

CHAPTER FIFTY-FOUR

Rhonda Uft was garbed in a smart, blue, linen dress, her hair newly frosted, even the back. She wore a bit of makeup, and a few of the older men on the jury watched her a bit more closely than before. She approached Dr. Milton Lustig, the defense's star witness, her head leaning slightly toward the jury, a warm smile on parade to that side of the courtroom.

"Dr. Lustig, thank you for taking time from your busy schedule at Stanford University to help us understand this case. First, may I ask, where did you go to undergraduate school?"

"Yale."

"And medical school?"

"Columbia."

"And residency?"

"Stanford."

"What is your medical specialty, sir?"

"Obstetrics and gynecology."

"Oh, so you stayed on at Stanford after you completed your residency there?"

"Yes."

"Is that unusual?"

"I don't know about unusual, but not many of us are lucky enough to work there."

"Well, how many from your residency class made the cut?"

"Two."

"Out of?"

"Sixty-three total residents."

"Did you do a fellowship?"

"Yes."

"In what field?"

"Obstetrics."

"Where was that?"

"Stanford and the NIH."

Rhonda Uft turned to the jury, "The National Institutes of Health. Doctor, I know you need to get back down to Stanford this evening to see your patients, so we will make your testimony directly to the point. Do you have any medical publications?"

"Yes. I am the co-editor of two textbooks..."

"Let me just stop you there. What are the two textbooks?"

"Both are on obstetrics. The first addresses abnormal pregnancies. The second is a surgical manual with the latest techniques in difficult deliveries."

"Any other publications?"

"Yes. Thirty-two journal articles."

"On what topics?"

"A broad field of obstetrical studies."

"Do you have experience in treating tubal, or should I say, ectopic, pregnancies?"

"It is one of the most common reasons I am called to operate on a patient."

"What do you mean by, 'called on'?"

"When a staff obstetrician is uncomfortable with the all the traps involved in an unusual type of tubal, they often call me. It's only because I do them all day long. The more you do, the better you get."

"Thank you. In regard to this lawsuit, have you reviewed the records of the plaintiff's present medical situation?"

"Yes, meticulously."

"Did you happen to review the ultrasound image of the plaintiff's pelvis as part of your review of records?"

"Yes."

"You see, one of the plaintiff's arguments is that she only began bleeding in the Mitchie-Sterling Hospital Emergency Room. The ultrasound image you reviewed was taken nearly two hours before the plaintiff claims the bleeding started. We are trying to put this question to rest." She exhaled like an 18-wheeler clearing its air brakes. "Finally. So, let me ask, do you read ultrasounds of tubal pregnancies as part of your medical practice?"

"Every day."

"Do you have special training in reading ultrasounds of patients with tubal pregnancies?"

"Yes. That was what I did at the National Institutes of Health."

"Please remind us just what the National Institutes of Health is, the NIH."

"The NIH is in Bethesda, Maryland, just outside of Washington D.C. Basically, it the main U.S. agency for medical research."

"Is going there for training open to every doctor?"

"No, it's pretty selective."

"But you did go there as part of your obstetrics training?"

"Yes. I was lucky enough to."

"Back to the ultrasound you found in the plaintiff's chart. Did you notice any abnormalities?"

"Most evident is the collection of fluid in the pelvis."

"What is your opinion of the source of that fluid?"

"Given that we now know the patient suffered an ectopic pregnancy, that is the source of the fluid."

"What is that fluid?"

"Clearly, blood."

"How much, would you estimate?"

"That is hard to state with certainty, but I would say between two and three units, depending on the size of the patient."

"Can we tell just when that blood collected there?"

"No, but we know it was there when the patient had the ultrasound that night. There had definitely already been very serious bleeding."

"Is it likely that much blood had been in the plaintiff's abdomen for days and days?"

"You cannot tell. Sometimes, these leak blood for many days."

"Is it possible that the plaintiff was on the cusp of a disaster when she delayed coming directly to the emergency room?"

"Yes."

"Is it probable?"

"Yes."

"Is it possible that the plaintiff was bleeding when she was sitting in the emergency room?"

"Yes."

"If you had sent this patient to the emergency room, would you have expected her to go to the desk and tell them she was there?"

"She's a PhD? For goodness sake, yes."

"Let's say she was too sick to walk to the reception desk; would you expect her husband to announce himself?"

"A high school math teacher, a former NFL football player? For goodness sake, yes."

"So, would you sum up what you have established so far?"

"Yes. First, the patient was certainly bleeding when she arrived at Mitchie-Sterling Hospital. And, next, a terrible mistake was made by the family in their failure to go to the emergency room immediately, when told to do so by the general practitioner. Finally, it is inexplicable to me that they did not insist upon immediate care."

"Thank you. Another urgent issue in this case is that the plaintiff's ectopic pregnancy was a result of a congenital malformation..."

"Objection." Jennings took a step toward the bench. "Your Honor, Ms. Uft is testifying. The main issue in this case is not if the plaintiff's ectopic pregnancy was a result of a congenital malformation. She is out of order feeding the jury her bias."

"Sustained."

"Yes, Your Honor. Dr. Lustig, you testified that you have read the records thoroughly. Is that correct?"

"Yes."

"Do you believe you are sufficiently familiar with this case to discuss the most important aspects of it?"

"Yes."

"What, sir, do you see as the main issue in this case?"

"From what I have read of this case, there was a clear anatomic irregularity in the fallopian tube. There is absolutely no medical reason to doubt the intra-operative observation made by the general surgeon who did the surgery to save her life." Rhonda Uft lifted her hand waiting for Jennings to object, but his head was buried in a three-ring binder.

"Go on, sir," she hummed.

"If you have a major malformation of any part of the adnexa—that's the ovary, tubes, and uterus—you can assume there are more malformations."

"Let's not assume. Let's say there is just the one malformation, that is, the sharp dogleg in the tube. How does this affect a doctor's ability to treat this patient?"

"That's the most important question of all. How the patient is going to act, I mean how the ectopic is going to act, is unpredictable. All the rules for ectopics are out the window when there are malformations."

"Let me stop you there. You say there was more than one malformation?"

"Yes, the deformity in the spine, the deformed fallopian tube, and the bifid uterus. That's a lot, and I'm sure there are many more lurking within this patient."

Harrison Jennings was on his feet. "Objection. There is no evidence, not a single fact, that there are," he spat, "many more lurking."

"Sustained. Doctor, we can do without the melodramatics. Thank you."

Rhonda Uft went on without acknowledging the judge. "But, if you get the patient in time, as an experienced surgeon, can't you treat anything that comes your way, right?"

"Wish I could. The truth is, we have certain rules about how we treat a particular medical problem. We don't experiment on our patients. When something out of the ordinary appears, we must not try to invent new treatments..."

"Let me stop you there again, Doctor. How could an out-of-the-ordinary problem result in an outcome that is not good for the patient? You see it and figure out a way around it."

"With malformations, we can't predict, for example, when the patient will start bleeding, or even where the bleeding is coming from. How can you guarantee a successful outcome when you are faced with a problem you can't see, or that no doctor has ever before seen? We are working through a tiny hole. We expect to see certain structures as we move down toward the problem. We check them off in our minds, often out loud, just to be sure. If something is missing or not where you expect it, that raises the stakes. And that is very dangerous for the patient."

"Can you give us an example in real life to demonstrate how dangerous unexpected malformations can be?"

"Of course. Take your kitchen sink drain at home. The side that has the waste disposal unit. Your bracelet breaks and drops in. You make sure the switch over the sink is turned off, and in goes your hand. You've done it a hundred times. Problem is, at the factory ten thousand miles away, the worker making thirty cents a day left a bare wire exposed. That's like a malformation, isn't it? So, your hand hits the wire, it pushes the bare spot against the metal body of the disposal unit, circuit's inadvertently activated, and on turns the motor. There go your fingers. How can you fix it, that is, get the bracelet out safely, if you don't know what to expect?"

"Thank you. I think it's time to share with the jury the diagram you studied to help lead us to the truth." She nodded for an underling to flash a detailed, anatomic illustration onto the screen. "Doctor, would you orient us to the anatomy."

"Yes, of course." Without being asked, he stood and walked to the screen. Using the laser pointer pulled from inside his suit jacket, he went over one obscure ligament after another. Then it was the blood vessels, the ovary, the fimbriae, the flawed fallopian tube, and, finally, the bifid uterus.

Lustig stopped and looked directly at the jury. "Ladies and gentlemen, here you see a distortion of the fallopian tube. No normal tube in the body has a kink in it. That defeats the whole purpose of a tube, doesn't it? This is not normal. It means the egg cannot possibly have a free path from the ovary to the uterus, which, itself, in this case, is also deformed. There can be no argument about that. It is common sense. If you're drinking soda through a plastic straw, and you bend it until it kinks, no more fluid gets through." He looked to Rhonda Uft.

"Thank you, Doctor, you can take your seat, if you don't mind." She smiled at the jury. "If this had been your patient, would you have been able to promise a perfect ending to the treatment?"

"Sadly, no. I wish I could make the jury understand that there are times when nature throws a curveball, and the best-trained physician on Earth can't do a thing. And I wish the jury members never have to feel that sadness—that despondency—that, even after a sacrifice of twenty years at twelve to sixteen hours a day preparing for that moment, you are powerless to stop the inevitable. I hate it."

"Thank you, Dr. Lustig. That's a lot to think about." She turned to the bench. "Your Honor, I have no further questions for Dr. Lustig."

CHAPTER FIFTY-FIVE

Harrison Jennings walked, posture firm, toward the witness stand. He fired his first question. "Dr. Lustig, how much do you charge per hour?"

Lustig mocked, "How much do you charge per hour?"

"Sir, I ask the questions here. But I will go along with you: $225/hr. And now back to you, Doctor."

He spoke softly. "Five-seventy-five."

Several of the jury members raised eyebrows. It was not lost on Rhonda Uft, whose head dropped and fingers trembled. Jennings noticed and turned back to the witness. "You told us you read the records; I think you said, 'meticulously'."

"Yes."

"How many pages of records did you review?"

"I don't know the total number."

"Were you told you had all the records?"

"Yes."

"Well, I have three Xerox boxes stuffed with notes. That's 5,000 pages per box, and three boxes is 15,000 pages; and let's say you spent, and I'll be kind, 30 seconds per page. That's, let's see, 7,500 minutes, or," Jennings looked up to the ceiling, his lips pulsating as fast as a sign-language interpreter at a presidential news conference, "or a hundred-twenty-plus hours. At $575 per hour, that's," the lips now moved like a machine gun, "that's around $70,000. Is that correct?"

404

"Of course not. I only charge three-twenty-five for record review."

"So that's," Jennings' eyes drifted up again, "$45,000, not including the travel time, the actual testimony, and..."

Rhonda Uft was out of her chair. "Objection. This is what all experts charge. Counsel is trying to obfuscate the quality of Dr. Lustig's testimony with his own prejudices."

"Sustained. Move on, Mr. Jennings."

"Yes, Your Honor. Doctor, tell us, when did you get the records?"

"I don't remember the date."

"Give us an approximation."

"First of March."

"When did you forward your results to Ms. Uft?"

"About three weeks later."

"Were you on vacation during that period?"

"No."

"In fact, Doctor, were you at a medical conference during the second week of March?"

He looked up and thought for a moment. "Yes."

"Were you one of the organizers of that conference?"

"Yes."

"Where was the conference?"

"Rome."

"Lovely city. What is the time required to fly by commercial airliner from San Francisco to Rome?"

"When it's all said and done, about a day each way."

"Did you work on the plane."

"Exactly."

"How many records did you actually carry with you to Rome?"

"The major file."

"How big was it?"

"Five hundred pages."

"That left 14,500 pages sitting on your desk in San Francisco, and it left you eleven or twelve days to read those records, 'thoroughly'. Is that correct?"

"Technically. But your presumption is flawed."

"And how is that, Doctor?"

"Thousands of pages were hospital records that just listed routine blood pressures and basic nursing notes."

"Fair enough. But we lawyers are such sticklers for detail. Do you know why?"

"It's a way to bill more time?"

Galanter growled, "Try to remain professional, Doctor. Mr. Jennings."

"No, it's because we are in the business of finding the truth. Finding that one hidden little fact that upsets the applecart, that shows that all the posturing and empty words we listen to all day in court are false, just red herrings. We uncover lies."

Rhonda Uft groaned, "Objection. This is not law school. Counsel is wasting the court's time."

"Overruled. I want to see where this is going. Mr. Jennings."

"Thank you, Your Honor. Let me ask, Doctor, do you remember reading hospital notes from a Dr. Evans, a consultant obstetrician who requested the ultrasound several times but never did get it?"

"I'll be honest, I read every page, but I do not have independent recall of each word. Much of the data is superfluous. Please be reasonable."

"Well, this superfluous data was important." He asked for the notes from Dr. Evans to be projected. "Now, Doctor, what is this?"

"This appears to be a short consult from Dr. Evans, as you mentioned."

"Please read the part about the ultrasound."

"The doctor says, 'I would like to review the ultrasound of the patient's adnexa before commenting further about any underlying congenital or acquired malformations.'"

"This was dated five days after the surgery. Yes?"

"Apparently."

Jennings went to his desk and lifted another sheet of paper from the current binder. "Now, please look at this document." He turned to the defense table. "Ms. Uft, Bates 0336." It was flashed on the screen.

A minute later, both parties looked up. "Doctor, what is this?"

"Another note from Dr. Evans."

"Please read the part about the ultrasound."

"'I would still like to review the original ultrasound of the patient's adnexa. It has been promised but not delivered. I reserve comment about the patient's pelvic anatomy until I peruse that imaging study."

"Does it appear to you that Dr. Evans is frustrated?"

"A bit. On the other hand, it is common for there to be delays in document delivery in the hospital. The wheels of medicine churn slowly. Surely, you've heard that about how slow the law moves."

"Indeed, I have. It seems all of the defense's witnesses are acutely aware of the deficiencies in the legal system. But the point is, this doctor had, yet again, asked for, and been promised, the pictures of the ultrasound, and still no joy. What are the usual possibilities for that discrepancy?"

"Objection. Calls for speculation?"

Galanter thought for a moment. "Sustained, but I'm still interested in where this is going. Please rephrase, Mr. Jennings."

"Thank you, Your Honor. Doctor, in your long experience, have you ever had to wait for the delivery of records you requested?"

"Yes, of course."

"Please name one issue that caused the delay."

"I am not able to do so, but everyone in this courtroom is well aware the world is far from perfect, even at Stanford, and we're pretty well regarded in the world of medicine."

"That is, more highly regarded than Mitchie-Sterling Hospital in McKinley, Washington? Withdrawn." There were smiles in the jury box. Jennings asked, "Doctor, do you remember any further consult notes from Dr. Evans?"

"I have no independent recollection of any notes from him."

"In fact, it is a her, as noted when she writes in the chart that she was sorry she had not been able to help the Maddinglys, but that she and her husband were relocating to the East Coast. Did you see that in your meticulous evaluation of the record?"

"I have no independent recollection of that entry."

"Now, sir, did you review that ultrasound?"

"Yes, in detail, but if that doctor left the hospital, it is very likely that she was busy getting ready for her move, not all that interested in walking down to radiology and getting the study herself. That's all it would have taken."

"Did you know Dr. Evans?"

"Of course not."

"Then how do you know what was on her mind?"

"Just throwing it out there."

"Sort of to see if it sticks to the wall, huh? In court, we deal with facts, not wild guesses. A woman's future life depends upon what the jury is given as facts."

"Objection. Counsel is testifying."

"Sustained."

"Let's talk about the image, particularly the date it was taken. What is the date imprinted on the image?"

"November 25th."

"Several weeks later, Dr. Evans still hadn't, despite having asked to see the image, been able to review it. Is that true?"

"It appears so."

"Is it, in your expert opinion, unusual for an imaging study that is dated and filed in the first few pages of a patient's chart not to have been available to a consultant weeks later?"

"I can't answer that. It's not my hospital."

"But you've had a lot to say about the superior nature of Mitchie-Sterling Hospital, haven't you?"

"Objection. Argumentative and not probative."

"Sustained."

Lustig blurted, "It's a fine institution."

Galanter exhaled volubly, "The jury will ignore the witness's last statement. There was no question pending."

"Doctor, let's look at the ultrasound on the big screen." The grainy picture was projected. "Sir, is this the one image from the ultrasound you reviewed in regard to Dr. Maddingly's ectopic pregnancy?"

"It might be."

"Look, if there's any doubt, please say so before we go on."

"It appears to be the ultrasound I reviewed. I have no reason to believe this is a trick."

"Okay, but the instant you have a single reservation about its authenticity, please alert us."

"I will."

"Were you aware that there was more than just this one view from the ultrasound study that night?"

"Yes. But it is customary that only the critical images are forwarded to the expert witness."

"Wait a minute. Are you telling this court that someone other than the expert decides which images are critical?"

"Look, you can't forward every scrap to the reviewer."

"Sir, are you telling the court the images were just scraps?"

"Not at all. They forwarded what was important."

"So, you have not seen the other views?"

"That is correct."

"Do you know if there are other views?"

"I assume there are."

"You assume? At $575 an hour, you assume? Withdrawn. Let me ask, how many views are in a typical ultrasound?"

"A couple of dozen."

Harrison Jennings went to his desk and pulled a sheet from his binder. He sent it to Rhonda Uft, the judge, and back down to Dr. Lustig. Jennings asked, "Sir, what is this?"

"It appears to be a letter from Ms. Uft to you."

"Please read the short note."

"Mr. Jennings. In answer to your letter of September 10th, I advise that my clients are in possession of only one view of the ultrasound on Ms. Maddingly performed on the night of November 25th. It has been forwarded to you in your previous demand for production of documents. Sincerely, Rhonda L. Uft."

Jennings acknowledged, "Thank you. So, you only have that one view. Is that correct, Doctor?"

"That is correct."

"Okay, in the interest of time, what did it show?"

"I see free fluid in the pelvis."

"How can you be so sure?"

"It's right there, at least to the trained eye."

"Oh, that's right, you have special training in reading OB-GYN ultrasounds. Remind us, where was that training done?"

"The NIH, the National Institutes of Health."

"Very impressive. By the way, did you happen to cross paths with my client, Dr. Maddingly, while you were both working there?"

"I don't think so. It's very large."

"Well, she was there for six months. And how many months was the course you did there?"

"It was several weeks."

"In fact, it was just two weeks, wasn't it, doctor?"

"I don't remember the exact number of days."

"Well, according to their records, you were there for nine and a half days. Let me ask, how long does a radiologist study ultrasounds of the pelvis before taking professional boards?"

"I have no idea."

"Well, it's over a period of years."

Rhonda Uft's voice was so subdued in her objection, "Introducing facts not in evidence," Jennings turned to the defense table. Her eyes seemed locked on the courtroom window.

Even Galanter hesitated before speaking softly, "Sustained."

"Thank you, Your Honor. Doctor, do you see a possible distortion of the fallopian tube that might be an ectopic pregnancy?"

"No. Doesn't mean it isn't there. Just as I said to Ms. Uft, the answer to this case is not in the ultrasound. It is, like most things in medicine, in the quality of the physician who interprets that bit of information."

Jennings turned to the judge. "Move to strike as unresponsive. I have no idea what he is talking about, Your Honor."

"He answered the question with a clear 'No.' Overruled."

"Thank you, Your Honor. Doctor, in your lengthy career, have you ever seen a mislabeled x-ray?"

"I have to tell you no; I have not. If it happens, it is exceedingly rare."

"Well, Mitchie-Sterling Hospital does in excess of 100,000 imaging studies per year. I imagine Stanford does far more than a million. Is that fair?"

"I have no idea."

"Just for fun, your children's hospital, by itself, sees half a million patients a year. So, you folks probably do millions of just pediatric imaging studies a year. But let's be conservative and say a million. Do you believe Stanford is 99.9 percent accurate in radiology paperwork?"

"I don't know."

"You know it isn't. Even with this ridiculous level of accuracy, that leaves twenty studies per week that are mislabeled or lost at your institution. That's 1,000 per year, and you have been there for twenty-five years, so that's 25,000 messed up studies; probable more like a couple hundred thousand. Are you telling this court, as one of the Stanford's leaders, that you never heard of such a thing?"

"Never have."

"Well, would you agree that if, and this is only a hypothetical, a doctor is looking at an image of patient that really isn't that of the patient they think it is, there can be no way to determine by that imaging anything about bleeding or any other problem regarding that patient?"

"Objection." Rhonda Uft was back in full throat. "As in the past, counsel is trying to poison the jury without a single speck of evidence. He thinks if he repeats his lie over and over, people will start believing it."

"Overruled. It was a hypothetical. The witness will answer the question."

"Given your hypothetical, you are correct, but you certainly have not shown me to my professional satisfaction this ultrasound image is not from your client."

"Okay, given the image we have, and given your expertise, you estimated that there were up to three units of blood in the pelvis. Is that correct?"

"Yes."

"And, given your expertise, would you say that three units of blood connotes serious bleeding?"

"Yes."

"And, given your expertise, once the bleeding started with a flow that caused three units to be lost, would you expect the bleeding to suddenly stop?"

"It might. And, as you know, it could have been from a slow leak over several weeks."

"But the fetal age was barely three weeks. Do ectopic pregnancies bleed immediately after conception?"

"Not usually, but there is no way to tell, with all her congenital malformations."

"And you are basing the presence of congenital malformations on a sketch by a general surgeon who had not done a single obstetrical surgery in over twenty years, not since you began as a doctor?"

"He's a professional, and I believe his observations, and I can see the abnormal bifid uterus on the image."

"Are you telling this court a bifid uterus causes abnormal bleeding?"

"No, but it is yet another abnormality in this woman."

"Are you telling this court a neural tube defect causes abnormal bleeding in the reproductive organs?"

"No, but we don't know what else is going on, do we?"

"If we don't know, then we have to guess, and we don't guess in a court of law. Do you guess when you are treating patients?"

"Sometimes you have to."

Jennings was silent for thirty seconds, long enough for the jury to absorb the witness's statement. He went on. "In which textbook have you seen a picture of a fallopian tube with a dogleg in it?"

"There is no picture. It's a malformation. We list them as we discover them. This was new. It isn't in the books yet."

"So, you are saying it will be in the next edition of your textbook?"

"I plan to publish this finding."

"Even though all you have in the way of objective proof is a drawing by a non-OB surgeon."

"A note will be made of that."

"Will you also note that the patient had been exposed, second generation, to Agent Orange?"

"I will."

"You will? Yet you don't have a shred of scientific evidence that this was in any way related to Agent Orange?"

"I think it is."

"So, when you get up in the morning, what you decide is solid scientific evidence becomes solid scientific evidence by sunset—just because it is your guess?"

"After twenty-three years, several textbooks, and innumerable papers, I have earned the freedom to consider the etiology of unusual medical presentations."

"Again, I don't know what you're talking about. And let me tell you, after fifty-some years practicing law, I have never heard a statement of that hubris spewed in a court of law."

"Objection. Badgering. And Dr. Lustig is an acknowledged thought leader in the field of obstetrics."

"Sustained."

Jennings smiled. "Yes, Your Honor. "Doctor, can you give us a scientific, biologic explanation for a massive flow of bleeding prior to getting to the hospital that suddenly stopped long enough to allow the patient to walk all over the hospital, up and down stairs?"

"First of all, I did not see anything in the notes to suggest this wasn't a gradual buildup. She might have been fine, just a slow leak, the pelvis filling gradually, but constantly, until she was sitting in the emergency room, and the final blood vessel ruptured. This means she was on the verge of suffering a catastrophe at any moment."

Jennings had risen. "Let me stop you there. So, you are testifying that the final blood vessel didn't rupture until she had been sitting in the ER for an hour and a half. Is that correct?"

"I wasn't there. I don't know when it ruptured."

"But it was after she was walking around the hospital? Yes or no?"

"I can't know that."

Jennings sighed. "Okay, then why are you testifying in this case if you don't know anything? Withdrawn. Let's agree, just for a hypothetical, that there were three units of blood in her abdomen. The radiologist knew the patient was to be escorted to the ER after he read the film. I mean, he knew the patient wasn't leaving the hospital for, say, the University of Washington. Shouldn't the radiologist have notified the ER that there was a potential tragedy walking around the hospital, basically attended by only an x-ray tech?"

"I do not know that the ER wasn't advised."

"Is that written on the radiology report?"

"I need to review it again."

"It wasn't, but let's say it was. Even more reason to ask why Dr. Cardozo wasn't informed, or was informed and did nothing.

The voice was suddenly more strident than usual. "Objection! Calls for speculation.

Galanter mumbled, "It's okay, Ms. Uft. Let's settle down. Sustained."

Jennings went on. "Doctor, what could cause there to have been bleeding that suddenly stopped to allow Dr. Maddingly to seem normal?"

"If there was fresh bleeding that night before they arrived at the hospital, vasoconstriction could account for a slowing of the flow."

"What is that?"

"The blood vessels clamp down to stop the bleeding."

"Is it likely?"

"It is possible. The body always tries, tries very hard, to stop abnormal bleeding."

"Let's say, hypothetically, that that is possible. The patient sat in the emergency room for over an hour. Actually, it was a lot longer. Would the clotting system have taken over in that period of time?"

"Perhaps, but at best it would have been pretty precarious. I mean mild trauma, something as simple as walking to the restroom, could cause the blood pressure to go up and the clot to be blown out of the torn vessel. Then the bleeding starts all over again."

"Okay, but given that Dr. Maddingly was just sitting in the waiting area, her head on her husband's shoulder, is it likely for the bleeding to start again?"

"Look, I don't know if it is likely. Maybe she coughed, sneezed, twisted in her chair, whatever; maybe just her normal blood pressure opened the internal wound. Look, one way or the other, it happened."

"Can you tell the jury when the massive bleeding suddenly started again?"

"Of course not."

"Well, the clerk who walked past Dr. Maddingly, the one who alerted the triage nurse that Dr. Maddingly was desperately ill, was good enough to testify in deposition. Have you been informed of her testimony?"

"No."

"Well, to recap, she told us she had passed Dr. Maddingly several times over the hour-plus she sat unattended in the waiting area. She had noticed her because she was so pretty, and also because she was so taken by the way Dr. Maddingly and her husband seemed to be one soul." The doctor rolled his eyes. "Excuse me, Doctor, but that is the testimony we heard from the young clerk who essentially saved a life that night. Would you like to hear it word for word?"

"No. I believe you."

"Well, I am flattered. And an hour and a half later, just minutes after her last pass through emergency room waiting area before going home, she became concerned about the sudden loss of color in the patient's face and her sudden lethargy. The rest, what went on in the treatment area of the ER, well I'm sure you read in the patient's medical records. Is that correct?"

"Yes."

"Is it your opinion, knowing the natural history of tubal pregnancies, that Dr. Maddingly walked on her own, without help, into the emergency room waiting area, having fairly recently bled three units of fresh blood into her abdomen, and sat there—alert, for ninety minutes—and then suddenly nearly died"

"Yes."

"How is that possible?"

"We've been over and over this. She bled slowly for a week, and her body was able to make enough new red blood cells to allow her to function normally, at least on the outside."

"What do you mean on the outside?"

"She could have appeared normal, but her blood count would not have been normal.

"But given your expertise, and basic common sense, what is your opinion?"

"It is possible."

"But is it likely?"

"What do you define as likely?"

"A greater than fifty-fifty chance that she had been bleeding for weeks, her abdomen filled with old blood when she arrived at the hospital."

He smirked, "It may be less than your fifty-fifty chance that she had early massive bleeding, but it is nowhere near beyond a reasonable doubt."

Jennings glanced quickly at Rhonda Uft. Her head dropped, and her fingers began to tremble. He hid a smile as he turned back to the witness and sighed. "No, sir, beyond a reasonable doubt is the standard only in criminal cases. And for right now, this is still a civil matter. So, knowing that, do you still feel it is more likely than not that Dr. Maddingly bled three units of blood before she got to the emergency room waiting area?"

"I cannot give you specific numbers."

"But you are testifying about this woman's medical condition during those hours, aren't you?"

"I am, and, again, the records point to the fact that your client came to the emergency room after a delay, during which there was significant bleeding."

"Significant? I ask again, how much did she need to lose before she would not have been able to walk into the hospital from the parking lot, then walk down a flight of stairs to the lab, and then back up to radiology, and then get off the table and walk into the ER?"

"I was not there, and it depends on her size and the amount of blood she had before the bleed."

Jennings' mouth tightened as he spat, "You didn't have to be there to know she suffered a Class III hemorrhage. It was in Dr. Gauthé's operative report, which you, of course, read carefully, didn't you?"

Rhonda Uft groaned, "Objection. Asked and answered. We've been over this for the past hour. Counsel is badgering the witness. He is wasting this man's time. He has a plane to catch."

"Let's cool it down a few degrees, Mr. Jennings."

"Very good, Your Honor, but I don't give a hoot about his airplane. For what he's getting paid, he could have a private jet waiting for him."

"Objection."

"Sustained."

"Thank you, Your Honor. Now, Doctor, have you ever examined Dr. Maddingly?"

"No."

"Have you ever met Dr. Maddingly?'

"No."

"How tall is she?"

"I don't know."

"How much does she weigh?"

Lustig shifted his eyes toward Sabrina for the first time since entering the courtroom. "I am guessing 160 pounds."

"Did you note her height and weight before you came here to testify about the rest of this woman's life?"

"Yes."

"Well, her height and weight appeared dozens of times in her records, the ones you told us you studied so thoroughly. But just to let you know, she is five-foot-nine and weighs 133 pounds. That's about eight units of blood, total. According to you, she lost 3 units, or..." up went Jennings' head and so began the vibrating of his lips. The jury sat, holding its breath. waiting for the next set of astonishing numbers. "That's nearly forty percent of her total supply. I ask again, is it likely that she was able to walk into the emergency room waiting area and remain conscious for an hour and a half with that percent loss of blood?"

"No, it is not likely, if the bleeding had just taken place."

"Thank you."

"My last questions concern your interpretation of the drawing Dr. Gauthé made of Dr. Maddingly's anatomy." He walked to the easel and flipped over the cover sheet to reveal the primitive illustration Gauthé had made for the court at Jennings' insistence. "Let me ask, if you looked at this sketch of Dr.

Maddingly's anatomy, would you have made the same conclusion, that she suffered from a serious defect that led directly to her ectopic pregnancy?"

"Yes."

"Yes? You stood in front of the screen when Ms. Uft put up a slide of Dr. Gauthé's real depiction and pointed out a number of peculiar anatomical features. Actually, you spent a lot of time demonstrating your expertise in diagnosing extraneous blood vessels and ligaments, and now you say you could have just taken a quick gander at this child's sketch that Dr. Gauthé made for the jury and given us the same answer?"

"No. I needed all of that information to convince the jury."

"Convince!? Convince? Is your job to provide expert facts for the jury, or to sway them to find for your employer?"

"Of course, it is to provide facts, but it just so happens I believe in my conclusions. Can't you understand that?"

"Yeah, especially about the amount of blood loss Dr. Maddingly suffered and stayed perfectly awake."

"Objection. Is there a question in there?"

"Sustained."

"Fine, but Doctor, didn't you one minute ago tell this jury that on a more probable than not basis...No, strike that. May I ask the Court Reporter to read verbatim the testimony in which Dr. Lustig quoted the odds that the bleed had taken place before Dr. Maddingly got to the ER?"

The woman rewound her tape. "'It may be less than your fifty-fifty chance that she had early massive bleeding, but it is nowhere near beyond a reasonable doubt.'"

Jennings stopped for a moment before thanking the reporter. "Doctor, given your expertise, would you agree, from Dr. Gauthé's diagram, that the egg had travelled well beyond the so-called impenetrable kink? Is that true?"

"Yes."

"Given that Dr. Maddingly had no other risk factors for ectopic pregnancy, why do you surmise she suffered an ectopic pregnancy?"

"Sometimes it just happens, and we don't know that she didn't have other risk factors for ectopic pregnancy."

"What other factors did she have? List them, please."

"We don't know."

"So, you are, again, just assuming she had problems?"

"Where there's one problem, expect others. And, sure enough, there is no question she has a bifid uterus."

"But there are no facts in this case to show the bifid uterus caused bleeding, are there?"

He thought for a moment, glanced at Rhonda Uft surreptitiously, then mumbled "Well, there's the spinal problem."

"Are there any other proven malformations this patient has that are medically known to cause abnormal bleeding?"

"I still think it was due to the Agent Orange exposure."

"Move to strike as unresponsive."

"Sustained."

"Have you ever read a scholarly journal or textbook that tied ectopic pregnancy to second-generation exposure to Agent Orange?"

"Yes. There is a group in Japan that has linked Dioxin, one of the poisons in Agent Orange, with a disruption of nitric oxide production in rats. And we know for a fact that nitric oxide disruptions are one of the dangers of taking DES. And we know for a fact that DES causes malformations in the daughters of women who took it during pregnancy. Maybe the jury doesn't remember DES, but it was given to pregnant women from the Thirties through the Sixties in the belief that it would decrease complicated pregnancies. It turned out to be poison and was banned in 1971. What it did do was cause vaginal cancer and malformations of reproductive organs in their daughters, especially the uterus."

"Very good, but is there a single shred of evidence that links DES and Agent Orange?"

"I'm just throwing it out for background that both poisons have constituents that cause disruption of nitric oxide production."

"Are DES and Agent Orange two very different chemicals?"

"Yes, but..."

Jennings stopped him. "Doctor, we happen to be aware of that recent research from Japan. In fact, ..."

Rhonda Uft jumped from her seat. "Your Honor, please let Dr. Lustig finish his answer."

Galanter nodded. "Go ahead, Doctor."

Jennings was going to object that Rhonda Uft had herself refused to allow Khai Weathersby finish her answers, but he was too excited that Lustig was just diving deeper into the trap. He nodded at the man to go on.

"I was only trying to show that poisons in both DES and Agent Orange cause a disruption of nitric oxide production. That's good enough for me."

Jennings smiled subtly toward Rhonda Uft. "Good enough for you. Doctor, are there other poisons in DES and Agent Orange besides Dioxin?"

"Yes."

"Name them."

"It's very complicated."

"I asked you to simply supply names, not to discuss the biochemistry. The names, sir."

"I would need to examine a reference text."

"Okay. At least, tell us what these poisons do?"

"I would have to refer to a reference text."

"So, you have no idea if the poisons in DES and Agent Orange really affect the body in the same way. Is that correct?"

"I would have to refer to a reference text."

"Well, we have here the article from Japan you referenced." He walked to his desk and pulled several papers from a deeply buried binder. He handed it to the doctor. "Is this the research you are referring to, sir?"

Lustig read the first few lines and nodded. Jennings spoke quietly. "Doctor, we need you to speak the words, 'yes' or 'no'."

"Yes."

"Well, you said we're talking about nitric oxide. Correct?"

"Correct."

"Actually, it was nitric oxide synthase, NOS, wasn't it, Doctor?"

"Yes, the synthase."

"And nitric oxide synthase sounds like nitric oxide, but it is a completely different chemical, as different as butter and dirt; isn't that right, Doctor?"

"They are different chemicals."

"What is the synthase, Doctor?"

"A chemical that assists in making nitric oxide in the body."

"Are there different types of nitric oxide synthase?"

"Yes."

"How many?"

"Several."

"In fact, there are four. Now, please tell us the name of the specific nitric oxide synthase they isolated from the Dioxin victims."

"I don't remember the specificity."

"Well, please read from the paper as to which oxide synthase they isolated from the Dioxin victims."

"nNOS."

"Nnnnn NOS. Neuronal NOS. Now, please..."

Rhonda Uft jumped to her feet. "Objection. Your Honor, this is a waste of the jury's time. Counsel is muddying the waters with esoteric chemistry that has no bearing on this case."

Judge Galanter looked to the jury. Several of them were sitting on the edges of their chairs. "Mr. Jennings, where are you going with this?"

"Your Honor, DES and Agent Orange are two completely different toxins that poison the body in two completely different ways. Another red herring, the witness dragging the term nitric oxide into this courtroom. The witness is using his so-called expertise to introduce not just misleading but completely false scientific data into this proceeding. I'm trying to give Sabrina Maddingly a fighting chance for a fair trial with facts, not sham science."

"Overruled. Go on, Mr. Jennings."

Half the jurors smiled and nodded.

"Doctor, please tell us the specific type of nitric oxide synthase that causes birth defects in DES daughters."

"I have to be honest and say I don't remember which one."

"Well, does iNOS, Iiiii NOS, Inducible NOS, sound right?"

Lustig's face wilted. "Yes."

"You're the expert. Are nNOS and iNOS the same chemical?"

"All I can say is that they are both involved in the production of nitric oxide."

"Each type of NOS works in a different part of the body. Is that correct, sir?"

"It's far too complex to go into here."

"Believe me, sir, this judge and this jury, and even I, can tell the difference between a womb and a lung. Do they affect different parts of the body, yes or no?"

"Yes."

"So, in the end, is there any scientific connection you can present to this jury to link the poison in DES and that in Agent Orange?"

"More research is needed."

"More research is needed, and you had the gall to bring that up as fact in a court of law. Withdrawn. At this moment, the only connection between iNOS and nNOS is they happen to sound similar, like Douglas and Donald. No similarity in the cause of genital malformations, is there?"

"More research needs to be done."

"Did you ever, in your twenty-some years of practice, ever see the child of a person exposed to Agent Orange?"

"Not to my knowledge."

"Do you have a colleague who ever saw congenital malformations of the ovaries and fallopian tube due to second-generation exposure to Agent Orange?"

"I have no way of knowing that. And I don't need to know it. As soon as you see her spinal deformity, you know there will be other problems. A kinked tube is not normal. And, after so many tens of thousands of patients, I can tell you that my impression, my gut feeling of Dr. Maddingly's reproductive organs—from her ultrasound, the surgeon's report, and her hospital course—is that things were far from normal, and not just in those organs. Don't ask me for specifics. Like I said, it's what my gut tells me. Ever heard of the art of medicine—going beyond the textbooks? That's why, and I'm not trying to be arrogant, I am sought by doctors who have patients with bad problems."

"Sir, perhaps the court is not as evolved as medicine, but we use facts in court, not gut feelings. I have no further questions for this witness. After all, he has a plane to catch."

"Ms. Uft, re-cross?"

"Just a few questions, Your Honor. Dr. Lustig, given the kink in the tube, would that qualify as a strong predictor, on a more likely than not basis, that there was some problem in the function of the tube?"

"Yes, absolutely."

"Why?"

"The fallopian tube is so delicate and perfect, any deformation makes it very unlikely the tube will operate normally."

"Doctor, do you see, in your practice, patients who need immediate surgery for ectopic pregnancies."

"Thousands and thousands over the years."

"Sir, as an expert, did you feel comfortable telling us you were sure there was something wrong with plaintiff's reproductive anatomy?"

"Bet my reputation on it."

"Thank you, Doctor. That is all I have."

Judge Galanter looked wearily at Harrison Jennings. "Do you wish to re-cross?"

"One question, Your Honor." Dr. Lustig glanced surreptitiously at his watch. "Not to worry, Doctor, this won't take long. Since you brought up actually seeing sick patients in your office, let me ask, does your private office have an operating room?"

"No, of course not."

"Have you ever started a central line in your office?"

"No."

"Do you even have a central line kit in the office?"

"Probably not."

"Tell the jury, please, what you would do if a patient of yours, a healthy, young woman, had sudden, what she thought was, menstrual cramping? She tried to get ahold of your office, but there was only a message telling her to leave a message.

"Like the majority of women, she sees you as her primary care doctor. Her husband gets antsy and brings her into your office as a walk-in. What would you do?"

"My medical assistant would have my receptionist tell her to go the emergency room."

"Emergency room? She has menstrual cramping. Sit for four hours waiting to be seen in an ER—for menstrual cramping?"

"We don't have the capacity to see walk-ins."

"Wouldn't you examine her first?"

"Well, no matter what it is, I cannot do emergency treatment in my office, and a patient who shows up at my door with a possible life-threatening problem is a huge potential risk for malpractice, and..."

Harrison Jennings' palm was in the air. "Are you telling this jury of laymen and women that fear of a malpractice suit would make you turn away a patient in need?"

"Not at all what I'm saying."

"Then what are you saying?"

"I can't help her in my office, so I send her to where they can help her."

"You can't at least take a history from an established patient? Eyeball her?"

"It will turn into an hour visit. That's what the ER is for."

"Would you call ahead to advise the ER doctor that you are sending over a potential problem?"

"No. That's what triage is for."

"Thank you, Let's say you have a really astute MA, and she brings the woman into an exam room and does a blood pressure. It is fine. Pulse is fine. She briefs you. Do you still send her to the ER?"

"Yes."

"How fast?"

"Immediately."

"Why?"

"She could have an ectopic pregnancy that was ready to rupture."

"But you wouldn't call ahead and advise them?"

"Like I just said, that's the responsibility of the ER staff."

"Was it the responsibility of the ER staff at Mitchie-Sterling Hospital to screen Dr. Maddingly?"

"The family screwed that up."

"How?"

"By just sitting there."

"Your fifty-thousand-dollar fee later, that's the best answer you can come up with to hide obvious malpractice?"

It was so late in the day, the stale air so sullen, the crash was a bit softer than Harrison Jennings had presaged. "Objection in the strongest terms."

"Sustained."

"Oh, and by the way, Ms. Uft misspoke. Mr. Maddingly did, indeed, check in at the ER reception desk, just like every other patient. Did you not see that document in your *meticulous* evaluation of the records?"

"I have no independent recollection of that document."

"And what makes it worse is that the ER doctor, himself, knew she was there. No triage nurse or staff member ever approached Dr. Maddingly to check on her well-being, despite the stark warning from a licensed medical doctor. There isn't a soul in this courtroom buying your story. I have no further questions for this witness."

"Ms. Uft?"

She spoke quietly, without emotion. "No, Your Honor."
And court was adjourned for the weekend.

CHAPTER FIFTY-SIX

On Saturday morning, Khai saw Mike at the Safeway in Evanston. She took a step toward him but stopped, remembering the mandatory sensitivity training she'd attended for all health providers in the county: classes on AIDS, racial sensitivity, and the proscription about a doctor ever initiating contact with a patient in public. That had become, in the present social climate, foundation for a breach of confidentiality lawsuit. It was up to the patient to initiate contact in the out-of-office setting.

At that moment, Mike detected movement and looked up. His smile was radiant. "Hey, Dr. Weathersby, is that really you?"

"No, it's my twin sister." She laughed aloud but lowered her voice and smiled. "How's the trial going? Mr. Jennings said it wasn't a good idea for me to show up. I'm to appear detached, not supposed to have a dog in the fight."

"Talk about dogs and fights. They're assaulting each other like animals; one makes a point, the other rips at it with honed canines. Trial hangs over our heads like a giant stone. Can't sleep, can't seem to forget it for a second. That Rhonda Uft, the hospital's lawyer, you remember her..."

Khai laughed stiffly, "A real humanitarian."

"Yeah, she's been threatening Mr. Jennings that she's going to ask the judge to make us pay the hospital's legal fees if we don't drop the lawsuit."

"She can't do that. Just more lawyer BS. Don't you worry a bit. You're going to win no matter what. The hospital will finally sit down with Mr. Jennings and offer a settlement. Sometimes the skunks wait until the last minute—courthouse steps on the way into to the last day of the trial. Lawyers squeeze every last minute of billable hours out of the parties, and then, poof, it's all over in seconds. To hell with the client's sanity. You just need to drive into your head that you will come out on top. You will win. But, first, tell me about Sabrina. How's the counseling going?"

"The counseling is going..."

Khai stopped him. "This is no place to be talking, over the flank steak and sausages. There's a Starbucks around the corner. I mean, if you're comfortable with that."

"Are you?"

Khai laughed. "What are they going to do to me? Kick me out of the county medical society that I still haven't joined, and never plan to?"

Mike put the package of pork chops back in the cooler, and Khai replaced her loaf of whole wheat bread. They laughed.

Each paid for their own coffee. At the back of the shop, Khai spoke softly, "Please go on about Sabrina. Does she have any more movement?"

"We're trying external electrical stim. Insurance pays for that. She can hold a fork in her right hand and just grasp a knife in her left. She lets the knife kind of sit on top of what she wants to cut and moves the food underneath it with the fork. Sort of works. It's not pretty. PT is pushing coordination. Each week, there's a tiny bit of difference. May move on to the legs in a few months."

Khai smiled. "That's so encouraging. How about the depression?"

"Well, she gave in and started taking the atypical antidepressant. Took about a week, and she was not as depressed as before. Still not dancing in the streets, but at least we talk every night during the cocktail hour. Memory is still a problem. Dr. Darling says it may be more a function of the actual depression and the stroke than the ECT. You know, for all her life, she had such a sharp recall of the tiniest details. Birthdays, exactly how old people were, telephone numbers—like a savant, but with a beautiful personality. Never had a bad word for anybody. Now, the sharpness is gone, and, sometimes, she's even a little callous. I mean, she's the best friend I ever had, and her brain's so far above mine; still does things that blow my mind. She's become a Seahawks fan. Knows everybody's number, season schedule, stats from last year.

"But it seems she doesn't want to do any more than she has to. Doesn't read her journals anymore. They just pile up in the corner."

"I know that feeling."

"She's wants to start going to the U to see patients a few days a month, but her boss hinted it isn't the best continuity these patients need. The lady's right, and Sabrina knows it, but she chafes at the thought someone's telling her how to be a doctor. Grumbles about it. Sometimes, she can be unreasonable. Isn't the same Sabrina." He sighed and shook his head. "Killing the both of us because she knows what's happening." He suddenly looked up and smiled. "But I ain't givin' up on her. Not for one second. Never will."

"Can't imagine you would. Tell me, how's the trial actually going?"

"You really want to hear this? I can go on forever."

"Not working today. Just came up to collect some charts. I'm all ears."

"Okay, here goes. I think Mr. Jennings believes he can smoke out the truth about the ultrasound. Somehow, they destroyed it or doctored it, or so he says. Still can't prove it. You heard about the Supreme Court thing, didn't you?"

"Not much. Lawyers from the state did come up and grill me before one of the hearings. Didn't give 'em a crumb. I don't believe a thing the state says, or, especially, what the hospital says. I don't believe a thing the county medical society says, or the state medical society for that matter. It's all money, even the doctors. Wonder why I ever put in ten years for free. Let me rephrase that—paying out of pocket for most of it, to get here."

"Dr. Weathersby, all I can say is that you have been a godsend for us. Thank you for paying for ten years. And thank you for testifying for us. Mr. Jennings said you waived your fee."

"Not so fast, Mike. I told him I'd drop all but twenty-five dollars. He said it would take about three hours. I figured that I'm worth minimum wage—at least."

"You told us you were making minimum wage in residency."

"Barely. Twenty-four thousand a year for a hundred hours a week. I guess it was close."

"Yeah, but I read where you guys are allowed to pick clean the trays of the guests who don't make it through the night. That counts for something."

"Oh my God, don't remind me. We actually had a guy who did that. Meatloaf. Enough. Back to the story."

Mike drew a deep breath. "Okay, okay. A month after Mr. Jennings received the records from the hospital, like three Xerox boxes of 'em, all he could find of the ultrasound done that night was just the report. He told us that wasn't kosher; that imaging studies were routinely burned onto a CD, given to the patient, and, also, the hospital keeps the original images, like for ten years, at least, in Washington.

"So, he emailed Rhonda Uft asking for the disc, but two days later, she called back to tell him the files from that night had been corrupted because there had been a windstorm."

Khai muttered, "I remember it very well. Uft said the hospital had a second of power outage before the generators kicked in. Harmed the computers."

"But, all of a sudden, at your deposition, one image magically appears. Uft said she had not been aware it survived until the day before."

Khai interrupted, "Couldn't read it; just a bunch of black shadows on top of gray."

"I'm not sure if you know all that has gone on in the courts about the ultrasound since then."

"Just that the hospital has blocked every attempt to find other images."

"That's right. So, a couple of months ago, Mr. Jennings had lunch with his son at Sergio's. You ever been there? Nice place."

She paused for a moment. "Yeah, I have. Pretty nice."

"Anyway, Mr. Jennings' son is a computer geek. Told his dad whole thing sounds lame, that he needed to get the exact time of the outage. Mr. Jennings called the CUD. They wouldn't tell him, so he emails the legal department and threatens to sue them because the failure caused critical medical information to be lost. He gets an email half an hour later, says the outage wasn't until long after Sabrina's test, and the images should have been saved to the hard drive.

"Meanwhile, his son, Todd, like I said, a Microsoft game tester, but also a closet computer forensic buff, says the whole thing is a mound of bull scat because the hospital was able to rescue at least one picture. Told his father there were more images. He guaranteed it. Asked to take a look at the hard drive or server, or whatever it is. Apparently, his son's working on a data recovery program. Says if there's anything in the hard drive, he'll find it."

"So, Mr. Jennings submits a subpoena to the hospital demanding the radiology department's imaging files for that night. Rhonda Uft refuses that demand, and the next one, so Mr. Jennings took it to the judge for a hearing. The hospital submitted sworn declarations to the judge that there had been only one image rescued. The rest of the drive had no files pertaining to Sabrina. Then they tell the judge that, even if the files could be recovered by a forensic examiner, they would not release the hard drive because of HIPPA privacy rules. Other patients' files would then be compromised, they argued. But the judge ruled against them. He said the hospital was ordered to go through the files and filter out all but the data for the hours between 11 P.M. and 2 A.M. That brackets the time we were there, and the hospital admits there were no other ultrasounds done between those hours."

Mike had barely taken a breath, seething, grumbling with a pressure of speech that only intensified as the minutes passed. He hadn't even touched his coffee. He finally stopped and reached for his cup. As he glanced down, he saw that Khai had long finished hers. He grimaced. "I'm such a brute. I'm sorry. Can I get you a refill? Need to keep you awake for the rest of the story, if you can stand it."

"Thanks Mike, but I'll get it. You rest for a minute. This'll count for your workout today—maybe tomorrow, too."

"You ain't heard nothin' yet!"

When she sat back down, she locked his eyes. "You're hurting inside, aren't you, Mike?"

"Nah, happy we're gonna get this thing over with."

"Okay, but it's the doctor in me roaring again. Ever thought about talking to someone? I mean, well, you know what I mean."

"I'm fine. Really."

"Look, Mike, you have to be the best husband in history. Everyone at the hospital said it. Nurses used to giggle that they wished they had found someone like you. Even the guy nurses."

He laughed openly. "I hope so. I mean, I want Sabrina to know her life is the only thing that matters to me."

"I know. Please, if you need to do something to even off the stress, there are good ways. Really. Let me know, and I'll get you where you want to go. Okay?"

"Thanks. Huh, even the boy nurses?"

"Stop it, right now. Just go on with the story, though it sounds as if you're making it up for a book or something."

"No, really, it's true."

"I know. Let's hear it."

"Okay, the hospital called the next hearing. They had a bunch of sworn statements from the hospital IT experts that there were no files, period. Judge ruled against 'em again, ordered them to give us whatever storage devices had been in place that night.

"Again, they refused to comply. So, Mr. Jennings went to the Washington State Court of Appeals. Hospital even had lawyers from the Department of Health saying it was against Federal regulations to release what may contain other patient records to a third party. The appeals court said the same thing Judge Galanter did. Filter the files. They upheld Galanter's ruling.

"The hospital said, 'Fine, we'll appeal to the Washington Supreme Court.' Then the dogs sat on their butts until the last minute they were allowed to appeal. Another month wasted. Then they sat back and waited to see if the Supreme Court would take it. A few more months down the drain. Judge was forced to give us continuances, one after the other. Looked like the appeals might drag on for another year.

"While we're waiting, just to keep that Rhonda Uft on her toes, Mr. Jennings subpoenas the ultrasound tech from that night for a deposition. He said it was a fishing trip; no, no, he said fishing expedition. He told us there wasn't much we could do to a tech who says she didn't remember who or what she saw on some night better than a year before.

"You remember that radiologist who died on I-740, Thanksgiving Day? Well, it turns out he was the one who did the ultrasound study."

Khai stopped him. "Yeah, I knew that. Seemed so creepy, but it was coincidence. Hospital didn't even know there was a problem with the case until a few days later. Pretty weird, though. Now, Mike, please at least take a sip of your coffee."

He did, and his speech slowed for a minute as he told Khai about the tech's deposition. "Mr. Jennings thought maybe she'd get scared, slip up and spill that the hospital erased the images. But the instant he spoke the name of the radiologist, she burst into tears, writhing around like she was being tortured. She finally managed to squeak she didn't remember Sabrina and said she wasn't even working that night. But then Mr. Jennings pulled out her timecard. Sure enough, she was there for about six hours. Man, she went nuts. 'Why can't you leave me alone, blah, blah, blah,' then she jumped up and ran from the room. Almost tripped over Sabrina's wheelchair.

"This lawyer, the one representing the hospital at the deposition, couldn't have been twenty-three. Before the tech's butt was through the doorway, he snapped at Jennings, 'Satisfied now?'

"So, the next day Mr. Jennings received a call from Rhonda Uft. He always emails her, but she only uses the phone to call him. He says it's so there's no record of what she says. Anyway, she threatens him that if the Washington Supreme Court ruled against them, the hospital was prepared to take the matter to the U.S. Supreme Court. They were willing to go to any lengths to protect the privacy of their patients."

Khai huffed. "My ass. What a bunch of lowlifes."

Mike nodded, took a sip of coffee, and went on. "Mr. Jennings' brother, he's a retired lawyer down in Seattle, had been following the case. He told Mr. Jennings that he'd do the legal legwork for any Federal appeal, and it would be pro bono. What a family."

"Part of that World War Two and Korea generation. Not many of them left. We got lucky."

"We did, for sure. Anyway, when the Supreme Court of Washington upheld both lower courts, eight months had gone by since the suit had been filed, and Jennings sat down with his brother and us and said that if the hospital continues pushing the appeal, it was going to cost them a million more in legal fees."

"Who cares about their fees?"

"That's just it. If we continued to fight, and, somehow, they won at the Federal level, and they could convince the court there really aren't anymore images, and maybe there aren't, they could ask the court to rule that we have to pay their legal expenses. He said it could happen; he'd seen it more than once. He said what usually happens is they bluff for a while, and when they have us shaking in our boots, they come and offer to drop the demand for legal fees if we drop our malpractice case. Mr. Jennings said the sensible thing to do was move on without the files and wait for them to screw up. He thinks they will.

"He and that Rhonda Uft met with the judge the next morning and came up with a date for the trial. And here we are."

Khai sighed, "What a saga. You deserve better, Mike, the both of you. But you stay tough and beat 'em without crawling around like snakes. They are such bad people. A hospital, doctors.

"Anyway, thanks for telling me. That's the longest I've sat in one place with one person and talked for years. Thank you."

"No. Thank you. I feel so much better."

"You think about what I told you, about talking with someone, please."

431

"I will."

They stood, shook hands, and she turned to leave but stopped. "Hey," Khai brightened, "I told Mr. Jennings I have an old pal back on the East Coast, radiologist, specializes in ultrasound. We went to medical school together. It's time to ask him to take a look at the one view they've turned over. He's got no dog in the fight. We dated a few times, but I got engaged, and he was good enough to back off..." Her eyes reddened, and she stopped speaking for a moment then groaned an empty laugh, "But it is what it is, or some such aphorism. Is that an aphorism?"

"You're asking Henry Wadsworth Longfellow?"

"Hey, I'm going to send that image off to him today, and the radiology report, and I think the discharge summary. Let's see if he can find something to embarrass the hospital..."

Mike jumped in, "At a minimum."

She tapped his arm gently and left.

CHAPTER FIFTY-SEVEN

K hai received an email reply from her radiologist friend, Tom Campbell, that afternoon. He asked Khai to send her phone number; he enclosed his. She sat in her tiny apartment fretting over contacting a guy who had once been more than a friend, but with whom she'd broken up and, soon thereafter, married another man. Done with her third light beer, and with a fresh one in front of her, she grabbed her phone and punched in his number.

He pretended to sound surprised. "Damn, Khai, it's been, what, two-hundred years?"

"Doesn't seem that long, Tom—maybe a hundred-and-fifty."

"At least. Hey, thanks for the email. I wondered what happened to you. Last I heard, you left Mass General and didn't tell anyone where you were going. Figured Perry got reassigned, secret mission or something, and you pulled up stakes to hide from the KGB." When there was no answer, he asked guardedly, "You okay?"

Khai took a while to answer. "Long story. Better some other time when the Rooskies aren't listening in. They're tapping my phone you know. Also the CIA and the Gestapo."

He gushed, "Me, too. At least I know where you are. It's somewhere with a 617 area code, which, by chance, is right here in Boston. Were the rumors false? Are you here?"

"Nope, I'm in Seattle. Backward fishing village on the other coast."

There was another hush until he couldn't stand it. "Hey, I was flattered to hear from you."

"Thanks. That's nice of you to say."

"I was. You were the class rock star. Golden genes—that's what we used to say behind your back. Gees, a fighter pilot marries a fighter pilot. Nothing out of the ordinary about that. And you guys were so good together; taught me a lot."

Khai forced a smile and asked, "So, Tommy, married, three kids?"

"Wow. You nailed it."

"Do I know your bride?"

"Nah, I'm fibbing. Just got out of residency. Mine was five years, remember? First job. Only nights and weekends for three years until I'm eligible to make partner. Sucks."

"You know, I never understood that; five years for a radiology residency, and you rads come up with the exact same conclusion on every patient. 'Recommend an MRI, CT,' fill in the blank, 'to better delineate what might,' only might, mind you, 'be a tissue density in what might be the right adrenal...' Just dawned on me how you guys work. Add another test and hope like hell you get chosen to read it and line your pockets while we in the trenches work for Medicare rates. I know you people!"

Tom laughed. "Hey, Khai, you and Freddie Flyboy got kids? Bet they're gorgeous."

This time, he could feel the bitterness of the pause. "I'm sorry Tom, we're not together."

"Oh, Khai," he wheezed, trying to hide the tremor in his throat. "I was always afraid you guys, you know, two alphas. Figured that's why you left the East Coast—to get away."

"Well, you're right about the second half. Look, I just can't talk about it right now. I'm sorry."

"Whatever is best for you. Seems like it's still pretty raw."

"Yeah, really hard, but here we are. We'll talk about it sometime. Just want you to know you're also a gem, Tom, a really great friend during that stupid medical school."

She began to sob, and Tom whispered, "Do you want me to come out."

"Oh, Tom, that's sweet, but it's okay. I'm getting stronger. Told so many patients there's a reason for everything—all the good and the bad—I've started to believe it myself. I mean, I thought I had, but..." And her voice trailed off.

He could not speak for a full minute, and the sadness that flowed from both coasts grew until he squeaked, "Please tell me what I can do."

Khai drew in a deep breath, then released it slowly. "Well, the reason I emailed you was not to extend an invitation to my pity party, but for a selfish favor."

"You're the least selfish creature I ever met."

"Thanks, but you haven't heard the favor yet."

"Lend you money, again?"

"Very funny, but yes. You're the rad. Okay, enough idiocy. We need help with the patient records I sent you."

"We?"

"Yep, the malpractice attorney and the family."

"OMG. You've gone over to the dark side—consorting with the enemy."

"Yeah, but don't you think there are times when we gods screw up?"

"For sure, but not on purpose." He stopped, but only for a moment. "And this patient—you get too close?"

"Maybe. But you don't know her."

"Okay, but remember what they drilled into us in med school, right? 'You young doctors need to remain aloof. You'll last a year if you get involved with your patients.'"

"I remember it well, but this one has gotten under my skin. Did you read through the discharge summary?"

"Rough post-op course."

"Yeah, and pre-op, too. But that's not the problem. It's the hospital."

"Did they screw up?"

"To be honest, I don't really know if they're responsible for what happened. Maybe I am, but that's another story. Thing is they, the hospital, whether it's their fault or not, got themselves several meters deep in the kimchee by screwing around with the medical records. They're hiding something."

"They alter documents? That's the death knell, ya know. They get caught, they lose the case that day, whether they did anything wrong or not. They must know that."

"For sure, but it's complicated. Maybe insidious, maybe not. We just don't know. See, they claim the patient was bleeding internally long before she got to the hospital, but that doesn't make sense. I mean, did you take a look at the ultrasound?"

"Yeah, not the best quality. Embarrassing, to be honest. They're using that image to defend themselves?"

"Yep. See what I mean?"

"Well, yes and no. If that's all they have, then that's all they have. Even radiology isn't perfect."

"Okay, Your Honor. But you saw the free fluid, right?"

"Yeah, looked like close to three units, maybe more. Amazing she was upright."

"And that's the point. Sure, she could have had a slow leak, but other than a few cramps during the week, she was totally asymptomatic until ten minutes before showing up on my doorstep, which was just a couple of hours before the ultrasound. Took her blood pressure and pulse—both totally fine—had good color, and mentating well, sharp as a tack. Saw her again forty-five minutes later. Same vitals. She got to the hospital half an hour later, went for a pregnancy test—lab was down a flight of stairs—and the tech had no problem drawing blood, i.e., no vascular collapse. Ten minutes later she walked back upstairs and across the hospital to radiology for the ultrasound. When that was done, she and her husband were escorted, on foot, to the emergency room. No one looked at her for ninety-minutes, but, apparently, she was fine until right before they finally took her back. Actually, the only reason they took her back was because she crashed in front of their eyes, right there in the ER waiting room. So, again, the ultrasound doesn't make sense. And they won't let us see the computer files to search for other images."

"Did you ask the radiologist who read the films?"

"Tom, you're not going to believe it, but all of this took place on Thanksgiving Eve. Radiologist left the next morning for Bellingham, up on the Canadian border. Got into an accident two miles from here. Drunk came all the way across the median on I-740 and killed the whole family."

"Oh my God!"

"Yeah. Hospital claims he dictated a report that night, but we didn't get the report until a year later. They also said in court that all the other images were destroyed."

"Destroyed? How can that be? Once they're in the server, they're in there for good unless someone erases them, which is really hard to do with the new software even the worst hospitals are using. They're in there somewhere."

"Hospital went to the courts to plead that the files were corrupted so they wouldn't have to turn over the hard drive or whatever it is."

"Then, where did they get the image you sent me."

"Claimed that was the only one they could rescue."

"Oh, I see. And by the way, are you sure her ectopic was on the left?"

"Absolutely."

"Well, the image you sent me shows the large collection of fluid in the pelvis, a thickened left fallopian tube, probably, and an unremarkable appendix that happens to be on the left side. If the tubal was, in fact, on the left, only thing I can think of is a situs. Also saw most of a small, barely bifid uterus, garden variety, if you ask me. But I don't know what any of that has to do with being left alone in an ER to bleed to death."

Khai groaned, "Exactly my point. Everybody knows the corporation's lying through its teeth. They swear there was bleeding before the ultrasound, but it doesn't make medical sense. But the lawyer says they might be able to get the jury to buy it because we can't prove the ultrasound image is phony."

"Khai, of all people, you should know that's SOP. Lie, lie, lie, do anything to cover your ass, no matter the cost. You once told me that's how the military lives."

"On the whole, I would tend to agree with you, but some of these guys put the colonels to shame. Not a whole lot of honor amongst some of these thieves, and they're doctors!"

"OMG, are you daffy or something? What does being a doctor have to do with it? This is the business of medicine, young lady. No different than the corporate pencil necks we sit around and trash. Medicine laid the golden egg, and you need to do whatever it takes to guard your share. Not every single one of 'em, but enough to keep you looking over your shoulder when you sit in meetings with the board of directors. All driven by the bottom line. All that BS about the patient coming first. Corporate profits come first. That's not breaking news, Ms. Khai."

"Tom. I'm not going to live that way for the next thirty years. I can't."

"Not who you are or who you will become. Anyway, we're probably not gonna solve the world's ills before midnight. So, tell me what I can do. Craft a friend of the court statement? They can videotape me under oath. I can say they're flat wrong if they claim she would have been able to walk around with that much free fluid in her abdomen."

"I'm not sure yet, Tom. Let me talk to the lawyer. He's really a decent guy."

"Yeah, I'll bet."

"You know, people say that about us, too."

"Okay, Khai, I'll take your word for it. You're the straightest shooter I ever met."

After a long pause, she answered. "Thank you, Tom. That means something coming from you. Lemme get back to you. It'll need to be pretty soon. The trial's getting close to the end."

"Okay, I'll be here waiting with bated breath. And why don't you get me the actual image from the hard drive printed on photo-quality paper, not the Xerox of the Xerox. Let me see if there's anything, a tiny clue. Sounds like we should be helping your patient—and you."

"As soon as I can twist their arm for it. Break off their damn arm if I have to."

CHAPTER FIFTY-EIGHT

After she hung up with Tom, Chris Gauthé called and talked her into spending the night at his condo. By eleven, the beer buzz was long gone, and she drove to his condo in Soundview. She couldn't fall asleep, though, thinking about the past couple of days, the conversations with Tom, with Sonya Laureano, and the caustic taste lingering as she thought about the yogurt and how smoothly Chris had explained it away. Finally, she fell off into an uneasy sleep, but it could not have been fifteen minutes before she jumped up.

Chris rolled over and whispered, "Are you okay?"

"Yeah, yeah. I'm gonna go get a cup of tea and sit out in the living room for a few minutes. You want anything?"

"No, just for you to be happier."

She did not answer and left the room to brew a cup of chamomile tea, then sat on the couch wondering why her insides were twisted in such painful knots. It suddenly struck her that Tom had said all he'd seen on the ultrasound was free fluid, a normal appendix, and the bifid uterus, which he had described as garden-variety. She took that to mean it was not the kind produced by teratogens, poisons that cause malformed babies. He had also mumbled the word "situs," to explain why the appendix appeared on the left, but Khai had gone through half of the fourth beer and not absorbed the significance of what he'd said. She startled, thinking back to the first time she'd seen Sabrina, and the barely visible, hair-thin scars on her right abdomen. In the process of trying to figure out what was happening in her patient's belly, Khai had posed questions she thought might lead to a diagnosis of an unusual appendicitis. She'd asked if the tiny marks had been made by a surgeon or were just healed cuts from toppling off a bicycle, maybe a fall in the backyard.

Sabrina reported she'd had a routine appendectomy when she was a kid but did not remember the details. She'd never had another twinge in her tummy, not even a bladder infection.

Why, Khai scolded herself, hadn't she reacted the instant Tom made the comment about there being an appendix on Sabrina's ultrasound? She wondered if Sabrina could have been born with two appendixes, one on the left, one on the right.

She opened her laptop and went to the internet. There was no such thing as two separate appendices on opposite sides of the body, but there was such a thing as situs inversus totalis—an unusual congenital finding in which all of the organs of the chest and abdomen are reversed. Yes, that was the term Tom had used, a word that had passed into one ear and out the other.

She read on. With a situs inversus totalis, the appendix is found on the left side of the abdomen, the heart is on the right, the liver on the left, on and on. She had a distant memory of having heard about the syndrome in medical school, but she'd certainly never seen it. That did not matter; the National Institutes of Health had. The woman whose ultrasound the hospital was pawning off as Sabrina's had several malformations, not just the bifid uterus. She wondered if the person who'd chosen the false film had not noticed the appendix, or maybe just taken what was available on the internet, gambling that Harrison Jennings would not waste the money to call a proper radiologist. After all, everyone knew Sabrina Maddingly had a bifid uterus. Maybe that was what their expert had been referring to, his gestalt that this was damaged anatomy.

Khai opened Sabrina's chart on her laptop and searched for x-ray reports of the lungs. She knew very well there had never been a mention of the heart, stomach, liver, or anything else residing on the wrong side, but she wanted to be sure. Had there been a situs, that would have been the meat of the defense's case—a totally damaged human being. So, the only real abnormality Sabrina had was the bifid uterus, and that was present in more than one in two hundred births, probably even more often, for most were so benign, the patient never knew she had been born that way.

Khai was excited and jumped up to wake Chris and ask if he had ever seen the rare anatomic finding of situs inversus totalis. After a few steps, though, she stopped short, pondering how he would react if he learned of the hospital's ruse. Her next thought was that it was not beyond reason to imagine he had been co-opted into the ploy; perhaps he had himself suggested it in the first place to smooth his way back into the fold. She shook her head, trying to imagine how a seasoned surgeon could have missed the scars on Sabrina's belly. Then it struck Khai there had to be more to the hospital's blackmail than just a surgeon's disintegrating marriage—far more.

She stole into the bedroom and gathered her things, pretending she was going to the bathroom, but then slipped out and left the condo. It was ten miles down the highway that she began to snivel, soon sobbing that she had been taken, fooled, humiliated. A few miles later, her cell phone rang. It was Chris. She turned the phone off.

The next morning, she called Harrison Jennings. "Sir, I don't know if I'm allowed to call you directly, or even indirectly, but I've discovered a major mistake in the records Mitchie-Sterling Hospital gave you. Can I come up to your office and look through the charts they sent you?"

"Dr. Weathersby, I'm so glad you called. I wanted to talk to you about the testimony Dr. Gauthé gave at trial. He sort of surprised us."

"Actually, I heard. Do you think it hurt the Maddinglys?"

"You can never tell how a jury hears what witnesses say. Some of them are smart enough to read between the lines; most are not. And, maybe, that's the beauty in the system. Yeah, it was not what I expected, or hoped for. I was thinking of recalling you. Jury was very impressed. They felt you were professional. Probably the only witness who they trusted. I could tell by the way they reacted to your testimony."

"That's very flattering. Thank you."

"Just being honest. So, Doctor, what have you discovered?"

Khai outlined the obvious mistake but warned that she needed to review the records with her own eyes to see if mention of the abdominal scars was ever made, and, particularly, if any one of Sabrina's treating physicians, who each supposedly took a fresh history when they first met her, ever asked if she'd had any history of abdominal surgery, no matter how remote. What usually happens, she explained, was that once a complete-looking history finds its way into the chart, the next doctor just copies that one. Generally, it makes not a bit of difference, but in this situation, it might be vital to the case. If all the subsequent doctors used the original history, which was given by her husband, considering she was essentially comatose for the first few days, all of them missed the appendectomy. If she remembered correctly, several of specialists dictated they had read the actual ultrasound. That was not hard to understand. As a consultant, you charged the insurance company a fee for reviewing imaging studies. Some of the consultants, she was sure, just read the report; she wondered how many actually dug around for the film when it was finally added to the chart.

Khai told Jennings, "You could make the argument that the lot of them failed her miserably. But I have to see if the doctors who said they took a history, and claimed to have done a physical exam, mentioned the scars. If they missed them, that's embarrassing. If they charged Sabrina for reading the ultrasound, and didn't mention the appendix, that was shoddy work. But if they charged her insurance company for a reading they never did, it's insurance fraud. I don't know, but to me, that seems to make all the records suspect. Also compromises the quality of the care she received at Mitchie-Sterling Hospital."

Jennings agreed but added, "We don't have time to hire someone to do a forensic examination of the financial records. Take months to subpoena all the records and private bills the consultants submitted to the insurance company. Have to cross-reference who claimed to have read the ultrasound and charged the insurance company full freight to peruse a single image before the hospital reported they rescued the lone image. Can of worms. We're going to have to live with what we've already got regarding the crooked ultrasound. On the other hand, I think we're getting close to proving it was bogus."

"Mr. Jennings, I can come back and testify about the left-sided appendix on the ultrasound and that Dr. Maddingly does not have a reversal of her organs. I need to go over the op report for the first night, and when Gauthé took her back to surgery the next day. And, do you have a report from the expert witness they brought up here?"

"Yes, but it's not terribly complete."

"May I take a look at it? Let's see if he says a word about an organ that suddenly appears on the ultrasound, and he has no idea what it is. Let's see if he mentions an extraneous loop of bowel or something."

"Dr. Weathersby, I think you may have missed your calling. Yes, you may have all the records—anything you need. Look, I have to go to court but please come by, and I'll leave the charts on my desk. Take all the time you need."

He thought for a moment before adding, "Okay, Doctor, let's say all this falls into place, and I'm not being disparaging to you, but if I put you back on the stand, the first thing Rhonda Uft will establish is that you are not a radiologist, and she will use that to exclude your testimony. The only way this is going to work is if we put a proper radiologist before the jury. And even if we could find a board-certified, ultrasound-trained radiologist not on the staff at Mitchie-Sterling Hospital, there's still, as you can imagine, a Seattle-wide boy's club. Nobody wants to rock the boat and testify against a colleague. Who knows, maybe tomorrow your radiology practice will merge with the guys up in Redmond.

"And that also means a surprise witness. That can get tricky, legally."

"Mr. Jennings, how much time do we have?"

"How much do you need?"

"I'll call you back. When are you going to be free this morning?"

"I think the defense still wants to put on another expert, one that's a researcher on congenital defects, to explain why Sabrina wound up with meningitis. All part of their argument that her spinal defect was the cause of all bad things in her past and her future. And, as we know, they may have something. My only refuge is the 'but for' argument."

"Sir?"

"But for the awful bleed they failed to recognize and treat, Dr. Maddingly would never have had to have such urgent surgery; she would not have had the stroke; and probably, on a more likely than not basis, not have been so compromised by her near death that she would have been susceptible to the infection in her brain. But for the problem not having been recognized in the emergency room when she first walked in, like it should have; but for Dr. Cardozo acting like a jerk, she would have undergone earlier, but routine surgery, been home the next day, and back to work a week later. That 'but for.'"

"Well, will it help if we prove they provided a forged document? I certainly know that if a doctor changes a chart note to cover up malpractice, and the plaintiff finds out, that's the end of the case. The defense folds, offers the plaintiff a big settlement, and the doctor gets in Dutch with the state medical commission, and worse, with his malpractice carrier. Is that not the same for a hospital?"

"My knee jerk answer is you are correct. But you can never tell with a jury. They may be mad at the hospital but may also believe it was a mistake, and I can't take back that I made such a big deal of there being a certain percentage of mistakes that just happen in life.

"Bottom line is that while the hospital may be less than perfect, that doesn't change the fact that the patient's underlying problem is not the hospital's responsibility. They did the best they could, given the circumstances, the most important of which is that she did, indeed, have a terrible congenital problem. That can easily appear, at least to the layman, as the precursor of more of the same. In this case, you can be sure that in her closing argument Ms. Uft is going to be nearly in tears for the tragedy of Sabrina Maddingly, but she's going to tell the jury that her hospital is not responsible, and that there is still time for Dr. Maddingly to sue the VA. Why, she may even offer to give all her pleadings to Dr. Maddingly for her case against the government. A real Christian, that one."

Khai laughed. "Okay, but back to how much time do we have?"

"Rhonda Uft is going to be calling your ex-nurse, Sharon. It's out of the order of the usual witness parade. Should have put the expert OB on last, but he had all these critical board meetings to attend. Or so he says. It turns out good for us.

"Your former nurse is going to testify that you didn't express the urgency of the matter sufficiently, that Sabrina was already nearly in shock, and that you let her leave AMA."

Khai tsooked, "Unbelievable. Do I get to defend myself?"

"No need. Like I said, I'll take care of it. Not much of a challenge. Surprised a little that Uft is putting her on the stand. Toxic lady, and that's being kind. Jury'll see it a few seconds after she sits down. Not to worry. It'll backfire, allowing the jury to see her last.

"That should only take an hour, but I can drag it out for a day if you need the time to work on the records. And, by the way, do you know a radiologist who might be willing to testify for us? They'll be paid well, I promise."

"I do."

CHAPTER FIFTY-NINE

K hai spent her day off at Harrison Jennings' office. No one, except Khai and a physical therapist, had noticed the surgical scars on Sabrina's belly. She called Tom that night. Before they were done, Tom was on the computer booking a flight to Seattle. Khai fought back half-heartedly and finally promised to be at the airport to meet him.

She took a sick day and was there when he arrived the next afternoon. They went out for dinner, and Khai described the case. Tom rubbed his hands together excitedly and grinned.

Khai teased, "You won't do that in court, will you?"

"May not be able to help myself."

They drove back to her apartment, and she begged him to take the bed, but he refused, had a couple of beers, and drifted off on the couch.

Khai had tried to call Harrison Jennings all that day, but he did not answer his phone until after six. He was speechless as Khai told him that a board-certified radiologist was in town and ready to testify. "And he won't accept a penny for it, but I think we should cover his plane fare."

Jennings laughed.

By seven that night, Chris Gauthé had called Khai four times. She did not answer and erased his messages without listening to them. At nine-thirty, she heard a car stop abruptly outside her apartment. When the door slammed, she peered out the window of her bedroom to see Gauthé's Porsche in the no-parking zone directly in front of the building. She did not answer the door until the knocking became so insistent, an elderly neighbor stepped into the hall and asked if there was an emergency.

Khai chained the door and opened it a crack. "What is it, Chris?"

"Khai," he pled, "what is wrong? Is it that I didn't give up my career for a patient? What, you don't want my daughter staying with me?"

"No, Chris, the whole thing is wrong. You know it, and I know it."

At that moment, Tom startled awake and, hearing the tremulousness of Khai's voice, got up and stood behind her. "You okay, Khai?"

Gauthé sighed. "All you had to do was tell me. I never tried to control your life or who you want to sleep with."

"No, Chris, it's not what you think at all," she raised her voice, "at all. And you should be going now."

Tom took a step closer to the door, and Gauthé's face tightened as if ready to attack, but he wheeled around and bristled down the hall." She undid the chain and watched as he disappeared into the elevator, then she spoke to the neighbor who was still standing in the hallway. "Thanks, Mrs. Valente. Don't worry; he's harmless."

She smiled at Khai, "Oh, I understand how they can be, these boys. I was young once, you know." She giggled and disappeared into her apartment.

Tom sighed, "I hope I didn't have anything to do with that."

"Not at all. Long story. Tell you in the morning. Meanwhile, if you want to shower, let me get you a towel. I'm such a poor host." When Tom went into the bathroom, Khai remade her bed then went back out to the couch in the living room, covered herself with a blanket, and pretended to be asleep. Tom came out in his towel, shook her gently, and when she didn't stir, he laughed and went to the bedroom.

Khai called Harrison Jennings at 5:00 the next morning. She could hear the smile in his voice when she told him Tom was up, ready to take the witness stand. He warned, though, "Our friend Rhonda Uft is going to fight this like a mad momma grizzly. And she might be right. Surprise witnesses haven't been deposed."

Khai asked, "But she'll be able to cross-examine him. She can ask anything she wants to. Isn't that good enough?"

"Not really. She won't know what's coming. Won't have had time to confer with her medical sources to see if what our witness says is true. She's smart, no doubt, but she's not a radiologist, and she has no idea what to ask to have the witness admit there could be another explanation for what he is going to claim is unquestionable proof of an appendix and other malformations that Dr. Maddingly obviously does not have."

"But the truth is the truth."

"Doctor, you do this long enough, and you realize there is no such thing as the truth. For every so-called clear fact you throw up against the wall, the chances of it sticking are less than fifty percent."

"I imagine it's up to the judge. Do you think he'll let Tom testify?"

"You can never tell that, either. But let's see if we can organize this thing, make it as bulletproof as we can. Doctor, do you happen to have a copy of his CV?"

"I've got it right here on my phone. I'll email it to you as soon as we're done."

Jennings was silent for a moment. "Suddenly an idea springs from the ether. Do you feel comfortable giving me his email address? If I contact him, that's not out of the ordinary. I mean, when a lawyer needs an expert, you don't go to the phone book. Someone in the know suggests a name, and the attorney contacts him. That's the way it's done."

"Good. I'll give you his cell number."

"No, I think it's better to email first. Looks more professional, less set up."

"And, Doctor, I think it's better if no one sees you and Tom together. Would you mind dropping him off a couple of blocks, say from the Denny's on 29th and Atlantic? If he's willing to meet, we'll do it there at the restaurant. If someone sees you and Tom and me together, it'll get back to Rhonda Uft, and she'll find some way to tell the jury. Make it look like you, a supposed unbiased, or, let's say, only mildly biased witness, is in this thing up to her teeth. Take some of the sting out of your excellent testimony. That make sense?"

"Yes. I'm glad I do what I do and not what you do. I may be pickled in hospital politics, but you're drowning in it."

Jennings laughed. "Maybe not much longer, but on the other hand, that's part of the fun—always on your toes, always trying to think a move or two ahead of the game."

Khai mumbled, "I guess so. And, by the way, Mr. Jennings, what did my superior former nurse have to say on the stand?"

"Oh, her. No surprises. Rhonda Uft had her tell the peanut gallery just how cavalier you were about what she, Sharon, tried to tell you all along was an emergency. To hear her side of the story, you were going to send the Maddinglys home and have them come back in the morning for a recheck. But she, Sharon, was so upset, she brought you an AMA form. And you were so embarrassed that you took it out on the patient—started yelling at Sabrina—and Sharon had to calm things. And then you yelled at her, in front of everybody, just like you always do. That's why she quit."

"That's a fairy tale..."

Jennings interrupted, "I know, and now the jury knows. We worked backwards—with the so-called quitting. I introduced the sworn statement from your receptionist. You know, that Sharon refused to pick you up from the hospital the day you went down there with the little girl who lost her leg. Poor Sharon; turned white first, then a lovely shade of crimson."

Khai laughed, "Must have really set off her yellow teeth."

"Looked like the flag of Spain. I asked her flat out why she had refused to come get you. She said that wasn't true. I have to admit I was getting annoyed; said to her, 'You are under oath, madam. Are you aware of that?'

"She snapped back so hard at me, 'Yeah, I know,' I thought my head might blow off."

"Well, what did happen?"

"Her first excuse was that you always yell at her, and she couldn't bear sitting with you in a car for the fifteen-minute ride back to the clinic. Then I asked her why the receptionist put in her sworn statement that she, Sharon, refused to go because she was afraid the owners wouldn't cover her gas.

"She got very quiet then mumbled that everyone in the clinic was jealous of her because she was a real nurse, and they were just secretaries and lab techs. I said, 'But what about the gas story? Is it just another lie from the stupid people you're forced to work with?'

"She said, 'Yeah, but that's only part of it.'

"'So, what's the other part, I mean, specifically, about not being compensated for your gas?'

"She went on that you are so high and mighty just because you went to Harvard med school. When I asked her what she meant, she said, 'Ya know, a highfalutin snot. They're all the same.' When I asked her if she knew where you really went to medical school, she finally allowed she didn't know about Yale, or even what it was, and really wasn't aware of the difference between medical school and residency. Pretty sad. Then I pushed her until she admitted she only had a two-year nursing degree from a junior college in North Dakota.

"I smiled and spoke softly. 'I think we all understand how some employers take advantage. Rip you off on hours and don't talk about overtime. They fire you if you claim five minutes. Everyone knows that.'

"So, Rhonda Uft snorts, 'Objection. Is there a question in there?'

"Anyway, I withdrew my statement, though I had to sneak in that that the bottom line was, she left a medical doctor stranded ten miles away in the middle of an urgent care shift over fifty-cents worth of gas. Rhonda huffed and puffed, but she couldn't help seeing the jurors' faces. Shut her right up, and it was late enough in the day that I knew the judge would end court as soon as I was done with your friend. Rhonda just wrote off that nurse as another check in the bad column.

"But I simply had to ask one final question. 'Madam, after you left the clinic in Evanston, where were you hired?'"

"She stuck her nose in the air and cackled, 'I work for Mitchie-Sterling Hospital.'

"Told me she was, of all things, an ER nurse. Asked her what she thought of Cardozo. Told me he was 'interesting.' Asked what she meant by interesting, but she perseverated, 'I don't know.' Asked her six times before Galanter told me to move on.

"She couldn't remember if he had ever used profanity during work hours. 'I don't know.'

"When I asked if she still worked there, she said, she had quit to be with her family, to raise her kids. She didn't want them coming home to an empty house.

"I said, 'How old are you, again, Ms. Fritzer?'"

"'Forty-seven.'"

"'And how old are your children?'"

"'Early twenties.'"

"I looked to the jury. Their jaws were hanging. 'No further questions for this witness.'"

"Galanter glanced at Rhonda. 'Ms. Uft?'"

"She muttered, 'No, Your Honor.' Barely heard her. And that was the end of court for the day. I was so exhausted, I turned off my phone off and took my grandkids to McDonald's. Sorry you couldn't get ahold of me."

CHAPTER SIXTY

Before court convened that morning, Jennings and Tom Campbell met at Denny's. Jennings asked, "Doctor, how sure are you that shadow is an appendix? I heard that can be hard to define on an ultrasound."

"True, but I'll stake my professional reputation on it." He took out his I-pad and showed Jennings the ultrasound from Mitchie-Sterling Hospital and compared it to a slide show of ultrasound situs inversus totalis appendix images from the internet.

Jennings shook his head. "How the expert could have missed it is beyond me."

Tom wagged his head. "Actually, not so hard to understand. First, we have to assume the guy didn't do it on purpose. I would hate to think there was even the slightest chance that a well-respected doc would do that. Then, it is a situs inversus totalis, which is very unusual. Not the sort of thing an OB GYN sees very often—probably never in a career.

"In medical school, they teach us over and over you only see things you're looking for. The guy may have had a special short course in ultrasound for OB/GYN disease, but that means all he's going to see in this patient is OB/GYN things. I mean, he already knew the diagnosis of ectopic pregnancy, so he's not looking for anything else. I'm not trying to be smug, but he's not a radiologist. So, the appearance of a totally unexpected, rare finding is not something he'd reasonably be expected or able to find.

"Also, he didn't examine the patient, and there were no records of her diagnosis, except the history Dr. Weathersby did on the patient, and the

450

mention of the remote history of an appendectomy by, of all things, a physical therapist. Good for her. Look, the expert surely ignored Dr. Weathersby's notes. After all, she's the demon. And who looks at PT notes? Makes you wonder, doesn't it?"

Jennings spoke quietly. "Doctor, are you willing to say those very words, 'Stake my professional reputation on it,' when you are testifying?"

"Of course. That's why I'm here."

"Thank you. But we also need to do a little housekeeping. What is your fee for the trip here, your other expenses, and your professional time? Dr. Weathersby said you were not going to charge us. I can't allow that."

"Mr. Jennings, do you know how much I make a year?"

"That's not the point. What matters is that you're providing a priceless service. And anything that comes for free does not work. You know that in medicine, and I know it in the law. You must bill us for, at the very minimum, your flight, and some hours for your professional time."

"Well, sir, my dad's a captain with United. I fly for free. Free is good. He even got me upgraded to business class on the way out here. Maybe get first class on the way home, too. My professional time is salary based, so I'm getting paid for my time—took a sick day. A doctor with a sick day. As far as I can see, we're square."

Jennings twisted his mouth. "Is that all? Are those the only reasons?"

"You are very insightful. I'll be honest. Khai Weathersby was the class gem. I loved her, and when we stopped dating, we stayed friends. Wasn't surprised when she married Perry. He was a great guy, and they were a great couple. Such respect for each other. Taught me how a man should treat a wife. Have no idea what happened, but I know she's hurting real bad. Anyway, I'm not taking bread out of the Maddinglys' mouths. If Khai isn't, I'm not."

"Doctor, I don't know what happened either. She is incredibly disciplined. Compartmentalizes. I guess none of us will know anything more about her until she decides it's time. If she ever does.

"I will, though, honor your wishes about the fee. How about this: I will make a personal donation to the charity of your choice, out of my own pocket, not out of my clients' settlement, even if there isn't one?

"And we have one more issue. That is how you came to be involved in this case. If it comes out that you know Dr. Weathersby as a friend, her testimony on behalf of the Maddinglys will lose some of its muscle. What I thought was, perhaps, we could argue that she was looking at the ultrasound before her testimony and noticed a shadow she did not recognize. She knew she couldn't ask any of the local radiologists for the obvious reason that all of them are associated with Mitchie-Sterling in McKinley. She knew you from medical school and remembered that you had done a radiology residency. Hadn't been in touch with you for years. She gave me your email, and here we are. I can assure all of this, and the subsequent arrangement you and I made, are the standard process by which an attorney hires an expert witness. Is that within the realm of what you are willing to say?"

"You bet I am. But, Mr. Jennings, do you think I could meet with the patient before court to talk to her and see if the abdominal scar jibes with an appendectomy? Sure make a difference if I can say I met with the patient, and the expert didn't."

Harrison Jennings called Rhonda Uft from the law library at the courthouse to tell her he was filing a motion to allow a surprise, rebuttal witness. He offered to send her Tom's CV and tell her exactly which questions he was going to pose, and how Tom was going to answer."

She did not speak for a moment, and Jennings relaxed, preparing to provide the entire story. Then came a strident intake of air, and, by reflex, he braced for the paroxysm of rage. "Who the hell do you think you are? You aren't going to trick the court into allowing this nonsense to be fed to the jury. There is not going to be a witness on that stand that I haven't had the opportunity to depose. No way."

"Well, Ms. Uft, it sounds as though your shoes are a bit tight this morning. I was wanting to handle this like professionals, but I see that was too much to hope for. So, I am going to the courthouse, and I'm going to file the motion, and you can do as you please. I think the judge will find the weight of this evidence outweighs your bluster. Good day, madam." He hung up.

At 9:00, Galanter convened court. Before he called for the jury, he snapped, "Mr. Jennings, I see you have surprised the court with a very tardy motion."

"Yes, sir, tardy, indeed, but of such far-reaching significance to this case, and the general veracity of statements made by Mitchie-Sterling Hospital, it seems well within the realm of your authority to allow the witness.

"Further, sir, it isn't as if this is a bolt of lightning out of the blue."

Rhonda Uft growled, "Your Honor, please, this was completely unforeseen. Mr. Jennings had a deadline to notify the court of his witness list. We met the deadline, and supposedly he did as well. But now he wants another bite of the apple. I object most strenuously to the request for special privileges."

Before Galanter could answer, Jennings raised his hand. "Your Honor, Ms. Uft's expert witness claimed to the court that he was specially trained in ultrasonography at the prestigious NIH. I am not saying it is suspect that he happened to miss, as I explained in my motion, a normal appendix that just happened to be on the left side of the abdomen. To be forthright, he likely did not even know that Dr. Maddingly had had an appendectomy as a child, but it was even in her records from Dr. Maddingly's time at Harvard. Surprisingly, the only mention of it in the records Mitchie-Sterling Hospital forwarded to us was from a physical therapy note. And who reads physical therapy notes? Perhaps not even experts who testify that they read every single page of the records so very carefully."

He paused, and the judge put up his hand to stop Rhonda Uft. "Here's what we are going to do. First, today is only a half-day as my afternoon calendar has me in criminal court. I don't want to, but I will cancel the whole day if, Mr. Jennings, you would you be willing to make your expert available to Ms. Uft for a deposition. Further, it seems that if we are just arguing about a very clear-cut medical finding—either it's there or it isn't—is it too much to ask the defense to find an expert of her own to rebut a single finding on one image of an ultrasound in one day? What do you say, Ms. Uft?"

"Your Honor, it is too much. It's not just the presence of an appendix, it is my ability to demonstrate that an appendix on the left is even more proof of severe underlying anatomic abnormalities. Maybe she had two. There's a lot of research I need to do."

"Now, Ms. Uft, you have a stable of lawyers standing behind you at this very minute. Surely, two or three of them can contact the hospital to corral someone to testify on your behalf. Yes or no?"

"Your Honor, that is unfair. Then Mr. Jennings is going to cry that he didn't have time to depose my witness. Where does it end?"

"Good point. Mr. Jennings, if Ms. Uft finds a rebuttal witness, would you be willing to forego deposing that physician?"

"No problem, Your Honor. I do reserve the right, though, to cross-examine him or her if they get on the stand in this courtroom."

"Of course, you will be able to do a cross. Ms. Uft?"

"I suppose so, Your Honor, but I maintain my objection."

"Well, Ms. Uft, if you do not agree, I will make a judicial decision on what I feel best serves the interest of justice. You have the right to delay the case once again and submit an appeal to a higher court."

Jennings laughed inwardly. Rhonda Uft had lost the appeals she had made in the case before it came to court. The appellate judges, everyone in the courtroom well knew, were human beings, and grouchy ones at that. Yet another appeal from Rhonda Uft over an issue that the judge had handled fairly meant that if she appealed this and the judges ruled for the judge, again, an appeal of the final verdict was dead in the water before the ship took to sea.

With her body coiled as tight as a spring, she muttered, "I accept the plan."

Galanter raised an index finger. "And, Ms. Uft, that means you may not appeal my decision on this point. Appealing anything else in the trial will be fair game, but not this decision. Are you in agreement?"

"Yes, Your Honor."

"Good. Before I adjourn court, Bailiff, please bring the jury in. When they were seated, he smiled at them more gently than he had in the past. "Ladies and Gentlemen, as you know, court was supposed to be in secession only for the morning. A significant matter of law has been raised. Solving it requires the attorneys spend the day in deposition. I apologize, but please understand that resolving the matter is crucial to the outcome of this case. You've done yeomen's service so far. I hope this last twist in the path will not be too hard to deal with. We are very close to the end. Thank you. You are dismissed until 9 A.M. tomorrow morning."

CHAPTER SIXTY-ONE

Rhonda Uft bristled into the courtroom the next morning, her face more twisted than usual. Jennings turned to Sabrina and Mike. "Looks like her shoes are now three sizes too cozy." When she shot a glance at Sabrina, Sabrina covered her mouth with her right hand to hide the smile. Mike didn't bother to cover his.

With court convened, the judge turned to the jury. "Ladies and Gentlemen, though the plaintiff rested several days ago, the court is going to allow him to call a final witness. We do this in the spirit of insuring justice. Thank you for your patience. Counsel, please call your witness."

With Tom sworn, Jennings questioned him about his CV, stopping at the board certification in radiology. "Doctor, would you tell us just how long you spent in your residency to learn how to read and interpret x-rays?"

"Five years."

"Well, sir, we had another witness in this trial, an OB/GYN, who told us he spent two weeks, actually nine and a half days, learning to read ultrasounds. Could you please tell us if, in your professional opinion, that is sufficient time to make pronouncements to this jury about a critical ultrasound?"

"Without trying to be funny, I would submit that in my residency, I took a six-week course in obstetrics. I would dare say you would not let me deliver your baby."

"Are you saying that even six weeks is too short a period of time to learn the subtleties of reading ultrasounds?"

"Yes, sir. You can ask any reasonable doctor in this country about those short courses. They are fine for learning to read an imaging study when everything is normal. Not so good when a life is at stake."

"Thank you. Now, Doctor, would you tell us what you found on Dr. Maddingly's ultrasound?"

"Very simply, a normal-appearing appendix, but located on the left."

"Well, what is so special about being on the left?"

"We all start out in life with an appendix, but as everyone knows, sometimes the appendix becomes unwell and has to be taken out."

"Could you show us on the screen what you mean?"

Tom played the laser pointer on a diagram of the abdomen. He stopped at an elongated pouch the size of an index finger sticking straight off the side of the large bowel. "This is the appendix. There is a tiny hole connecting it to the large bowel. Inside the bowel is stool. Sometimes, a bit of that stool gets pushed through the hole into the pouch. But, say, it is a dry, hard bit, like the seed of a small fruit. The hole gets clogged. There are bacteria in the stool, and they will cause an infection if they are not constantly moved along and out of the body as part of the feces. If something gets stuck in the hole, the bacteria carried along with it into the empty pouch of the appendix continue to grow and give off gas. But the gas can't get out because the hole is clogged. Then the swelling caused by the gas closes the hole off even smaller. In a couple of days, the appendix swells like a balloon. That swelling cuts off its blood supply and, in a day or so more, the tissue starts to die. Very painful. Just like if you put rubber bands around the base of your index finger. Turns blue, and pretty soon the flesh starts to die. Gangrene sets in. Gangrene produces even more gas, more pressure, and soon the nearly-dead appendix finally bursts like an overfilled balloon. Now, all that infection gets dumped into the abdomen. Naturally, we try to take the appendix out at the first sign of infection, days before it bursts."

"Thank you, Doctor. Now, sir, would you please return to witness stand and look at this binder of medical notes." He held up the binder with which the jury was so familiar. With Tom reseated, Jennings asked him to turn to Page 7 in Section B. "This document has been introduced into evidence as Number 502. Doctor, what is this document?"

"It is a chart note from Dr. Khai Weathersby."

"I know you are not an expert in these matters, but on the stamp in the top right corner, what do you see?"

"Law Offices of Uft, Cooper, and Linegarth."

"When is the stamp dated?"

"September 10th of this year."

"So, they had this document long before this trial. Does that appear to be correct?"

"Yes."

"Now, if you would look down to the heading Past Medical History in Dr. Weathersby's chart note. Please read it."

"Number One: Spinal cord defect with high grade, though partial, paralysis of left upper extremity/secondary to father's exposure to Agent Orange; Number Two: Appendectomy, laparoscopic as toddler, uncomplicated; Number Three: No other pertinent history."

"Now, under Physical Examination, please read the portion after the subheading 'Abdomen / Inspection'."

"Three barely visible, well-healed, laparoscopic scars on the right lower abdomen at McBurney's Point."

"What, sir, is McBurney's Point?"

"That is the usual spot under which we usually find the appendix." He lifted in the chair and pointed to the spot on his right lower abdomen.

"Now, for the other document I handed you. Who is it from?"

"Darly Hauser, Licensed Physical Therapist."

"What does it say under Patient?"

"Sabrina Maddingly."

"What is the date of the document?"

"May 16th of last year."

"Please read the date stamp on the top right."

"The date is May 27th."

"Does it have the name of a law office below it?"

"Yes, Uft, Cooper, and Linegarth."

"Again, of course, you are not an expert in legal documents, but do you believe this is the date the law office of Uft, Cooper, and Linegarth received this document?"

"Yes."

"So, it appears they had this document long before this trial as well. Is that correct?"

"Yes."

"Doctor, please read the one sentence under Past Surgical History."

"Appendectomy-remote."

"What does remote mean?"

"Happened a long time ago."

"Under Physical Examination, the sub-section Abdomen, what does it say?"

"Healed, small surgical scars in right lower abdomen associated with appendectomy per patient."

"Thank you. Now, Doctor, did you go through the discharge summary for Dr. Maddingly from Mitchie-Sterling Hospital?"

"Yes."

"Was there mention of an appendectomy?"

"No."

"Was there mention of old, surgical scars on the patient's abdomen?"

"No?"

"Okay, I have one more medical chart note to go over." He handed Tom a few sheets of paper."

"What is this?"

"This appears to be the op note done by Dr. Gauthé on the night of admission."

"Under history, does it mention appendectomy?"

"No."

"Is there any mention of healed surgical scars on his patient's abdomen?"

"No."

"How is it possible that a surgeon who is operating on a patient's abdomen does not see and note healed surgical scars?"

"Objection. Calls for speculation."

"Sustained."

"Thank you, Your Honor. Okay, let me ask if it is unusual, in your opinion, for a surgeon to fail to mention the presence of surgical scars in the very area he or she is about to open on a patient?"

"Yes."

"Okay. Let's get down to business. Why is it so strange for us to have you up here talking about appendectomies and appendix shadows on ultrasound?"

"Very simply because Dr. Maddingly had an appendectomy decades before this ultrasound of her abdomen was done, and now, on this ultrasound, she still has an appendix."

"Does the appendix ever grow back?"

"No."

"Is it possible only a partial appendectomy was done?"

"Not on purpose, but sometimes a 'stump' is left behind. It is harmless."

"Is there any chance we are simply seeing that 'stump'?"

"No. Look at the slide of a normal appendix." An ultrasound image appeared on the screen. "It is long, well formed, and quite normal. A stump is a stump. Small and like a skin tag. This is not a stump. This is." He flashed five slides of small stumps on the screen.

"Is it possible that we are seeing something other than the appendix? For instance, a bit of fat or a different organ that looks like the appendix?"

"No."

"Are you sure, Doctor?"

"I will bet my reputation on it. In fact, I'll bet my medical license on it."

"In your expert opinion, as a board-certified ultrasound specialist, is there any explanation why you found an apparently normal appendix in a patient who had an appendectomy?"

"There is no medical reason. The only explanation is that this is not the ultrasound of a patient who has undergone an appendectomy."

"Are you telling us this is not an ultrasound of Dr. Maddingly?"

"I am telling you this is an ultrasound of woman with an intact appendix on the left side of her body."

"And, again, you are absolutely sure?"

"Yes, certain."

"But wait a minute, Doctor; you said on the left side. Is that possible? I thought you told us the appendix is on the right side. What is happening here, sir?"

"This is a clear example of situs inversus totalis."

"And what is that in English?"

"It is a rare malformation in which all the organs of the chest and abdomen switch sides. Heart is on the right, liver on the left, and so on."

"Does Dr. Maddingly have a single remark in her chart, with all the x-rays and CT scans that she has undergone, that a single organ is misplaced, on the wrong side?"

"No."

"Is it possible that only the appendix is on the wrong side?"

"No."

"Does it follow that we cannot use this ultrasound to determine if Dr. Maddingly had been bleeding into her abdomen before she got to the emergency room?"

"Objection. This does not mean that the plaintiff wasn't bleeding before she reached the emergency room."

Jennings jumped in before the judge could rule on the objection. "Excuse me, Your Honor, but I asked if we could use this ultrasound to determine if there was bleeding before Dr. Maddingly entered the emergency room. If Ms. Uft wants to convince us there was bleeding, she is free to do so, but," he growled, his face growing scarlet, "she isn't going to use *this* ultrasound anymore. Not one more time. That's for sure."

"I'm sustaining defense counsel's objection because, regardless of the veracity of this particular ultrasound, we still have not determined if there was bleeding before the plaintiff arrived in the emergency room. It will be up to the jury to determine the facts."

Jennings sighed and turned to Tom. "Thank you, sir, for your professionalism. I have no further questions."

Sabrina, who had been increasingly trying to stifle a cough during the trial, suddenly began a spasm of hacking that shook the room. She broke into a sweat and began shuttering so, her wheelchair was vibrating. Mike's eyes grew wide as he stood and wrapped his arms around her from behind. He whispered, "I'm here, Sweetheart. Always."

The judge locked his eyes on Sabrina. "Mr. Maddingly, is Dr. Maddingly okay?"

He looked up and mumbled, "Just a moment, sir."

Rhonda Uft leaned back and shook her head less than subtly. The judge noticed and asked Mike, "Would you like to take a break."

Jennings now spoke. "Your Honor, we would ask the court for a ten-minute break?"

Galanter banged his gavel, and the jury was dismissed. "Mr. Jennings, shall I summon the medics?"

"Your Honor, let's see what's going on. I don't want any excuses that the defense wasn't able to cross this witness. Just give us a minute."

Mike wheeled Sabrina to the ladies' room, where one of the female deputies took her inside. Before the door closed, the cough became violent, and Jennings took out his phone to call 911. Sabrina was put on a breathing mask, lifted onto a gurney, and taken to the first floor.

Jennings stood in between the medics and the ambulance that sat right outside the door. He snapped, "She may not be transported to Mitchie-Sterling." One of the technicians began to grumble, but when Jennings explained they were suing the hospital and that taking her there would be clear malpractice, the medic twisted his lips in annoyance but stopped protesting. "She is a patient at the U, and that's where she's to be transported. Anywhere else is going to land you in court—I promise." The man looked as if he was going to spit on the ground near Jennings' feet, but climbed into the driver's seat of the aid car and pulled joltingly from the building. Mike followed in his car.

Sabrina's oxygen saturation was eighty-six percent on the trip to Seattle. She was admitted to the intensive care unit. Despite a mask with one-hundred percent oxygen, her saturation continued to fall, so she was put to sleep, and a breathing tube was inserted.

Mike had been asked to leave the room and stood in the waiting area, numbly gazing into the parking lot six floors below. He watched a petite blond in scrubs walk peacefully toward her Subaru, keys in hand, though a Porsche that had been idling in a corner of the lot suddenly screeched forward and came to a skidding stop behind her. The driver sprang out and hovered menacingly. They spoke without obvious emotion for a moment, but the man suddenly tensed and grabbed her elbow. She pulled away forcefully and broke into a jog for her car. When he caught up with her, he slapped the keys from her hand so hard, they flew across the lot toward the hospital. As she turned to look at them, Mike realized it was Krystal Kaywood. She was crying. There were more shouted words until the man reached for her again. She ducked to the side then broke into a sprint toward the hospital. When the man turned to chase her, Mike' jaw dropped at the apoplectic hue of Chris Gauthé's face.

Krystal made it into the hospital before Gauthé could grab her, and he stopped short as she disappeared into the emergency room vestibule. Gauthé bristled back into the parking lot, stooped to pick up Krystal's keys, looked about furtively, dropped them in his pocket, and tramped to his car. His lurch from the parking lot left deep black tire marks on the macadam.

Within seconds, the parking lot was filled with hospital security, and, minutes later, seven Seattle Police cars were at the doors, several with their sirens still blasting long after the emergency was over, cops standing about, gabbing with buddies.

Mike was called back to Sabrina's room. He wanted to tell her about what he'd just seen, but she was still asleep, the ventilator hissing every few seconds, her color returning to normal.

Shortly after Sabrina's ambulance left for Seattle, Harrison Jennings returned to the third floor. Court resumed. As the judge opened his mouth to recall the jury, Rhonda Uft stood and asked for a mistrial on the grounds of theatrics."

Without a reply, Galanter had the bailiff reseat the jury. His only utterance was a curt, "Counsel, do you wish to cross-examine?"

"Yes, Your Honor," she cried out, "I certainly do."

"Proceed."

Rhonda Uft marched to the witness stand even more brusquely than usual, but her gait was marked with a new hitch that caused the toe of her left pump to catch on a lifted seam in the linoleum. She caught herself just feet from her witness then stood for several seconds, staring, her lips moving in mumbles without producing any sound. Galanter took a breath to address her, but she snapped at Tom, "Doctor, have you ever heard the medical truism that, 'If there is one congenital defect, look for others'?"

"Yes."

"Therefore, it is likely that the plaintiff has more than just one congenital defect, correct?"

"Incorrect."

"Incorrect? Let's take a step back. Does the plaintiff have a congenital defect?"

"Yes."

"And didn't you just testify that if the plaintiff has one defect, then there are others."

"I did not."

"Shall we have the court reporter read back your testimony?"

"What you asked was, 'Doctor, have you ever heard the medical truism that if there is one congenital defect, look for others?' I've heard that statement, but it is not a truism, as you called it. It is simply a saying, which carries as much objective truth as saying, 'where's there's smoke, there's fire.' Correct sometimes, but far, far from always."

"Well, let's get down to the meat of the argument. You said in your testimony that there is no possibility that a person who has had an appendectomy can have a normal-appearing appendix on ultrasound. Is that correct?"

"Yes, I said that."

"Sir, I am sure, in all your studies for board examinations, that you learned there is such a thing as a duplex appendix. Is that correct?"

"Yes."

"Could you tell the jury what that means."

"It means that a person has one more than one appendix."

"So, it is very possible the plaintiff has more than one appendix."

"Yes."

"And, given that she has a known congenital abnormality, isn't it within reason to allow that she might have a slightly better chance of having another congenital abnormality, specifically, a duplex appendix."

"No."

"But a duplex appendix happens. You have already admitted that. Can you prove that is not the case here?"

"I can say only that the chance of a duplex appendix is vanishingly small—about point-zero-zero-four percent."

She stood, absorbing the number, until a manufactured cough rose from the defense table. She spun around irritably to see one of her underlings motion her over with his head. She walked to the table and snatched a sheet of paper from the assistant's legal pad. She read it, nodded to herself, and went back to her witness. "Doctor, did you just say, 'vanishingly small chance'?"

"Yes."

"Well, sir, point-zero-zero-four percent out of the three million births per year in the U.S. in the Seventies, when the plaintiff was born, works out to one out of 2,500 births. One in 2,500 isn't so small, is it? Do you still want to use the words vanishingly small in front of this jury?"

Tom pulled a pen from his suit jacket and wrote slowly in the margin of the records sitting before him. Rhonda Uft crowed, "Are you going to give us an answer?"

He did not look up for another moment, then smiled, "Excuse me, ma'am, but your arithmetic is wrong. Decimal place mistake. It's one in 25,000. That's all of 120 people in the whole U.S. born with an extra appendix. And, further, the two different appendices *never* appear on opposite sides of the abdomen. They are always near each other, very near. This has been the source of malpractice cases, surgeons missing a second appendix. You always look around to make sure there is nothing else involved."

"Objection, speculation."

"The judge muttered, "Sustained."

"Thank you, Your Honor. Just a couple of questions. Doctor, how did you learn of this case?"

"I learned the specifics from Mr. Jennings."

"How did Mr. Jennings find you?"

"Mr. Jennings was looking for a radiologist with a specialty in ultrasound who did not live in the McKinley area. He was afraid no one locally would be willing to testify that there was a questionable document generated by Mitchie-Sterling Hospital."

"Objection. He's stating facts not in evidence."

"Sustained."

"Let's try again, Doctor. How did Mr. Jennings find you all the way across the country? Are you a nationally known and respected radiologist?"

"No, just a board-certified one."

"So, tell us again, how did plaintiff's counsel discover you?"

"A medical school classmate recommended me to Mr. Jennings."

"Who was that classmate?"

"Dr. Khai Weathersby. She was older, so was I. We elderly stuck together in med school. Is there something untoward about that?"

"I will ask the questions here. So, what was your relationship with Dr. Weathersby in medical school?"

Tom stopped and looked down, hoping Harrison Jennings would rescue him, but Jennings was reading from his notes. "We were classmates and friends."

"So, this was a social, not a professional, relationship?"

Tom inhaled deeply, ready to lash out, but forced himself to smile. "Social, professional, she was a fellow medical student. Hadn't heard from her in years, not since we all graduated, but she remembered that I was going to a radiology residency. Suddenly, an attorney contacted me directly about a patient who had an ultrasound that was clearly bogus. He told me Khai Weathersby had given him my name. Period."

"I object to the witness's characterization of the ultrasound as bogus."

"Sustained."

"I have no further questions for this witness."

The jury turned to Harrison Jennings, expecting a fiery re-direct, but he sat poker-faced. Galanter thanked the witness and excused him. He looked down at lawyers. "Are there any further matters for the court to hear before we begin closing arguments?" Both attorneys said no. "In that case, as it is late in the day, we will begin closing arguments tomorrow morning at 9 A.M. sharp. I remind the jury not to discuss this case amongst yourselves, or with any other person, until the matter is turned over to you for deliberation. Thank you. Court dismissed"

CHAPTER SIXTY-TWO

The next morning, Judge Galanter convened court and spoke gently to the jury. "Ladies and Gentlemen, we are now going to hear what we call closing arguments. You will remember that both attorneys told you in their opening statements, the second phase of the trial, what they intended to prove to you. The third phase of the trial was testimony from witnesses to actually give you the facts you need to make a decision. But, as in all trials, there was so much information thrown at you in so short a period of time, it must have been hard to remember even the key points. So, now, we enter the fourth phase of the trial, where the attorneys will sum up what they believe are the most important facts. We call it closing arguments or summation. The fifth phase of the trial will be your deliberations as you determine who presented the most convincing arguments.

"I know that on TV, summation is just a minute or two. In real life, that is impossible. Each side must be given sufficient time to go over the facts and what they mean. On the other hand, sometimes these remarks can go on far too long. As such, I am allowing each side forty-five minutes to deliver their closing arguments. Traditionally, the plaintiff goes first, then the defense, and then the plaintiff has one more chance to speak to you, but only to refute what the defense attorney said in her closing remarks. He cannot bring up anything new in the rebuttal, and he still only gets a total of forty-five minutes for all of his remarks. He may divide that time as he sees fit between his closing argument and his rebuttal.

"And then, I will give you instructions about what the law allows you to

466

consider in your decision. At that point, the trial will be placed in your able hands. So, let's begin with Mr. Jennings." He nodded toward the plaintiff's table.

Harrison Jennings had been looking intently at Galanter during the judge's remarks. He rose slowly, put his hands on the yellow legal pad in front him as if he was about to lift it, but nodded to himself, and pushed away from the table. Slowly, regally, he walked, head up, to a spot just two steps behind where Rhonda Uft had stood during the trial when addressing the jury. His tired blue eyes locked those of the jurors then paused until several of them craned a bit, waiting to hear from the soft-spoken man.

"Ladies and Gentlemen of the jury. Both Ms. Uft and I thank you for your patience and your public service. What an amazing system, that thirteen people willingly give up their lives for over a week to listen to two lawyers haggle. But what we both told you through our witnesses is like life. It seems there is no absolute truth—there are two sides to every story. One minute, you are convinced of one side's version; next minute, the other side seems more believable. All I can do is remind you of the inconsistencies in those stories and hope you can draw a conclusion as to which argument holds more water. Unfortunately, as I heard Judge Judy once tell disgruntled litigants, 'Hey, this is a lawsuit. One side wins; one loses. Get over it.'

"So, now I will give you the Maddinglys' perspective on just what happened on the night of 25th November. I will do this by comparing and contrasting that with what Ms. Uft laid before you with her witnesses.

"First, we never, ever pretended that Dr. Maddingly was a perfectly healthy woman. Dr. Maddingly was compromised in her left arm. She had an unquestionable defect in her spine, presumably from her father's exposure to Agent Orange in Viet Nam. But all she had was weakness in her left arm—period. She did not need a special parking pass for work; all she needed for steering her car was a strap she slipped her arm into to hold her hand in place. She did not need automatic devices for her left arm or for a now-useless left leg. She did not have the constant pain on the left side of her body that is so common after a stroke. In fact, she had no pain at all.

"Dr. Maddingly did not need to be humiliated every time she went to work by having an attendant come out of the University to help her from her car into a wheelchair, and then hand-carry her to her office, which has been entirely recreated to allow her to work, and then help her go to the restroom, the restroom of all things.

"Work? She has tried to do four days a week, then three, and was, when she finally had to stop, barely able to do two. She used to do six. She didn't have a wheelchair. She used to jog. She didn't need handmaidens to live.

"But now, she has suffered a brain injury, and there is no question that happened at Mitchie-Sterling Hospital on the night of 25th, 26th November. No one argues the severity of the brain injury.

"Ladies and Gentlemen, each one of you was chosen, not because we thought we could manipulate you, that's TV, but on the basis of your ability to think, to make an honest assessment of the facts, let those facts fall where they may, and then give us a just conclusion.

"Everyone in this room knows the difference between a massive brain injury and a birth defect of the spine. The defect in the spine caused some of the nerves coming from the spine to Dr. Maddingly's left arm to grow improperly. A stroke, on the other hand, kills nerves in the brain because a stroke cuts off the blood supply to that part of the brain. From a mile away, the result may look similar, but you have come here and sworn to look deeper. To tease out the real truth.

"In Dr. Maddingly's case, the spinal defect and the stroke could not be more different. Consider this example: If you run out of gas because there is a leak in a rusty fuel line, your car stops. If someone siphons the gas from your tank, your car stops. From a mile away, again, the result is the same, but the cause is entirely different. You can be sure the guy caught stealing your gas wants his lawyer to convince you, the jurors hearing his case, that the empty tank was a result of a hole in the rusty fuel line.

"While Ms. Uft has insinuated that all of Dr. Maddingly's problems are acts of God, I suggest this tragedy could have been avoided had Dr. Cardozo not been so angry at Dr. Weathersby. It all boils down to one man's personal behavior at work, and the hospital that knew of this behavior and still let him continue making life and death decisions.

"Let's talk about what happened with Dr. Cardozo. You witnessed his demeanor here in this courtroom, his arrogance, his convenient failure to remember any questionable aspect of his conduct that night. Do you think he's any different at work than he was here? Do you remember when he grinned at me and popped off at the mouth, 'I wondered how long it would take you to start screwin' with me'?

"Ladies and gentlemen," Jennings hissed, his face enflaming, "let me assure you, I am far too old to come into a court of law and screw with a witness. I do not need the money from this case. Not a penny of it. I'm here to right a wrong. What a lack of respect for you, for me, for Ms. Uft, and for Judge Galanter.

"And then there was his utter lack of interest in these proceedings. The only time he invested in this trial was when he was on the witness stand. I have been an attorney for nearly fifty-one years. This is the first time I have ever seen the major defendant in a major trial miss the entire proceedings, aside from his testimony.

"We heard that Dr. Cardozo was unable to start a central line IV. The excuse provided by the defense was that it didn't matter. We know the defense contends that as long as an IV was eventually started, the hospital did as they are required by law.

"We know from Mitchie-Sterling Hospital's own records that Dr. Maddingly's blood circulation did not collapse the first ten minutes she was in the treatment room. She was holding her own until over five minutes after she came under Dr. Cardozo's care. Then she started downhill, but, even at ten minutes, she still had non-life-threatening low blood pressure. Part of this is certainly because the emergency room personnel took so long to bring her back into the treatment area. It dramatically cut down the time they had to prevent this tragedy.

"And why was that?" He paused and raised his eyes to the ceiling. "That was because Dr. Cardozo had not alerted his staff that a patient with an impending disaster was sitting just feet away from them. And all because Dr. Cardozo was mad at a doctor who worked for a different company, one he did not like, one that was taking away his money.

"Ladies and Gentlemen of the jury, there had been more than ample time to start an IV in Dr. Maddingly while she still had good blood pressure and pulse, had Dr. Cardozo just sent a medical assistant into the waiting area to greet Dr. Maddingly and her husband. A one-minute assessment by a seventh grader would have brought Dr. Maddingly into the treatment area, and her life would have gone on, her ectopic pregnancy just a blip on the radar scope.

"By the time an alert receptionist on her way to the restroom saw what was going on, there was still time, but Dr. Cardozo didn't see the urgency and let several nurses fail repeatedly at starting a simple IV in the arm. I submit to you that within the first ten-minutes wasted on these botched attempts, Dr.

Maddingly was essentially gone. This was long before Dr. Gauthé arrived. Yes, he started the IV on his first try, but it was too late by twenty minutes. Defense argued it did not matter who did it as long as the job was done. Nonsense. Dr. Gauthé may have started an IV, but the job was not done, not by a long shot.

"We heard from Dr. Gauthé, himself, that he ran all the way to the ER the instant he was needed. But that was half an hour after Dr. Maddingly was taken into the treatment area. Please remember, we never heard a single witness confirm it was Dr. Cardozo who accepted he was in over his head and asked for help. Even Dr. Cardozo would not testify on the witness stand, after I reminded him he was under oath, that he made the decision to call for help. He told you he couldn't remember. That was the excuse he laid in your laps.

"Now, I'm going to read directly from the transcript of this trial. I hope it is not too confusing, but what can be more accurate than hearing words from the witness's mouth?

"I asked him, and this is from the transcript, 'How did you go about calling for help?'

"His answer, 'I certainly don't remember the specifics.'

"I asked if he called help. Answer, 'Obviously, I did.'

"'Why do you say obviously?'

"'He came to assist, didn't he?'

"I asked, 'Who came to assist?'

"'Gauthé.'

"'Who called him?'

"'Well, do you mean, did I get on the phone and make the call myself? That's not how it's done.'

"'No, I don't mean that at all. I mean did you, or did you not, initiate the call for help to Dr. Gauthé?'

"'I have no recollection of the specifics.'

"Ladies and Gentlemen, all this because he had had an argument with Dr. Weathersby? How dare he? Look, the great majority of doctors are caring, incredibly dedicated people. But, as in every walk of life, there are the deviations. You witnessed one here.

"Consider his answers to simple questions such as my request he recount his conversation with Dr. Weathersby. He remembered nothing of the encounter. Nonsense. Let me ask you. When was the last time you screamed obscenities at a stranger and you couldn't remember every word, every nuance?

Ladies and Gentlemen, the emotion of so intense an encounter stays with you for the rest of your life.

"And then the absurdity of him telling you to your faces that he trusts paramedics but not a board-certified medical doctor who is asking for teamwork in saving an innocent woman's life.

"He denied using profanity toward Dr. Weathersby, but we did hear from Nurse Tharker that Dr. Cardozo used incredibly unprofessional profanity that night, and did so on a frequent basis in Mitchie-Sterling Hospital's Emergency Room. This is who he is. Please do not allow the fact that Nurse Tharker was unable to control herself on the stand suggest her testimony wasn't crucial. I placed her in as uncomfortable a position as she had ever been in her life. I wish I could I say I was sorry for doing that to her, but there are truths in this world that must be brought out of the shadows into the light of day. We are adults, and we have adult responsibilities.

"Now, she resigned right after the night of 25th November. That was despite eighteen years at Mitchie-Sterling Hospital. Why? Because Mitchie-Sterling Hospital would not take definitive action to curb Cardozo's behavior. I'm sorry you had to listen to her racist outburst. She is no Mother Theresa, but no matter what all of us think of her, I hope you can see that she is a passionate woman who clearly would not lie to this court. What she told you about Dr. Cardozo's behavior was obviously heartfelt and accurate.

"Do you remember that Dr. Cardozo claimed he had not been told by Dr. Weathersby that a patient with a potentially fatal problem was being brought to his waiting room? When I pushed him, and asked what Dr. Weathersby had told him, he answered, 'I told you; I don't remember what she told me.' Then I asked if he knew she was a doctor. Again, he did not recall. A doctor who doesn't remember anything about the night a doctor came to him for help saving a life..."

Jennings stopped breathlessly in mid-sentence to stare out the window but abruptly restarted. "The lack of the slightest kernel of respect. Do you remember when Dr. Cardozo referred to Sabrina Maddingly as Mrs. Maddingly, and I said, 'Excuse me, Doctor, but that's Dr. Maddingly. Did you know she was a doctor?' Do you remember his answer? 'She's not a doctor. She's a psychologist.' And this from a board-certified emergency medicine physician who could not start a life-saving IV.

"I asked if he had personally reviewed the ultrasound report. 'I don't remember.' Well, did you see the actual ultrasound image? 'I don't remember, but I am sure I looked at it to orient myself.'

"Well, Ladies and Gentlemen of the jury, there was no ultrasound image, at least not for the next few months, probably a full year, until Mitchie-Sterling Hospital magically came up with one view of an ultrasound that certainly doesn't appear to be that of Dr. Maddingly."

Rhonda Uft sucked in an audible breath and rose an inch from her chair, but her eyes shifted toward the jury, and, ever so slowly, she dropped back into her seat, rolling her shoulders, pretending to have been just stretching.

Harrison Jennings paused until he was sure the jurors had seen Rhonda Uft's fizzled dodge then went on. "We demonstrated that Dr. Cardozo was disciplined by Mitchie-Sterling Hospital for his behavior and language during his failed attempt to start an IV in Dr. Maddingly. Discipline? A slap on the wrist? I don't know, and I don't care to know the specifics. We know that he was not punished with a suspension, or even a class on anger management. All we know is that he still works there, never lost a day, still on duty," he made quote marks with his fingers, "'ready' if your spouse or your children need life-saving care. Think of what they have spent on legal fees defending him. Why? Do they love him? I don't know. Do they respect him? I do not know that, either. But I do know Mitchie-Sterling Hospital spent an awful lot of money on this lawsuit to protect the corporation." He paused. "Let's think about that. What were their choices? They can't fire him, can they? That would admit they were remiss in keeping him on as a doctor. The corporation, the corporation, no matter the human cost.

"I asked him, 'Dr. Cardozo, did Dr. Gauthé start the central line on the first attempt?'

"His answer, 'I don't know. I had to leave the room and tend to the backup of patients.'

"'How did you know there was a backlog of patients?'

"'I don't remember.'

"'But you knew, apparently. Was that part of your decision to call for help, that there was a backlog of patients?'

"'Once Gauthé was there it probably was. The patient was being cared for.'

"Do you remember when I asked him, 'Is it possible that a staff member was so upset and concerned with your failure to do something to save Dr.

Maddingly's life that she made the call on her own?'

"His reply, 'That is highly unlikely—no matter what some people may claim.'

"When I asked what some people were saying, Ms. Uft objected that it called for hearsay, but Judge Galanter overruled her, and Dr. Cardozo told us there was an unfounded rumor that a clerk had called Dr. Gauthé. When I asked him if that was true, do you remember his body language, how his face paled?

"He mumbled, 'That's what I heard, yes, that someone else made the call. But you know, you believe half of what you see and none of what you hear.'

"That was his answer, a line from "I Heard It Through the Grapevine." Ladies and Gentlemen, please, Marvin Gaye was a great entertainer, but his lyrics don't count as fact in a court of law.

"I am not going to go over every inconsistent, arrogant, and inappropriate remark made by Dr. Cardozo. I will not waste your time and quote the twenty-four times he told us he couldn't remember what had happened that night. It is all available to you if you choose to ask Judge Galanter for the transcript of his testimony.

"I would, though, like to address one more thing—the ultrasound. I may not be able to prove, on the basis of beyond a reasonable doubt, that an ultrasound of a woman with an ectopic pregnancy and fluid in her abdomen was purposely substituted for Dr. Maddingly's actual ultrasound, but, please remember, the standard in civil court is, as you have heard many times in this trial, on a more probable than not basis, that is, better than fifty-fifty. What are the chances that the original ultrasound was lost? Fair, you say; but how were they able to rescue only the image that just happens to show free fluid, their misguided effort to convince you Dr. Maddingly was bleeding before she got to Mitchie-Sterling Hospital?

"Why am I bringing this up? So what? We know the ultrasound had nothing to do with Dr. Maddingly's medical care. Why? Why so much foofaraw over one picture? Why, because it is the very basis of Mitchie-Sterling Hospital's defense. If they can't show you blood in Dr. Maddingly's pelvis when she arrived at the imaging center at Mitchie-Sterling Hospital, then they can't put any reasonable argument before a court of law that Dr. Weathersby or Mr. Maddingly are responsible for what happened. She was stable when she got there. Period. There was still time.

"And on that subject, let us review the evidence regarding what we all learned about the human body and how it reacts to blood loss. We heard that, given Dr. Maddingly's height and weight, her body held a total of about eight units of blood. According to the specialist Ms. Uft put on the witness stand, the one who told us he was an expert on ultrasounds of the pelvis, Dr. Maddingly had lost about three units of blood into her pelvis. How did he know? Why, he looked at the ultrasound. He looked so closely that he didn't see the misspelling of the patient's name, or that the ultrasound did not jibe with Dr. Maddingly's medical history. But even he agreed that was nearly forty percent of her total supply. I asked him if it was likely that Dr. Maddingly was able to walk across the parking lot, downstairs into the hospital blood lab, back upstairs for an ultrasound, and then to the emergency room waiting area, where she remained conscious for an hour and a half waiting to be seen. Do you remember his answer? 'No, it is not likely, if the bleeding had just taken place.'

"And the only way he could determine if there had already been significant bleeding was by the ultrasound, which I hope we have shown is, at best, a clerical error, and at worst, evidence tampering, which, Ladies and Gentlemen, suddenly becomes a criminal matter, and a felony at that.

"And, then, he got so confused as to how he would have handled Dr. Maddingly's situation, he would have had her wait longer than she did that night.

"He was such an expert, he told you Dr. Maddingly's bifid uterus was caused by the poison DES. He told you it was similar to a chemical in Agent Orange. He was just so cocksure of himself, wasn't he? When I pushed him, do you remember how he sheepishly admitted the chemicals that he tried to convince you were the same, the ones that linked DES and Agent Orange, were actually completely different?

"So, I will stop here and just recapitulate that it would appear, on a more likely than not basis, again, better than a fifty-fifty chance, that Dr. Maddingly walked into Mitchie-Sterling Hospital Emergency Room with a good blood pressure, and over the next hour and a half, because of incredible negligence, essentially died. All of this because of a rogue doctor and a hospital that will go to any lengths to protect him so no one can touch their slice of the money pie.

"I'm not asking you to feel sorry for Dr. Maddingly. She doesn't feel sorry for herself. I'm only asking for a measure of justice. Thank you."

CHAPTER SIXTY-THREE

A rthur Galanter asked Rhonda Uft to come forward and address the jury.

"Ladies and Gentlemen, first, thank you for sitting here so patiently. Without you, there is no justice—for either party.

"Please let me remind you of what I promised in my opening remarks. First, the plaintiff's attorney admitted that the plaintiff was not a perfectly healthy woman who appeared out of the blue on the night of 25th November. I hope you can see that is, indeed, the case. She was seriously compromised. We knew about her left arm paralysis before the night of 25th November, but it wasn't until after the surgery that we learned of the multiple internal organs that did not form properly, particularly a deformed fallopian tube that was completely abnormal, and an abnormal uterus. Notice plaintiff's counsel did not try to dispense with the completely abnormal, two-part uterus. Never even mentioned it in his summation. How could he? All these malformations, Ladies and Gentlemen, it is no great surprise that it was nearly impossible to treat her as if she was a typical patient.

"Ladies and Gentlemen, I am so sorry her father was exposed to poison as he served our country. I am also sorry that she was so compromised that she had to have an automobile outfitted with special steering to accommodate the fact that her left arm and hand were incapable of driving a car. All of this decades before she came to Mitchie-Sterling Hospital asking them to save her life.

"It isn't fair that a young woman had to be issued a permanent disability sticker by the State of Washington, and one by the University of Washington. It isn't fair that on top of her neural tube defect, she also had a defect in her fallopian tube that led to an ectopic pregnancy. It isn't fair that that fallopian tube was defective to the point that no one can rule out the likelihood that it bled abnormally.

"This is the cause of her unfortunate state, not the exceptional efforts made by Mitchie-Sterling Hospital to save her life. Perhaps the family would be better served to seek relief from the U.S. Army, not an innocent hospital. The medical staff at Mitchie-Sterling Hospital was forced to work in uncharted territory, to go on a dangerous mission without a map, without vital information about where they were asked to go. No doctor here, in Washington State, or in Washington D.C., or in New York, or any place on Earth, would have been able to foresee the abnormalities they'd face saving her life.

"Quite the contrary to what the plaintiff's lawyer told you, we heard Dr. Gauthé, the plaintiff's own witness, for goodness sakes, tell you how the staff at Mitchie-Sterling Hospital provided Dr. Maddingly with lifesaving care. The only argument the plaintiff has put forward that could possibly be part of the conversation is that Dr. Cardozo did not start an IV fast enough.

"Not fast enough? Another of the plaintiff's own witnesses, Dr. Weathersby, told us that when someone is sick and their blood pressure is going down, the veins collapse and are nearly impossible to locate unless you are a trained surgeon. And what happened? A trained surgeon ran down to the emergency room the instant he was called, and he started the IV, just as Mitchie-Sterling Hospital protocol demands. Everything was by the book.

"None of the staff at Mitchie-Sterling Hospital claim to be gods or magicians, just as none of us claim to be at what we do. You met them, the caring, hardworking professionals who were put in an impossible situation by politicians who forced the plaintiff's father to go to war and exposed him, knowingly, to horrible poisons. These were mistakes made long before the plaintiff ever set foot in Mitchie-Sterling Hospital.

"At every single juncture, the plaintiff was treated by board-certified specialists who worked incredibly hard to save her. The sad truth, Ladies and Gentlemen, is that disease is inevitable. Everyone involved in caring for the ill has to do their part, that means the patient's family and the non-specialists out in the community.

"In that regard, the doctors and nurses at Mitchie-Sterling Hospital were up against the awful odds, not only because their patient had severe, underlying deformities, but also because, and I don't know how to put this nicely, of the dereliction of duty of the plaintiff's husband. We have shown, as promised, that he delayed bringing his wife to Mitchie-Sterling Hospital. How, I ask, can you folks make a decision about what Mitchie-Sterling Hospital did or did not do when the plaintiff's own husband willingly delayed bringing his wife there? It does not take a board-certified surgeon to understand that delay was instrumental in the unfortunate stroke and near-death suffered by the plaintiff.

"And what about Dr. Weathersby? She did not put the fear of God in these people. If she can't start an IV, then we expect her to get the patient to a facility which can. Why, she didn't even call an ambulance. You heard that from her personal nurse! Perhaps that is why the plaintiff's husband was so grievously cavalier. If any doctor should be defending herself in this case, it should be Dr. Weathersby. She is a maverick who has chosen not to join her colleagues in the local medical society that sets and maintains the standards for doctors allowed to practice medicine in *your* community.

"All of this has to be taken into consideration when we discuss the standard of care, the yardstick by which we measure the performance of the average, prudent provider in the local community. It is how similarly qualified practitioners would have managed the patient's care under the same or similar circumstances. As I mentioned at the beginning of this trial, here, in this court, the plaintiff must establish the standard of care, and then they have to prove to you, the jury, that the standard of care was not reached.

"Please find a single practitioner, aside from Dr. Weathersby, who didn't do as required. Again, you may say that Dr. Cardozo did not start the IV within a few minutes, but that is not the standard of care. The standard of care is that an IV was started in the ER. The question is not if every doctor is master of every procedure; that is an unobtainable and unreasonable yardstick. The question is if the doctor was smart and caring enough to put aside ego and call for help from a specialist. Maybe Dr. Cardozo doesn't remember calling for help, but that was a horrible night. There were two men with heart attacks waiting for him to save their lives. Yes, he was under a level of stress few, if any, of us will ever, thankfully, experience. Who the heck cares if he cursed? Who the heck cares if a racist nurse was offended by his words? We should be more offended by that woman's vile rantings. Dr. Cardozo was letting off steam in a horrible situation. She was preaching hatred in a court of law. She was not a competent witness. She has psychiatric problems of a profound nature, and it is good that Mitchie-Sterling Hospital relieved her of her duties. She has no place in a top-rated hospital.

"The bottom line here is, Dr. Cardozo was faced with an impossible challenge. For goodness sakes, who knows where the plaintiff's veins lie in her neck? Maybe, like her other organs, her anatomy in the neck is distorted. Again, the plaintiff's own witness, Dr. Gauthé, testified that it was just dumb luck that he was able to place the IV. And lucky for the plaintiff that an impossible job got done.

"We also need to address Mr. Jennings' character assassination of Dr. Cardozo, the man who worked so hard to save a life that night. First, whether you like Dr. Cardozo is not the question here. But, for just a minute, put yourself in his shoes. He gets a telephone call in the middle of the night from a person claiming to be a physician. Dr. Cardozo has practiced in McKinley for more than fifteen years. Ladies and Gentlemen, this is not a very big area. There are actually very few doctors locally, and he knows every one of them. Suddenly, at the beginning of the long weekend, he gets a call from a hysterical person claiming to be a doctor who has sent a dying patient to the hospital, not in an ambulance, but in her family car. Inexcusable. Then, this doctor does not provide a single fact to convince Dr. Cardozo he's to drop his dying patients and run around in the waiting room looking for the supposed patient to appear out of the ether.

"In fact, the failure of the plaintiff's husband to check in properly was just another of the family's poor choices that night. And then for him to just sit there in the waiting room when nothing was happening to get his dying wife into see a doctor—for an hour and a half?

"It is simply unreasonable to blame Dr. Cardozo or Mitchie-Sterling Hospital for the family's awful decisions.

"And a final note about Dr. Cardozo. How is it possible that a man as bad as plaintiff's lawyer has painted him has never been the subject of a lawsuit or any disciplinary action? He cursed when a frankly psychotic nurse made a stupid mistake. I felt like cursing at her when she played her little game with the court.

"Ladies and Gentlemen, we have no idea when the stroke took place. The plaintiff has not been able to prove a timeline, even on a more than likely basis, when the stroke took place. Was it before the plaintiff was brought into the treatment area? Most likely, I mean on a better than likely basis, the cascade of deadly factors was well on its way before she arrived at Mitchie-Sterling Hospital. And, even if it was after that, here again, both the plaintiff's husband and Dr. Weathersby are directly responsible for the delay. What reasonable doctor would not tell a dying woman to go to the hospital immediately? And, again, what kind of husband would just park himself in a chair in the ER and not demand his dying wife be seen immediately?

"And, finally, let's get this over with right now—the ultrasound. Again, it was the plaintiff's burden to prove the ultrasound was not that of the plaintiff. Perhaps it was a mix-up of records. We do not know; nothing has been proven, but this time, please put yourself in the shoes of the radiology department on that awful Thanksgiving. First, in the hours around midnight, there was a city-wide power outage. That is a possibly devastating occurrence in a hospital. Everybody was on edge. But the generators kicked in after the loss of power, just as they are engineered to. The result was that not a single patient was negatively affected. But, as everyone knows, that's not fast enough to save fresh computer files.

"It's not as if any doctor that day, or the next, or in the next weeks, needed that film. All that was needed that night was to provide emergency care for the plaintiff, which she got. Going through the protocol to rescue the ultrasound files could be left for the morning when the IT people came back to work, or even the next Monday, after the long holiday weekend. They simply weren't needed. They were taken only to provide the doctors with a tentative diagnosis before surgery. The diagnosis was completely known two hours later because a surgeon looked in there with his own eyes. Far better than an ultrasound. The film and the report were of no importance.

"So, let's go back to the situation at the hospital that night. After the power outage, the radiologist left the hospital for a Thanksgiving Day with his family in Bellingham. As you know, he was struck by a drunk driver on I-740, just north of McKinley. More than likely, and that is the legal standard here, there was terrible turmoil in the radiology department when they learned of his death, and that of his wife and two of his three children. That is to say nothing of the entire hospital's reaction. I'm sure you agree that it is reasonable that no one thought about the ultrasound for many weeks. Perhaps there was a mix-up when the ultrasound files were finally retrieved. I'm not saying that happened, but it is a reasonable explanation for the findings on the ultrasound. The radiologist was no longer around to correct the mistake. The tech, herself, is not trained to read the images, so she could not shed light on what they showed, certainly not in a court of law.

"And don't forget, since it was not ordered in the first place by a doctor with privileges at the hospital, no one was looking for it. Where were they supposed to send it? No one in the county knew who Dr. Weathersby was. She was not, and is still not, part of the established medical community. Further, she admitted to this court that she never asked Mitchie-Sterling Hospital for the film. I remind you again, the ultrasound was of no medical value. It would not affect the plaintiff's care a single iota. It is just a desperate red herring dangled in front of the jury to take the focus off the truth. Don't be fooled by a possible, insignificant clerical error. No harm, no foul.

"Mitchie-Sterling Hospital and its physicians and its staff, in fact, did yeoman's service to care for the plaintiff. Sadly, the plaintiff arrived at the hospital with an acute, deadly condition, and a long list of bodily faults that made treating her nearly impossible.

"Due to the professionals at Mitchie-Sterling Hospital, her life was saved. With time, she will recover sufficiently to return to her important work as a health provider at the University of Washington. In fact, this is the best outcome anyone could have hoped for. A sad case, yes, but it was God's will, not the fault of the caring doctors and nurses of Mitchie-Sterling Hospital.

"Thank you."

CHAPTER SIXTY-FOUR

Judge Galanter peered down at Harrison Jennings. "Sir, you have twelve minutes to present you rebuttal. Please begin."

Jennings rose slowly. He stepped even further from the jury than during his closing remarks. He could see the jurors' shoulders relax as the old man decompressed the space Rhonda Uft had usurped from them.

He was not at all hurried. "Ladies and Gentlemen, just a few thoughts. First, please ask yourself the most important question of your life: if one of your kids is badly hurt, would you want that child cared for in an emergency room where Peter Cardozo was the only person who stood between her life and her death?

"Next, please ask yourself the second most important question of your life. If your child suffered from a birth defect, would you allow some hospital to scream God's will because they screwed up?

"And, finally, would you allow some hospital, that appallingly harmed your child for life, to base its entire defense on a single x-ray that turned out not to be that of your child?

"Thank you for listening."

Judge Galanter was quiet for a moment then turned slowly to the jury. He spoke more solemnly than he had during the entire trial. "Ladies and Gentlemen, it is time for you to weigh the evidence in this case. It is your duty to come to a conclusion as to which side, on a more probable than not basis, convinced you more by their witnesses and their statements. Who presented the more believable arguments? That is the crux of the matter: who do you believe more?

"You must not allow sympathy or personal preference to influence your verdict on either the question of liability or the amount of damages. Remember that you are not champions or advocates for either side in this case. You are jurors, and you are responsible to this court and to your community for reaching a verdict that is not based on anything whatsoever except the evidence and the law in this case.

"You must not allow yourself to be influenced by the status of the parties in this case. All parties are entitled to equal justice in our courts, rich or poor, individuals or corporations. All persons are equal in the eyes of the law and must be treated as equals by you, as jurors.

In keeping with the oath that you have taken, interpret the facts and apply the law truly, correctly, and impartially. Your sworn duty is to seek the truth and to reach a verdict that is consistent with the truth.

"Open your minds to the views and opinions of your fellow jurors and share your thoughts with them, then vote your consciences."

CHAPTER SIXTY-FIVE

K hai was about to start the afternoon when she took a call from Mike, who filled her in on Sabrina's new pneumonia. She was off the ventilator but on a mask and still being pumped full of esoteric antibiotics. Just as Khai sat down to hear the rest of the story, the receptionist came to her and said Harrison Jennings was on the other line. She promised to get back to Mike during the afternoon.

The attorney sounded chipper. "Dr. Weathersby, I know you're busy, but just want to tell you we finished testimony an hour ago. Case has been turned over to the jury. You know about Sabrina, yes?"

"I was just hearing from Mike."

"He hasn't been in court. At the hospital with Sabrina. Just tried to call him, but he didn't pick up. Wanted to tell him, and you, that the case is over."

"That's nice of you to take the time to call me. How long do you think it will take?"

He laughed. "Easy to predict. Anywhere between one hour and eight days. But you need to know that you made a very important difference in the lives of two innocent people. You are a gem, my friend."

"Thanks. As are you, sir. You'll let me know, but, please, only after the principals hear."

The nurse tapped Khai on the arm and pointed to the wall clock. Khai nodded and ended the call.

In Room One, she introduced herself to a seventy-year-old man complaining that he'd felt a cold sensation in his throat for the past month. She had not heard of a complaint worded quite like that before and asked, "Mr. Post, you mean you've had a cold in the throat for a while?"

"No, I don't have a cold at all. It just feels cold, and for the past few days, my shoulders get cold. I was worried it was a heart attack, but thank God, it didn't go down my arms."

"You say cold, like tingly, like numbness?"

"I don't know. Like cold. Like someone holding an ice bag on the front of my neck. Doesn't hurt, so it's not a heart attack, thank God."

"Well, does exercise make it worse?"

"I have to admit, I should exercise, but I don't."

"How about climbing stairs?"

"My house doesn't have stairs. Mall has an escalator."

"Does it get worse when you get emotional?"

"I stay home pretty much. TV's been broken past two weeks. So, I don't have to watch the news."

"I know what you mean. Well, is it worse sitting up or lying down?"

"You know, I never paid any attention to that."

"Any shortness of breath?"

"Only when I go out to carry firewood into the house."

"Okay, that's exercise. Does it get worse then?"

"What, the shortness of breath?"

"No, the cold feeling?"

"Don't know, can't feel it over the breathing."

"Is the breathing harder than, say, a few weeks ago?"

"Now that you mention it, it could be, but it's gotten colder, so I have to carry more logs into the house. Can't really tell."

Khai's shoulders wilted, and she redirected her questions toward the man's medical history, He, though, remembered few illnesses. He wasn't sure but thought his parents died of old age in their sixties.

When Khai had him remove his shirt to do a physical exam, her jaw dropped at the sight of several surgical scars, the most obvious a thick, disfiguring wound over the breastbone. "What's that from?"

"That. Oh, I forgot. It was twenty years ago."

"What was it?"

"Roto rooter."

"Do you mean 'cabbage'?"

"Yeah, yeah, that's it. My brother had the roto rooter down below, on his prostrate. I had the new arteries in my heart...Come to think of it, he had a heart attack right after the roto rooter."

"How old was he when he had his heart attack?"

"'Bout as old as my old man was when he died. I don't know, sixty."

That keyed the algorithm in Khai's medical brain, and she asked for the EKG machine. She told the nurse to call 911 to transport him to Mitchie-Sterling Hospital Emergency Services. She gave him an aspirin, put him on oxygen via nasal canulae, started an IV, and crossed her fingers. The quick EKG showed what she already knew—a major heart attack. It was probably far too late for tPA, and she fretted the hospital would castigate her for not doing cardiac bypass surgery in the back room before sending him down. Then she giggled to herself as her middle finger surreptitiously extended next to her thigh.

She held Mr. Post's hand as he was wheeled away, gave him a little hug, and whispered, "You're gonna do great. Just a little speed bump, yet another one along the long road, huh?"

He clasped her hand and began crying softly. As they lifted him aboard the ambulance, he whispered, "Ain't you comin' along to be my doctor?"

"No, sir, gonna leave that to the real smart ones."

She turned to walk back into the clinic, shoulders sagging, her reverie pierced by the receptionist, who had rushed out toward her. "Dr. Weathersby, there's a guy on the phone yelling his back's killing him. Something about he needs more pain meds, or he's gonna come down here and make you, he said, 'understand'. Don't know what he means."

"Patty, don't worry about a thing. Let's let Ms. Margie in the lab handle this one. Her turn, I think. Would you wanna mess with Margie?"

"God, that's funny, Dr. Weathersby. But that's like the third madman on the phone today."

"We should be thanking our lucky stars it's less than usual. Next one calls, come and get me. It'll mean my turn's rolled around again."

The two walked into the clinic smiling, and Khai turned left to see the half-dozen patients who'd had to wait through Mr. Post. The first was a recheck on the woman from months before who had come down with genital herpes, the one whose elderly boyfriend, an ex-con, had been mortified when Khai suggested he had infected his lady with Herpes. She was back, this time limping.

"You know, doctor, that other problem is all better, but I fell two days ago. My ribs really hurt that night, so I went to the ER down in McKinley. Doctor said it was just a bruise, but he told me to follow up with some bone guy. Told him I was seeing a doctor up here. He got really mad when I said your name. Then he gave me a paper and told me not to come to you. 'I want you to go to a real doctor,' he said. Really, that's what he said. I didn't like him at all."

Khai smiled and put her hand on the woman's arm. "No problem. Let's take a look at the x-ray." She snapped it up on the view box and shook her head. "Not bad. May see a couple of little cracks, but nothing that needs a bone doctor. You'll be fine."

"But he told me nothing was broken."

"Ya know, sometimes it's hard to see these things. We'll get you better in a jiff. How 'bout down below? You sure it's all better?"

"You mean the virus from that bum? You remember he said he became a Christian? Well, that was a bunch of bull. Gave another neighbor lady the same thing. We tried to get him evicted, but the cops said we didn't have a leg to stand on. But, yeah, it's all gone. Hey, Doc, can I ask you about one more thing?"

"Of course."

"I got this thing on my tit. Really worried. Can't sleep. Could you tell me what it is?" She started to weep. "I know what it is, but they can do so much these days, can't they, Doc?"

"You bet they can. So let's take a look. Probably nothing."

"Oh, I don't know. Everything bad happens to me. I just know what it is, and I want you to do the surgery. Least you tell it the way it is. And you're a woman, and I don't want no more men pullin' and pickin' at me."

She lifted her food-stained sweater and out flipped an empty pancake of a breast. On the outside surface was a red blemish, less than a quarter of an inch in diameter. At the center was a tiny punctum of white—a pimple. She pushed the breast forward and wheezed, "Can you tell what it is?"

Khai pretended to study the lesion carefully, but only for three seconds until she smiled and put her hand on Mrs. Cooper's. "Oh, that's nothing. We see that all the time. Just let me flick the top off, the little white thing; you won't feel it at all, and it'll be gone in two days."

"Are you sure it ain't cancer? Sure?"

"I'm so sure, that if it is, I'll donate one of mine for an implant."

The old lady whooped in laughter. "That would be something, one pointing up, one down!"

Khai laughed. "Oh, you flatter me. What you mean is two in the middle. You'll look great."

Khai turned to get a needle out of a drawer, but the door flew open. The receptionist was pale. "That guy who wanted the pain meds is here. He's drunk. Got a broken bottle in his hand. Wants to see you."

"Patty, you go into the lab and call 911. Tell 'em there's an armed aggressor trying to take the doctor hostage."

"I'm sorry, aggress... what? I don't understand."

"No, Patty, I'll go out and talk to him."

As Khai entered the waiting room, a scruffy man sat, head forward, barely balancing in his chair. The reek of alcohol filled the room, and as she approached him, the spoor became so strong it stopped Khai in her tracks. She asked softly, "Sir, can I help you?"

The man looked up. "You ain't the one who told me I couldn't have no pain pills. Where is that bastard?"

He lifted the bottle, but his hand was shaking so, it looked like he was using it as a paintbrush. "Sir, look, let's get you into an exam room and figure out what's going on. Then we can talk about making you feel better. That okay?" As he wobbled to his feet, Khai spoke again. "But first, why don't you hand me the bottle, and I gotta tell ya, I don't like Jack Daniels all that much. Shoulda brought bourbon." His expression did not change as he turned and placed the bottle on his chair then followed her into the back. They spoke in the hallway for a moment. He groaned that he had a toothache that was killing him.

Khai shook her head. "They told me it was your back."

"My back tooth."

She took him by the arm into a room, sat him on the exam table, and looked into his mouth. "Jees Louise. That's gotta hurt." She pulled a key from her pocket and called for Margie. "Let's give Mister, Mister...?"

"Sims."

"Mr. Sims, two Vicodin from the narcotics safe. That'll cover you, sir, until we can get you to the ER down in McKinley. They'll get the dentist on call to see ya. Be all better in a couple of hours."

She walked him out to the waiting room. "Do you have money for the bus down to McKinley?"

He shrugged. At that moment, Margie came from the back with the two pills in a tiny paper cup, and a larger one with water. He swallowed the medication then wobbled back into his chair. Khai asked Margie to watch him as she went to the back to get her purse for carfare. Margie put up her hand. "No, Doctor," she whispered, "this one's on me."

Khai laughed quietly, "No, no, you got the last one."

"And you got the six before that."

Patty, who was walking past to her desk, murmured, "Dr. Weathersby, I'd like to help this time."

Margie interrupted, "Patty, you don't need to."

"Yes, I do."

Khai shook her head surreptitiously at Margie, who spoke quietly. "That's nice, Patty." When the receptionist turned to go into the staff room to get the money, Margie smiled at Khai. "You know, Dr. Weathersby, I hurt inside."

"Why, Margie?"

"Because you won't be spending the rest of your career here with us in this place. You're too good. Some real place is going to grab you up."

Khai hugged her, and both watched as the little man pulled the three dollars from Patty's hand and limped out of the clinic toward the bus stop. The receptionist stood shaking her head.

Khai asked, "Patty, what's wrong?"

"He never even said thank you."

"That's why he's where he is, and probably will be for the few years he has left. And they won't be good ones. The thanks don't come from our patients. They come from inside you—period. Promise me you'll remember that."

Patty smiled. "I'll try." A silence washed over the three, but the phone rang, and Patty ran back to her cubicle. She listened and held the phone up toward Khai. "It's a doctor. He says he has to talk to you. It's important, he said."

"I'll take it in my," she laughed, "in my office."

In the staff kitchenette, she pulled a chair toward the desk phone and lifted the receiver. She took a deep breath and pushed the flashing button. A voice blasted so brutally, Khai's body bolted upright. She recognized it immediately but held her tongue until the voice stopped for a breath. "Chris," she barked, "I'm working, and I'm not going to discuss it with you now...or ever." Her voice rose even further. "Choices, consequences. Ever heard of that?" She kept herself from hanging up as she delivered one more volley. "You are not to call here again. Just don't call me at all. Do you understand?"

Gauthé was silent for a moment, and Khai sighed in relief, but an instant later, he bellowed, "Who the hell do you think you are? You don't talk to me that way."

Khai placed the receiver in the cradle, leaned back into the chair, and sat there until Margie poked her head in. "Dr. Weathersby, I'm sorry, but there's a patient in Two."

Khai walked through the lab, took a sip of cold, bitter coffee, pasted on a neutral expression, and walked stiffly to the other side of the clinic. She took a deep breath and knocked on the door to Room Two before opening it. A mom with two little boys looked up dully. She groaned that one of the kids had a cough that was keeping the family up at night. The child had not had a fever or chills, not as far as the mom knew, and hadn't coughed up much at all.

Khai pulled the stethoscope from around her neck and wordlessly examined the child. She found, as usual, nothing to pin her hat on. Just another of the interminable coughs and colds that made up her workday. She smiled plastically at the mom and asked her to wait just a moment while she got a sample of cough medicine for the boy. Khai walked out of the room and closed the door. Three steps down the hall, a racket erupted behind her. She jumped back into the room, expecting to see children bouncing off the walls, but it was her little patient rebounding off the exam table, trembling, racked with paroxysms of cough, each ending with a high-pitched howl.

She had never seen whooping cough, never heard the whoop, never even known a doctor who had seen it, but this was whooping cough—there was no doubt. She asked the expressionless mom. "Are you sure he had all of his shots before school?"

She looked up. "I don't send him to school. I teach both of 'em myself."

"Okay, but did he have his shots, yes or no?"

"No. They're poison. And don't you give him any."

"Madam, I certainly won't, but I want you to know I believe your child has whooping cough." She felt herself dropping into a well of rage, one so deep there was no escape. She hissed, "This is exactly why your kid is supposed..." but she stopped herself and left the room to call the county health department. They suggested the boy be seen in the emergency room at Mitchie-Sterling

Hospital, for they had a quarantine room. Khai came back to the room and spoke softly but explained, unmistakably, the peril the boy and his family faced if they didn't go straight to the ER, and with no stops. She would call ahead and alert the staff.

She shooed the family out of the clinic through the back door, and as they finally pulled from the parking lot, Khai laughed to Margie, "That's three for three to Mitchie-Sterling Hospital. I'll be disbarred, or whatever they call it, by the close of business."

Margie laughed and began to reassure Khai when the screech of a car stopping in the parking lot caught the attention of every soul in the clinic. Khai growled, "Marge, get me an AMA form. Wonder if the woman can read and write. Their eyes rolled in concert, and Margie chuckled, "I'll get one and fill out the particulars. Why don't you take a break, Dr. Weathersby? Hide in a corner of the staff room, and I'll keep the evil vapors out here."

Khai patted Margie on the shoulder and took a step toward the breakroom when the backdoor crashed open, hitting the wall. She poked her head around the corner to see Chris Gauthé, face as tight as an animal trap, eyes maddened, searching left and right. Khai shot back around the corner, but the movement caught his attention, and he lunged toward her. As she tried to retreat, her back hit the wall, and Gauthé was upon her, gathering up her blouse in his fists.

"You need to come with me, now!"

"Chris, please, you need to turn around and leave. It's not too late. Nothing's cast in stone yet. Take your hands off me, and I'll forget this happened."

Margie peeked around the corner but darted back and disappeared. When Gauthé saw her leave out of the corner of his eye, he let go for a moment and seemed to be deliberating, though just a second passed before his right hand shot toward Khai's throat. As her head slammed against the wall, Margie reappeared, the office fire extinguisher held high over Gauthé.

Khai screamed, "Margie, don't."

"Yes, I will if he doesn't get his hands off of you!"

Gauthé spun around, and Margie began to pull the red metal cylinder forward, its trajectory set to end on the top of Gauthé's head. He ducked, yanked Khai, then shoved her against the wall, but as Margie set herself for another try, Gauthé blasted past her so hard, the woman's head thumped a dent in the drywall.

Gauthé thundered through the back door, ran to his family van, then sped out of the parking lot furiously, deep tracks left in the gravel. As the van swerved entering traffic, it nearly rammed a bicycle. Gauthé raised a middle finger at the cyclist before speeding off north. Marge tried to talk Khai into calling the police, but she shook her head. "He'll cool down. But I am going to file a complaint with the state licensing commission. Adding the cops to the mix will only get it screwed up. If the commission decides to make it a criminal complaint, well, then, we'll see."

"Dr. Weathersby, I'm sorry, but that man assaulted you. Jesus, he strangled you. You have a responsibility to stop him."

Khai thought for a moment. "He's a surgeon here in town; at the U, too. It'll be the end of his career."

"Khai, excuse me. You're the age of my daughter. If your father was here right now, what would he do?"

"The guy would cease to exist."

"I hope so. Would he be right? I mean would he have the right to use violence to stop him?"

Khai sighed, "Yeah, you're right."

"And do you think you're the first one he's done this to?"

"No, of course not. He doesn't like not getting his way."

"I'll ask again, what are you going to do?"

"Call the cops."

Khai did, and a chubby young officer came to take a report. When she asked if Gauthé was going to be arrested, the cop only muttered, "You don't live together, so this isn't really domestic violence. You got no marks on you. I'll give it to one of the detectives, but I can't promise you anything. I mean, he didn't use a weapon; you people did. Detective needs to look into that also. Probably best to drop the whole thing, if you get my meaning."

Marge jumped into the room from the hall. "You listen to me, young man; I am a witness. This was an assault with battery. You'll do more than just give it to a detective."

The office glared at her. "Is that a threat?"

Margie calmed and smiled. "You bet your ass it is." She turned to Khai. "Dr. Weathersby, can you spare me for a few minutes?"

"Yes, but what do you have in mind?"

"I'm going to take a little drive up to the Police Department. Let me talk to Ernie."

Khai laughed sadly, "Ernie?"

"Yep, Chief of Police. He's my brother-in-law."

The cop's hand began to tremble. "No problem. I'll take care of it. We'll get a detective to follow through, okay?"

Margie hissed, "Today?"

"I'll take care of it. We'll pick him up. Find out what's going on."

Margie spoke softly but with cast-iron rigidity. "Yes, you will."

The cop pivoted and bristled from the clinic. Khai shook her head. "Marge, you're quite a soul, aren't you? Not easily intimidated."

"My first husband assaulted me every time something didn't go right for him. I detest that behavior. Cops are men. Don't understand what that does to a woman. Only way to handle a slug like that cop is to threaten. Only thing they understand. Plus, I think I'm bigger than him."

"No, you're not. And you're beautiful. I didn't know the chief's your brother-in-law. That's handy."

She laughed warmly and put her hand on Khai's arm. "I don't have a brother-in-law."

Khai covered Marge's hand with hers. "Thank you. I'm probably going to be canned, so I need to see the few patients who didn't abandon ship. Make a few more bucks before the pink slip comes. Buy some fish heads and rice on the way home tonight. Fish heads are still cheap, 'least should be out here."

The receptionist had steered a number of the walk-ins to the hospital, and the few who remained were old folks with nowhere else to go, who'd spent an enjoyable hour kibitzing in the waiting room. Khai saw them, slowly going over the myriad complaints, but mostly just chatting, learning something from each patient.

CHAPTER SIXTY-SIX

K hai had turned off her cell phone before leaving the clinic that evening. At home, she had a glass of wine and sat trying not to relive every detail of the day. She finally turned on her phone to call her dad, but there were several messages from the Bellevue Police Department requesting a call back. Khai thought about refilling her wine glass, but she had a sick feeling she'd wind up having to drive that night, and that a cop would be at the other end of the trip. She was right.

A homicide detective answered. His first words were spoken gruffly. "I've been trying to get through to you for hours, Doctor." Khai thought about throwing herself at his feet in explanation and contrition, but a sudden spark jerked her mind back to the officers she'd had to placate during her years in the Army. That helplessness was one of the factors that drove her into medicine, and she swore during her awful residency that it would never happen again.

"Detective, what can I do for you? It's very late, and I have work in the morning."

He paused, and Khai could feel the heat rising. "Do you know a doctor by the name of Christopher," he stumbled over, "Gauthé?"

"Yes, sir." She had never dealt with the police for anything more than a couple of red-light tickets decades before, but her father had taught her as a little girl to speak to police only when they spoke to you, and then to say only, "Yes, sir. No, sir," and answer questions with no more than five bland words. And, above all, she was never to justify herself to a cop, no matter how friendly and accommodating the officer seemed. All they were trying to do was get enough verbiage from a confused, scared party to blame them, terminate the investigation, and get back to the doughnut shop.

He asked, "What was your relationship to him?"

She was struck by his use of the past tense. "Why did you say, 'was'?"

"Doctor, please, I asked you about your relationship with him."

"Colleague."

"What does that mean?"

"Fellow doctor."

"Did you work with him?"

"Occasionally."

"Did you have a have a romantic relationship with him?"

"Detective, respectfully, I have nothing further to say."

"Well, you are going to answer my questions, one way or the other..."

"Or what?"

"I've got a job to do, and it's going to get done."

"Officer, again respectfully, I have nothing further to say other than you may speak with my attorney. His name is Harrison Jennings." She pulled the phone from her ear, looked through her contacts, and read the number to him. "Good evening."

She ended the call and pushed the button for Mr. Jennings' cell before the detective had had time to pull the phone from his ear. Jennings was surprised but sounded happy to hear from her. She explained the situation and asked if he would help her.

"Dr. Weathersby, I would be happy to speak with this detective, but I have to warn you, I haven't done criminal law in three, maybe even four decades. You have nothing to fear from the police, though he'll bully you if you let him. I don't think he knows who he's dealing with."

"That's kind of you, Mr. Jennings, but, of course, I don't want or need to be involved with the law. I've got enough on my plate as it is."

"Yes, you do, but you stay alive long enough, you will deal with these people. It's okay. Believe me, it's nothing. They just want to get their ducks in order. Can't blame them, really, but it's the way they do it that gets good people upset. Anyone gets in their way, they morph into Sherman tanks.

"Now, let me call him. They're not so brave around lawyers. They know we can pull a law out of thin air and make their lives miserable, like they do to others. Sort of the Golden Rule, I guess. I'll get back to you as soon as I've talked to him. But please, in the interim, have a glass of wine, and just know you're not involved."

"Already had two glasses," she giggled.

"Well, have another half, and that's it!"

Khai did not touch the wine bottle. She sat down and thought again of calling her dad or Tom but was too nervous that she'd be on the phone when Jennings got back to her. She stood and paced about the apartment, laughing to herself that she could fly a million-dollar attack helicopter but always managed to drop both calls when she tried to switch over. Her head swam as she sat back in her tatty recliner waiting for the phone to ring. It did in less than three minutes. She leapt to her feet.

"Dr. Weathersby, Jennings here. Look, first, you're not involved in any criminal way, but I have to tell you that Dr. Gauthé committed suicide—just a block from his home on Mercer Island. In his car—shot himself in the head."

Khai gasped and fell back into her chair so hard, it nearly toppled to the floor. She whispered, "He has a family, kids. Oh my God. I didn't think..."

"If I may, Dr. Weathersby, I am going to recommend you cooperate with the detective. Look, in order for him to rule out that the death was a criminal act, he has to speak to the people who knew him. He has a job to do, and he's entitled under the law to question anyone he wants to. Just the way it is.

"One thing, though. Apparently, he already knows that Dr. Gauthé was down in Evanston today, and that he assaulted you. When he left the clinic, he was speeding on 740 and got picked up. He talked his way out of a ticket by telling he cop he was rushing up to the U to perform an emergency surgery. He said he was the only one who had privileges to do the procedure. I guess he took his cell phone out and showed him a hospital text calling him to Seattle. Probably was months old. Clever. They often are. By the time the dispatcher called the cop with the information about the assault on you, our friend was long gone.

"Doctor, that's all I know. Like I suggested, give the man a call and go along with the program for the next few days. He assured me he would protect your privacy and not drag you down there more than once."

Khai spoke with the detective, who now spoke softly to her. "Doctor, there's a lot you probably don't know about Dr. Gauthé. I'm not going to force you to come down here for an interview. There was a witness who made a statement that Gauthé was alone when he took his life. So, this is not really a criminal investigation, but I need to dot the i's and cross the t's. It will not be made public, at least your name won't. My chief has agreed—the word of God."

She drove to Bellevue the next day. The detective was young, hair close-cropped, uneven Van Dyke, and already carrying a police paunch. He seemed distracted and barely made eye contact with Khai when he asked, on his second question, if she and Gauthé had been intimate. She allowed they had dated, but she had stopped the relationship when it became clear he was still very married. The detective laughed cynically. "You and about six others, the six we've found so far." Khai was struck silent. "Then you must know about the drugs."

She finally mumbled, "No way. Drugs...I've never even seen an illegal drug. Not even weed."

"Doctor, I know that you are an Army officer. Served in the Middle East—twice. I believe you. This guy fooled a lot of folks. Good people, just like you. Before I put this one to bed, I'd like to ask if you'd help us find out who else he might have been seeing. Want to make sure there were no other assaults."

"Detective, if I knew, I would have popped him in the nose a long time ago. I will tell you, though, I think one was a blond. Found a hair in his bathroom. He tried to tell me it was from his nine-year-old daughter, but it was a little darker at the root, and the color was absolutely even the rest of the way up the shaft. Obviously bleached."

"That's probably the nurse he was seeing. I shouldn't tell you this, but he attacked her a couple of days ago in the hospital parking lot at the U. Didn't show up at the hospital for surgery the next day. Seattle PD was waiting for him there, and the local PD was in McKinley at the hospital. Didn't show up there, either. We looked for him all night. Didn't hear a word until he drove up to Evanston and assaulted you. Out of control..."

Khai interrupted him. "Been out of control for a long time. Smart enough to hide it from a lot of people."

"Yep, he did. Worst of all, jerk left behind two kids, and there's gonna be a lot of legal bills for his wife, rats crawling out of the woodwork to sue the estate. Selfish bastard." He paused and looked at Khai. "Doctor, you're free to go. Sorry to have taken up your time."

Khai drove to her apartment on Capitol Hill. It was as cold as usual, but a couple of glasses of wine fixed that. She crawled into sweats and sat by the phone until she gave in and called Tom. They talked for hours. When she was sure there wasn't anything left to say, she found some more.

The next morning, she gave notice to the owners of the walk-in clinic. They offered her a ten-percent raise. She thanked them and hung up before they could offer a few percent more.

The next call was from Harrison Jennings.

CHAPTER SIXTY-SEVEN

Jennings' voice was devoid of joy. "Dr. Weathersby, I'll just say, we won. And we did well, but I must leave it to the Maddinglys to fill in the details. I'm sorry I can't say any more."

Khai spoke softly. "Mr. Jennings, to tell you the truth, I don't want to know anything other than that the hospital has been held accountable."

"Didn't think you would." He stopped for a moment before going on, his tone even more sober. "I'm afraid it means very little to them. They detoxify it by telling the Board I'm just an ambulance chaser, and the Maddinglys are poor little victims; the price of doing business in the modern world. Actually, with the insurance company paying, there'll be nary a penny out of anyone's paycheck—little more than a nuisance for those involved. And it'll happen again, but no big deal. They just need to keep out of trouble for another three or four years, until the insurance cycle restarts. Like no accidents for three years, and you're back in good hands at Allstate."

Neither spoke for some time until Khai sighed, "You know, Mr. Jennings, I just quit the clinic. I'm going back home. I tried to run away by coming out here, but it didn't work. When I got off the plane at SeaTac, you know who was there to greet me? Me." When he said nothing, she sighed, "I am so sorry, sir, that I never told you what happened. It was completely selfish of me. I haven't told anyone, even Tom. All that drama in the trial about why I failed my boards. I feel so stupid, but I just couldn't bare my soul in that obscene courtroom. Rhonda Uft, that sick, sick person with the freedom to say whatever vomits into her mouth, ruining lives with her poison, hiding behind the fact that she's a professional woman, untouchable."

She stopped for a few seconds, and her voice hardened. "The reason I came out here was because my husband was shot down in Afghanistan. I got word a day before the boards. His parents insisted I still go to Chicago and take the test, 'That's what Perry would have wanted,' they said. I was mad as hell at them when I failed, but then I realized it was misdirected anger, actually all my anger at everyone, that huge chip on my shoulder, all of it was off course."

Jennings laughed, "Not all of it, Doctor."

"I guess. You know, sir, I'd always believed to bottom of my soul that God had been watching me, saw that I was a good soul; tried so damn hard to do right. Always believed in karma. Not so much, anymore. Do have to say, though, after meeting you, and the Maddinglys, some of the vitriol has been tempered. Thank you."

"Jees, Doctor, you do have a lot on your plate... You say you're going home? Where is that, if I may ask?"

"Well, first, I'm going to Hawaii, to the Punch Bowl in Honolulu—visit Perry's grave. That's the National Memorial Cemetery of the Pacific, where you can be buried if you were in the military. His remains were finally interred there. Took so long. At first, we were told he was shot down and captured; then that he had died in the crash, and that the government had his remains and would turn them over to Graves Registration the next day. That's what took a year. The bastards we put in office in Kabul made the Department of Defense pay a ransom to get them back.

"After that, I am going to return to Boston. I know, I know, horrible, dying East Coast city, but have you looked around Seattle recently? Drugs and crime and homelessness. All of it condoned, decriminalized, forgiven, encouraged by the Mayor and City Council. I hate it here. Combat Zone in Bean Town's safer. Good medicine there, too. Tom told me there are always openings at Mass General for internists. Says there a place just waiting for me. I guess some folks remember me. Maybe that's karma."

"He's a very fine man, that Tom. Smart, good looking guy, too."

"I know."

"Dr. Weathersby, may I say something?"

"Of course. You, I'll listen to."

"Flattered. Look, there isn't a family I know that hasn't suffered tragedy. And I don't mean losing a parent at eighty-five. I didn't tell you—it wasn't important—but my wife was killed by a drunk driver right here in McKinley. Son of a bitch was Chairman of the County Commission. Judge let him walk. Police said my wife was on her phone, drove into his lane. Lies. He drove into her lane, and she got hit so hard, her car came to rest on the other side of the road. She had her phone in her hand when the police finally got there. She was already gone, trapped, bled to death. She was trying to call me after the accident. Cell phone record proved it, but the judge ignored the evidence and freed the skunk. Went right back onto the Commission. Only punishment—he wasn't the boss anymore. So, my friend, none of us are safe from the poison. We need to get over it and move on because it's every one of us. What would your Perry have wanted? I think you know the answer."

Khai gathered herself and spoke over her tears. "Of course, you're right."

EPILOGUE

As Harrison Jennings predicted, the hospital announced their intent to appeal. At the first sit-down meeting, Rhonda Uft arrived late. She had lost much weight and was wearing a hairpiece. Her voice was slurred. It did not take her long to warn that if the Maddinglys didn't accept her offer of settlement, her firm would drag out the proceedings so long, they would not only lose their home, but their credit would be in shambles.

Jennings smiled at her. "Madame, you might want to revise your position. You see, I have loaned the Maddinglys enough to pay off their mortgage—oh, and the loan is interest free. And, better, because of the jury's finding, their medical insurance company has had to abandon their claim that all of this was associated with a prior condition, the lie you worked so hard to drum into the heads of the insurance adjusters. Suddenly, their medical bills have vaporized. Just like that. House was taken off the market this morning.

"Bottom line is, we urge you most strongly to file an appeal. I have an inkling that the court will assess the full twelve-percent annual compounded interest to the jury award. And I'll betcha ten bucks he'll award our legal fees, too. Please take as long as you like to delay. The Maddinglys, my wonderful children, all of us will be ever so delighted."

Rhonda Uft died several weeks later of a glioblastoma multiforme, a brain tumor that caused symptoms similar to a stroke, and, very commonly, marked personality changes. When Harrison Jennings had lunch with several of her senior partners to discuss how payment of the full jury award was to take place, the old men laughed cynically that Rhonda had been spared the latter symptom.

When the first check arrived, Sabrina and Mike drove to Jennings' office. They paid him much of the house loan he had tendered on their behalf, and asked that the balance be offered to Scott Bialek, to restart his case of wrongful death against the hospital.

As the weeks passed after the trial, the combination of the atypical antidepressant and the reduction in the traumatic stress of the case saw Sabrina's mood elevate to the point that she began to take graduate classes in the Department of Psychology at the U. She reopened the textbooks and started reading her journals. Six months later, she was teaching undergraduates; by the end of the next year she was seeing patients three days a week.

While Mike was offered the athletic directorship in Evanston, he chose to remain in the classroom but continued on as head football coach.

Khai and Tom married three years later. They named their first son Harrison.

TITLES BY
WILLIAM S. GOULD, MD

AT YONAH MOUNTAIN

B rand new Second Lieutenant J.W. Weathersby is on orders to depart for a combat tour in Viet Nam. At a West Point wedding, though, he commits a very public faux pas and is thrust as punishment into a class of 160 select young officers who sweat and freeze through months of brutal training at the United States Army Ranger School. J.W. joins an African American PhD candidate and a Rose Bud Sioux Harvard graduate, the three pushed together to trudge the mountains, forests, and deserts as Ranger buddies. As half the class is weeded out, they share their disparate lives and dreams. J.W. struggles to be cut from the program, and at the same time fights desperately to remain. At Yonah Mountain is a coming of age adventure, an examination of race relations in the military, and an authentic tale of Army Ranger training.

CAPTAIN IRON MUSTACHE

Captain Iron Mustache takes place in 1968 and 1969. United States Army lieutenant, J.W. Weathersby, just out of Ranger School, volunteers for duty in Viet Nam. It is not long before he changes from naïve youngster to hardened soldier. Something about rural Viet Nam, though, captivates him, and he convinces his commanding officer to allow him to live as the sole American in a remote rice-farming hamlet. His mission is to win the hearts and the minds of the peasants. J.W. forms a deep friendship with the village chief, and falls in love with the schoolteacher, Miss Lin. During a midnight battle, Miss Lin is arrested and tortured as a communist agent. At the same time, the chief is critically wounded, and disappears after being flown out of the village by an American medevac helicopter. J.W. and the chief's wife spend the last month of his tour driving the deadly roads of Viet Nam searching hospital after hospital for the man. Nearly half a century later, J.W. and his wife return to Viet Nam in a surreal effort to find the chief. He also wants to see Miss Lin, but the Vietnamese government is suspicious of his motives, and the days of his sojourn are fraught with struggle and frustration until a simple act of kindness changes his life.

IN BLACK GRANITE

In Black Granite is set in the decade after J.W. Weathersby returns from the war in Viet Nam. He eventually accepts the assessment of family, friends, and medical school deans that he will never become a doctor. He drifts without focus until the miracle of his first child's birth rekindles the craving to study medicine. This is a narrative of his dogged struggle to beat the overwhelming odds against a man in his mid-thirties gaining admission to an American college of medicine. In Black Granite scrutinizes the ruthless battle for places in medical school, and how the psyches of the chosen are sieved as they are herded through the decade as students and residents. The strain of endless days and nights away from family, of sleepless months, and of pervasive arrogance, distort the souls of even the strongest. Some find the path more treacherous than surviving a war.

C.O.L.A.

The day his father died, Dr. Solomon Forte promised his mother he would honor the man's memory by dedicating his years as a doctor to the treatment of injured workers. It seemed so clear a decision—his patients would be like his dad, stoic, honest, working class stiffs who sought nothing more from a doctor than an arm around the shoulder, a word of reassurance, and an ally in dealing with the state industrial insurance system. His life at the Whitaker Hospital and Medical Center is, though, the antithesis of his dream. He can't tell which of the roadblocks is most daunting: that posed by his medical colleagues, the threats of S.M.A.C., the State Medical Abuse Commission, the bureaucracy at C.O.L.A., the state's Commission on Labor Affairs, or the duplicitous patients, some of whom spend every waking moment trying to dupe him out of drugs and government benefits. Occasionally, a case is obvious–the worker really was devastated by an industrial accident. It seems to Sol, though, that those are the very patients C.O.L.A. torments. On the other hand, claimants skilled at ripping off the Commission run free for decades. C.O.L.A. also examines the specter of serious medical errors, and how they are so much easier to make on patients whose care is mired in the aggravation of government-sponsored insurance plans. Questions are also raised about the state-appointed morality commissions that determine which doctors relinquish their licenses for treating pain. Finally, it is a disturbing look behind the scenes of a modern, multi-specialty medical clinic.

A HEART WIND FROM THE DESERT

Dr. Solomon Forte has lost everything. There is little left but to offer himself to the wretched in war-torn Sudan. Arriving in the desert, heart brimming with hope, it does not take long to recognize that the social and political beliefs that have spawned the war and famine are the very forces that prevent him from carrying out his dream of caring for the dispossessed. At first, despite the warnings of the tiny European medical team left at the refugee camp in Darfur Province, he fights back with typical, strident, American resolve to save the entire population of refugees. The obstacles of central African life, however, soon draw the spirit from him, and he turns his efforts to preserving the lives of his Western companions. He falls deeply for a gorgeous, but outwardly hardened, British nurse. When she disappears from camp, he spends what strength is left searching for her. *A Heart Wind from the Desert* examines the need in all of us to accomplish something meaningful in the tiny fragment of time we are allotted, and the impossible hurdles faced when trying to change the way people have thought and behaved over the millennia. It is a tale of beautiful, warm children, but also of the stark life in the sub-Saharan Sahel.

RAPHAEL'S BLANKET

Raphael Blumenkopf is born clandestinely at the Bergen Belsen Nazi death camp on the 14th of April, 1945. His birth is an unprecedented miracle, as is the liberation of the camp by British forces that very afternoon. He has only his mother and a few surviving villagers from their home in Checzonovska, Poland. While the majority of the refugees leave Central Europe for Israel and the West, his band travels across Russia to China. A relative has promised jobs in Shang Hai's old Jewish settlement. The journey is fraught with threats from starving Russians, barbaric border guards, and destitute Chinese peasants. Just as the lives of the immigrants begin to normalize in China, the victory of Mao Zedong's communist army forces them to flee, this time to Hanoi. Five years later, the communist movement in North Viet Nam topples the French government, and the Jews run again. They settle in Saigon until the unrest there compels them to emigrate to America. Raphael's years in the U.S. are colored indelibly by the poison that follows him from the Holocaust, and he formulates a plan to extract revenge from a Federal judge with ties to the Nazis. Who could have envisaged the price he'd pay?

LINCOLN FRIDAY

Lincoln Friday is born into nothing, an obscure, dirt farmer's son, destined to live dominated by the jagged edges of two wars. His early years are an endless series of losses, yet he struggles back after each blow, and slowly, a strongbox of dreams emerges from the fog of his hopelessness.

The harshest test of Lincoln's life, though, comes when the effects of his exposure to Agent Orange devastate both his and his daughter's lives. While the Fridays fight back passionately, the courts, Congress, and the VA turn their backs on them.

In the end, his deeds were neither profound nor dazzling, but he left his mark on disparate people in disparate lands. The world he touched chafed less for his quiet dignity.

ABOUT THE AUTHOR

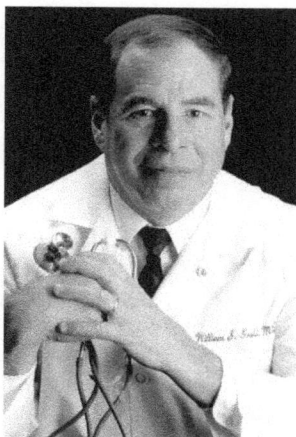

Doctor Bill Gould has practiced medicine in the Seattle, Washington, area since 1981. He has served as a volunteer physician in Darfur Province, Sudan, and in the underserved areas of Vietnam. He was recently a Visiting Professor of Medicine in China. He graduated from Cambridge and Harvard Universities in Asian Studies, and the University of Pennsylvania School of Medicine. He lives with his wife deep in the Cascade Mountains.

Visit his website at
www.billgouldmd.com